Expanded from Previous Editions by Barbara J Bain

Haematology

A Core Curriculum

Third Edition

Expanded from Previous Editions by Barbara J Bain

Haematology
A Core Curriculum
Third Edition

editor

Donald Macdonald
Imperial College London, UK

World Scientific

NEW JERSEY • LONDON • SINGAPORE • BEIJING • SHANGHAI • TAIPEI • CHENNAI

Published by

World Scientific Publishing Europe Ltd.

57 Shelton Street, Covent Garden, London WC2H 9HE

Head office: 5 Toh Tuck Link, Singapore 596224

USA office: 27 Warren Street, Suite 401-402, Hackensack, NJ 07601

Library of Congress Cataloging-in-Publication Data
Names: Macdonald, Donald (Hematologist) editor.
Title: Haematology : a core curriculum / editor, Donald Macdonald, Imperial College London, UK.
Other titles: Haematology (Macdonald)
Description: Third edition. | New Jersey : World Scientific, [2025] |
    "Expanded from previous editions by Barbara Bain." |
    Includes bibliographical references and index.
Identifiers: LCCN 2024045135 | ISBN 9781800616455 (hardcover) |
    ISBN 9781800616554 (paperback) | ISBN 9781800616462 (ebook for institutions) |
    ISBN 9781800616479 (ebook for individuals)
Subjects: MESH: Hematologic Diseases | Blood Physiological Phenomena |
    Hematologic Tests | Hematology--methods
Classification: LCC RB145 | NLM WH 120 | DDC 616.1/5--dc23/eng/20241227
LC record available at https://lccn.loc.gov/2024045135

British Library Cataloguing-in-Publication Data
A catalogue record for this book is available from the British Library.

For any available supplementary material, please visit
https://www.worldscientific.com/worldscibooks/10.1142/Q0485#t=suppl

Desk Editor: Nambirajan Karuppiah

Typeset by Stallion Press
Email: enquiries@stallionpress.com

Preface to the Third Edition

The first and second editions of the textbook *Haematology: A Core Curriculum,* were under the sole authorship of Professor Barbara J Bain. Generations of haematology trainees and students from the UK and further afield have benefitted from Professor Bain's dedication to haematology education, and in these editions, the clinical and laboratory features of blood diseases were presented in her characteristically clear and rigorous manner.

In the light of the scientific progress in haematology diagnostics and therapeutics, including next-generation DNA sequencing, targeted drug therapy, immune cellular therapy and gene therapy, Professor Bain decided in 2024, that a new edition was called for. It was proposed that this should be a multiauthor book, written by members of the Imperial College Centre for Haematology and affiliated hospitals.

This core textbook is based on the curriculum of our haematology teaching within Imperial College London, where the aim is to provide a foundation in the molecular and cell biology that underpins the pathology of blood diseases. Additionally, it discusses the clinical features of the common and important blood disorders seen in general and specialist practice.

I am especially grateful to Professor Bain for her advice on the preparation of this book and for permission to use the line drawings she created and many of the figures she collected. Our Imperial College colleagues in

Imaging, Histopathology and Molecular Diagnostics have been helpful in providing material for figures. Sue Katic and Julie Staves kindly reviewed the Blood Transfusion chapter. Finally I would like to acknowledge the help of Rosie Williamson, Nambirajan Karuppaiah, and the design staff of World Scientific Publishing.

Contributors

Editor:
Dr Donald Macdonald MD, PhD
Honorary Senior Clinical Lecturer, Centre for Haematology, Imperial College London, UK

Contributors:
Prof. Barbara J. Bain MBBS, FRACP, FRCPath
Centre for Haematology, Imperial College London and St Mary's Hospital, London, UK

Dr Edward J. Bataillard MA (Cantab), BMBCh (Oxon), MRCP FRCPath
Consultant Haematologist, Hammersmith Hospital, Imperial College NHS Trust, London UK

Dr Aristeidis Chaidos MD, PhD
Consultant Haematologist and Honorary Senior Clinical Lecturer
Hammersmith Hospital, Imperial College Healthcare NHS Trust and Hugh & Josseline Langmuir Centre for Myeloma Research, Centre for Haematology, Imperial College London, UK

Dr Fateha Chowdhury BSc (Hons) MRCP, FRCPath, FHEA, MSc
Consultant Haematologist, St Mary's Hospital, Imperial College Healthcare NHS Trust, London, NHS Blood and Transplant, UK

Dr Andrew Godfrey MBBS, BSc, PhD, FRCP, FRCPath
Consultant Haematologist and Honorary Senior Clinical Lecturer, Chelsea and Westminster Hospital NHS Foundation Trust, and Centre for Haematology, Imperial College London, UK

Dr Vishal Jayakar MD, MRCP, FRCPath
Consultant Haematologist and Honorary Senior Clinical Lecturer, Kingston Hospital NHS Trust, and Centre for Haematology, Imperial College London, UK

Frequently Used Abbreviations

2,3-DPG	2,3-diphosphoglycerate
ADP	adenosine diphosphate
ALL	acute lymphoblastic leukaemia
AML	acute myeloid leukaemia
APTT	activated partial thromboplastin time
ATLL	adult T-cell leukaemia/lymphoma
ATP	adenosine triphosphate
BM	bone marrow
CAR-T cells	chimaeric antigen receptor T cells
CCR	complete cytogenetic response
CLL	chronic lymphocytic leukaemia
CML	chronic myeloid leukaemia
CMML	chronic myelomonocytic leukaemia
CMV	cytomegalovirus
CNS	central nervous system
COPD	chronic obstructive pulmonary disease
COVID-19	coronavirus disease 2019
CPD	citrate phosphate dextrose
CRP	C-reactive protein
CT	computed tomography
DAT	direct antiglobulin test
DIC	disseminated intravascular coagulation

DLBCL	diffuse large B-cell lymphoma
DNA	deoxyribonucleic acid
DOAC	direct oral anticoagulants
EBV	Epstein–Barr virus
EDTA	ethylene diamine tetraacetic acid
epo	erythropoietin
ESR	erythrocyte sedimentation rate
ET	essential thrombocythaemia
FBC	full blood count
FFP	fresh frozen plasma
FISH	fluorescence *in situ* hybridisation
G6PD	glucose-6-phosphate dehydrogenase
G-CSF	granulocyte colony-stimulating factor
GM-CSF	granulocyte-macrophage colony-stimulating factor
GP	general practitioner
GVHD	graft-versus-host disease
H&E	haematoxylin and eosin
Hb	haemoglobin concentration
HBV	hepatitis B virus
Hct	haematocrit
HCV	hepatitis C virus
HDFN	haemolytic disease of the fetus and newborn
HDN	haemolytic disease of the newborn
HDW	haemoglobin distribution width
HIV	human immunodeficiency virus
HL	Hodgkin lymphoma
HLA	human leucocyte antigens
HPA	human platelet antigens
HPLC	high performance liquid chromatography
HTLV-1	human T-cell lymphotropic virus-1
IAT	indirect antiglobulin test
Ig	immunoglobulin
INR	international normalised ratio
IT	information technology
ITP	immune (autoimmune) thrombocytopenic purpura
LDH	lactate dehydrogenase

LIMS	laboratory information management system
MCH	mean cell haemoglobin
MCHC	mean cell haemoglobin concentration
MCV	mean cell volume
MDS	myelodysplastic syndrome
MDS/MPN	myelodysplastic/myeloproliferative neoplasm
MGG	May–Grünwald–Giemsa (stain)
MGUS	monoclonal gammopathy of undetermined significance
MHRA	Medicines and Healthcare products Regulatory Agency
MMR	major molecular response
MPN	myeloproliferative neoplasm
MPV	mean platelet volume
MRD	measurable residual disease
MRI	magnetic resonance imaging
mRNA	messenger ribonucleic acid
NADP	nicotinamide-adenine dinucleotide phosphate
NADPH	reduced form of nicotinamide-adenine dinucleotide phosphate
NAT	nucleic acid testing
NGS	next generation sequencing of DNA
NHL	non-Hodgkin lymphoma
NHS	National Health Service (UK)
NHSBT	NHS Blood and Transplant
NICE	National Institute for Health and Care Excellence
NK	natural killer (cell)
NR	normal range
NRBC	nucleated red blood cell
PB	peripheral blood
PCR	polymerase chain reaction
PCV	packed cell volume
PDW	platelet distribution width
PET	positron-emission tomography
Ph	Philadelphia (chromosome)
PMF	primary myelofibrosis
PT	prothrombin time
PV	polycythaemia vera

RBC	red cell count
RCM	red cell mass
RDW	red cell distribution width
RNA	ribonucleic acid
RT-PCR	reverse transcription polymerase chain reaction
RT-qPCR	real time quantitative PCR
SAGM	saline adenine glucose mannitol (suspension solution used in blood transfusion)
SARS-CoV-2	severe acute respiratory syndrome-coronavirus-2
TA-GVHD	transfusion-associated graft-versus-host disease
TACO	transfusion-associated circulatory overload
TRALI	transfusion-related acute lung injury
TT	thrombin time
vCJD	variant Creutzfeldt–Jakob disease
VTE	venous thromboembolism
vWD	von Willebrand disease
vWF	von Willebrand factor
WBC	white cell count

Contents

1

Physiology of the Blood and Bone Marrow

Barbara J. Bain

What Do You Need To Know?

☞ Which cells are normally present in the blood and their function
☞ The normal intravascular life span of erythrocytes, neutrophils and platelets
☞ Where and how blood cells are produced
☞ The production and function of erythropoietin
☞ The source and absorption of iron, vitamin B_{12} and folic acid and their role in haemopoiesis

Blood Cells and Their Functions

The circulating blood contains red cells, white cells and platelets suspended in plasma (Fig. 1.1). The cells in the circulating blood originate in the bone marrow.

Red cells, also known as **erythrocytes**, differ from most body cells in that they no longer have a nucleus. This is extruded when they leave the bone marrow. Normal mature red cells are disc shaped and, because they lack a nucleus, are flexible: they can deform and squeeze through

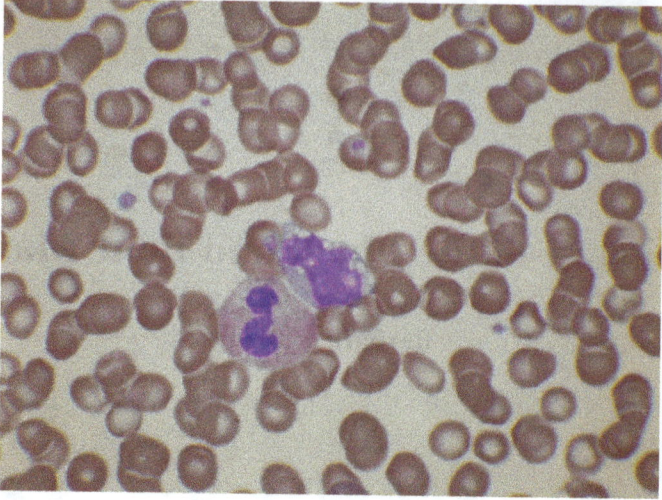

Fig. 1.1. A stained blood film showing erythrocytes, leucocytes (a neutrophil and a monocyte) and platelets. May–Grünwald–Giemsa stain (MGG).

capillaries. The major function of the red cell is oxygen transport from the lungs to peripheral tissues, but it also transports CO_2 from the tissues to the lungs and has a role in nitric oxide (NO) transport and metabolism, favouring generation of NO and vasodilation in conditions of hypoxia. The principle constituent of the red cell, responsible for oxygen transport and contributing to CO_2 transport and interactions with NO, is haemoglobin. It is an iron containing protein composed of four polypeptide chains known as globin chains, each of which has a deep pocket into which an iron-containing haem group is inserted. The tetrameric haemoglobin molecule is composed of two heterodimers, with each dimer in normal adult haemoglobin (haemoglobin A) being composed of an α and a β chain (Fig. 1.2). Oxygen for transport can enter the haem pocket and bind reversibly to haem. The globin chains can alter their relationship to each other in response to the uptake or release of oxygen by haem. Loss of one oxygen molecule from one haem makes it more likely that other oxygen molecules will be lost from other haems. This is known as co-operativity and is responsible for the sigmoid shape of the oxygen dissociation curve (Fig. 1.3). Co-operativity ensures that haemoglobin takes up oxygen readily as it passes through the lungs, becoming almost fully saturated, and that the oxygen is equally readily released when it reaches the tissues.

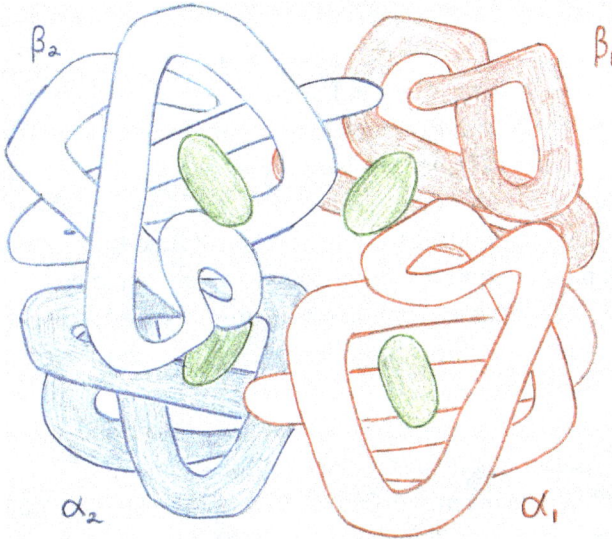

Fig. 1.2. A diagram of a haemoglobin molecule, showing two α and two β globin chains, each with a haem in the haem pocket. The $\alpha_1\beta_1$ dimer is shown in pink and the $\alpha_2\beta_2$ dimer in blue. The haem groups are represented in green.

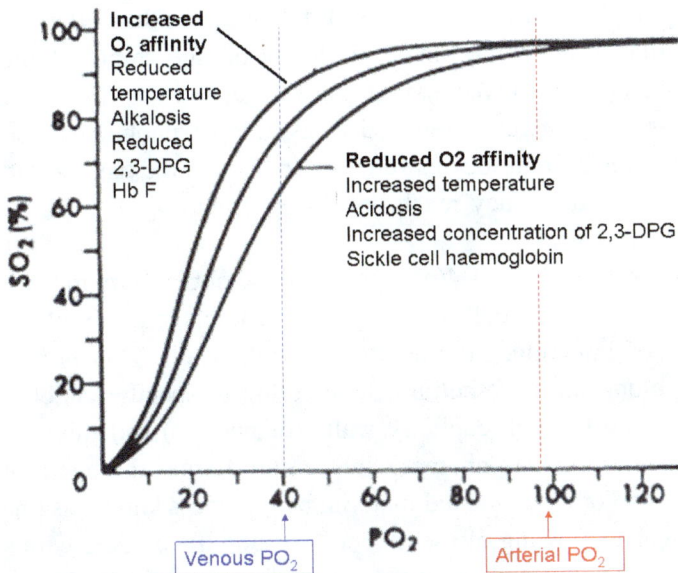

Fig. 1.3. The oxygen dissociation curve illustrating the sigmoid curve that results from co-operativity. 2,3-DPG, 2,3-diphosphoglycerate. pO_2 in mmHg.

Delivery of oxygen in the tissues is facilitated by a higher temperature and a lower pH so that more oxygen is available to metabolically active tissues. It is also facilitated by interaction with 2,3-diphosphoglycerate (2,3-DPG), a glycolytic intermediate that increases in concentration in response to anaemia. Higher temperature, lower pH and a higher concentration of 2,3-DPG thus decrease the affinity of haemoglobin for oxygen.

The surface membrane of erythrocytes is a lipid bilayer, supported by a cytoskeleton that maintains the biconcave shape of the cell. Erythrocytes contain enzymes of the Embden–Meyerhof (or glycolytic) pathway, which meets the energy needs of the cell and enzymes of the pentose (hexosemonophosphate) shunt, which protects the cell from oxidant damage. The erythrocyte life-span is about 120 days, and effete cells are removed by macrophages, particularly in the spleen.

The synthesis of haemoglobin is discussed further in Chapter 5 and the red cell membrane and enzymes in Chapter 6.

White cells, also known as **leucocytes**, defend the body against infection and participate in immune responses. Those that are normally present in the blood are of five types. Three of these are referred to as granulocytes, because their cytoplasm contains granules; depending on the colour of the granules in a stained blood film they can be divided into neutrophils (small lilac granules), eosinophils (larger orange granules) and basophils (large purple granules). They all have lobulated or polymorphous nuclei and thus are sometimes referred to as polymorphonuclear leucocytes or 'polymorphs'. Granulocytes function mainly in the tissues, rather than in the blood stream. They reach tissues by migrating through the endothelium of capillaries.

Neutrophils (Fig. 1.4(a)) spend only about 7 hours in the circulation. They are phagocytic cells that respond to chemotactic stimuli by migrating to sites of infection, inflammation or cell death. This process involves rolling along the endothelium by adhering to specific endothelial receptors, moving through capillary walls (diapedesis) and migrating through tissues in response to chemotaxins. Within tissues the neutrophils engulf bacteria and other unwanted material by a process known as phagocytosis. This involves flowing of pseudopodia around the particle with subsequent fusion so that the unwanted bacterium or other particle is enclosed in a phagocytic vacuole within the cytoplasm. The granules of the neutrophil (which contain proteolytic enzymes and myeloperoxidase) are then

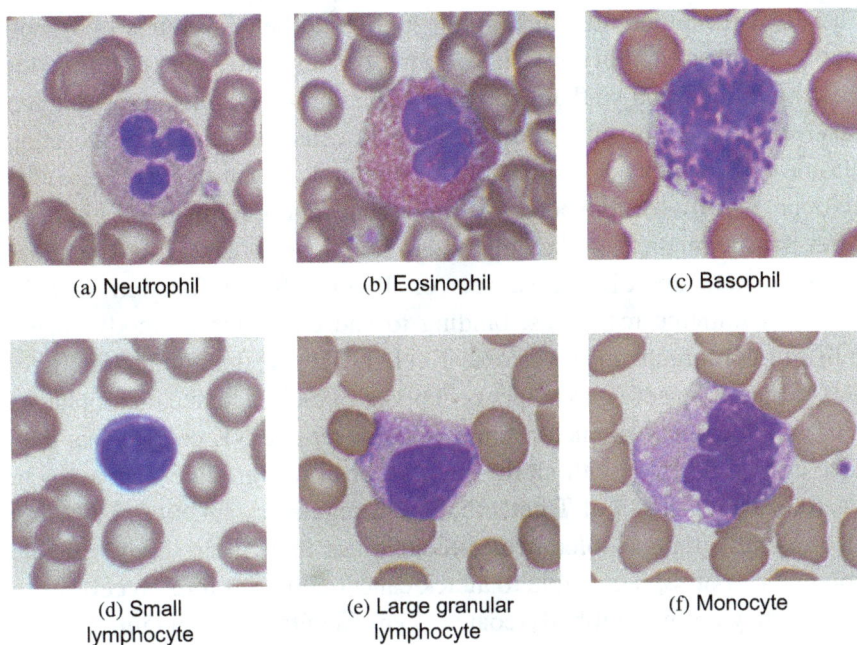

(a) Neutrophil   (b) Eosinophil   (c) Basophil

(d) Small lymphocyte   (e) Large granular lymphocyte   (f) Monocyte

Fig. 1.4. Normal leucocytes in the peripheral blood: (a) a neutrophil; (b) an eosinophil; (c) a basophil; (d) a small lymphocyte; (e) a large granular lymphocyte; (f) a monocyte. MGG.

discharged into the phagocytic vacuole, where H_2O_2 and other reactive oxygen species are generated; the result is killing of microbes and proteolysis of phagosome contents. Neutrophils spend about 30 hours in tissues.

The major function of **eosinophils** (Fig. 1.4(b)) is defence against parasitic infection. They are less efficient than neutrophils in defence against bacteria. In addition to these beneficial functions, eosinophils have undesirable side effects when they are involved in allergic reactions. **Basophils** (Fig. 1.4(c)) also participate in defence against parasites and in allergic responses.

Lymphocytes (Figs. 1.4(d)–(e)) are smaller than granulocytes and have a round nucleus. A minority of them have a small number of cytoplasmic granules. Circulating lymphocytes look very similar to each other but include cells of three lineages: B cells, T cells and natural killer (NK) cells. B cells are of bone marrow origin. They migrate from the blood stream to lymph nodes or other lymphoid tissues where they are exposed to antigens presented to them by dendritic cells (antigen-presenting cells).

They exit the blood stream through high endothelial venules of lymph nodes and post-capillary venules of other tissues. Antigen exposure leads to somatic mutation so that cells most capable of recognising the antigen survive and mature into both memory B cells and antibody-secreting plasma cells, which are responsible for humoral immunity. T cells are also of bone marrow origin but have undergone maturation in the thymus. After thymic maturation they migrate to lymph nodes and other lymphoid tissues. There are diverse subsets of T cells. Some function in cell-mediated immune responses, binding to and damaging antibody-coated cells or microorganisms (cytotoxic T cells). They also modulate the function of B cells by acting as helper or suppressor cells, activate macrophages and attract and activate neutrophils. Some resemble NK cells in that they have cytotoxic effect without the need for prior recognition of an antigen. There is also a subset of T cells that has a regulatory function, including maintaining immune tolerance. NK cells are part of the body's innate immune response, being able to attack cancer cells and foreign cells even though they are not antibody-coated. Lymphocytes that contain granules are either NK cells or cytotoxic T cells. Otherwise it is not possible to distinguish T cells from B cells by their appearance in the blood film. Lymphocytes recirculate between the lymphatic system and the blood stream. They spend a very variable period of time in the circulation. Their survival is very variable but in some cases is many years.

Monocytes (Fig. 1.4(f)) are the largest cells normally present in the blood. They have a lobulated nucleus and plentiful cytoplasm. They spend several days in the circulation, but their main function is in the tissues. There they mature into macrophages or histiocytes (collectively known as the reticuloendothelial system), capable of phagocytosing and killing microorganisms and breaking down and removing cellular debris. They present antigens to lymphocytes. Whereas neutrophils are most important in defence against acute bacterial infection, cells of the monocyte/macrophage lineage are most important in defence against chronic bacterial infections, such as tuberculosis, and chronic fungal infections. They secrete numerous cytokines that enhance the inflammatory response to infection as well as growth factors that promote the production of neutrophils and monocytes. In addition, macrophages remove parasites (such as malaria parasites) and other particles from red cells. They destroy red cells at the end of their life span and store the iron released from haemoglobin so that it can be recycled.

Platelets are small particles formed by fragmentation of the cytoplasm of bone marrow megakaryocytes. They function in the primary haemostatic response, forming a platelet plug at the site of small vessel injury. When activated, they also expose altered phospholipid on their surfaces, which interacts with coagulation factors to promote blood coagulation at the site of tissue injury. They survive for about 10 days in the circulation.

Bone Marrow Cells and Normal Haemopoiesis

All the blood cells are ultimately derived in the bone marrow from a pluripotent haemopoietic stem cell that is capable of giving rise to both lymphoid and myeloid progeny via a common lymphoid progenitor cell and a common myeloid progenitor cell respectively (Fig. 1.5). The common lymphoid progenitor gives rise to B cells, T cells and NK cells. The common myeloid progenitor is a multipotent haemopoietic progenitor cell

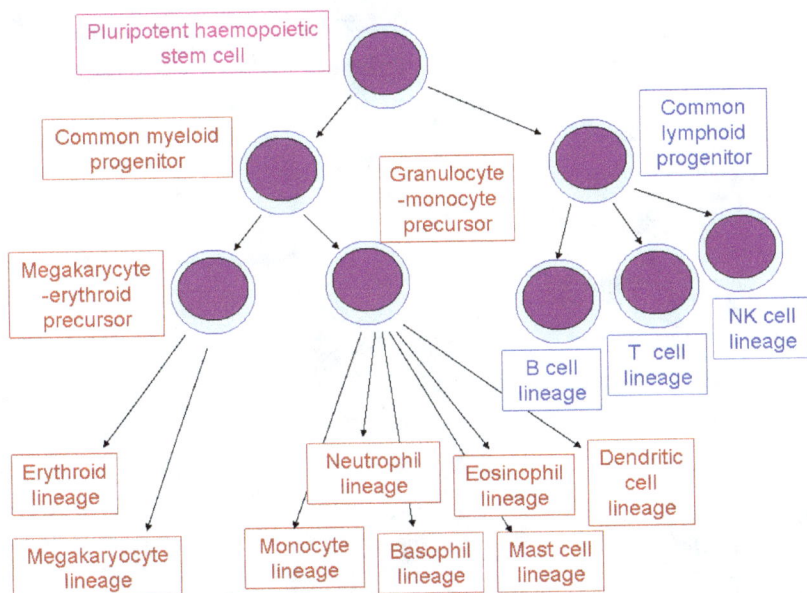

Fig. 1.5. The haemopoietic stem cell hierarchy.

(sometimes also known as a multipotent myeloid stem cell) capable of giving rise to cells of all myeloid lineages. It gives rise initially to an erythroid-megakaryocyte progenitor cell and a granulocyte-monocyte progenitor cell. The granulocyte-monocyte progenitor gives rise not only to monocytes and the three types of granulocyte, but also to the antigen-presenting dendritic cells and mast cells, which are tissue cells concerned with immune responses. The monocyte/macrophage lineage gives rise to many specialised tissue macrophages (e.g. Kupffer cells in the liver) and also to osteoclasts, which are giant cells needed for the breakdown and remodelling of bone.

Haemopoietic stem cells have as a defining quality the ability to reproduce themselves and to differentiate into progenitor cells of specific lineages that ultimately give rise to mature end cells (Fig. 1.6). Progenitor cells and their progeny undergo a series of cell divisions associated with maturation (Fig. 1.7). In the case of the megakaryocyte lineage, there is

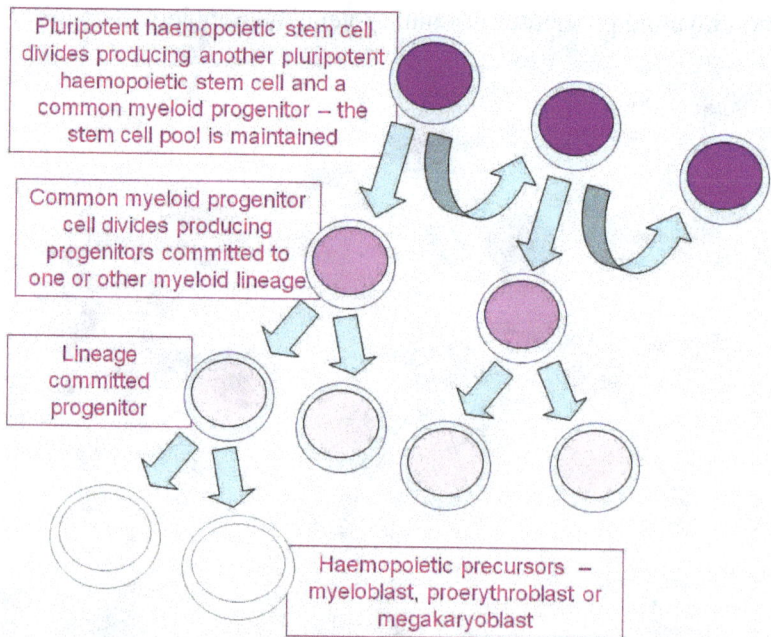

Pluripotent haemopoietic stem cell divides producing another pluripotent haemopoietic stem cell and a common myeloid progenitor – the stem cell pool is maintained

Common myeloid progenitor cell divides producing progenitors committed to one or other myeloid lineage

Lineage committed progenitor

Haemopoietic precursors – myeloblast, proerythroblast or megakaryoblast

Fig. 1.6. A diagram illustrating that stem cells both renew themselves and produce differentiated progeny.

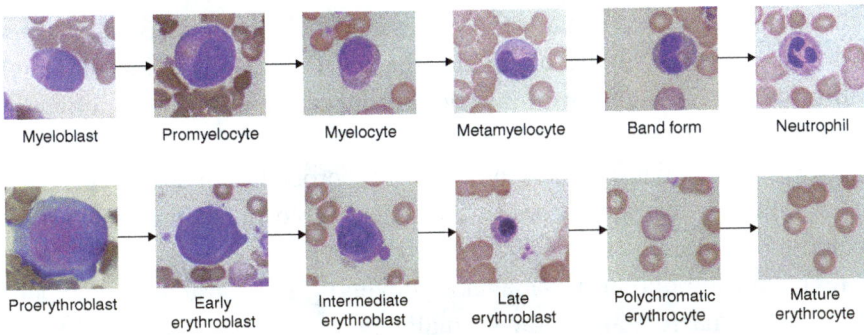

| Myeloblast | Promyelocyte | Myelocyte | Metamyelocyte | Band form | Neutrophil |

| Proerythroblast | Early erythroblast | Intermediate erythroblast | Late erythroblast | Polychromatic erythrocyte | Mature erythrocyte |

Fig. 1.7. The stages of maturation of erythroid and granulocyte progenitors to mature cells.

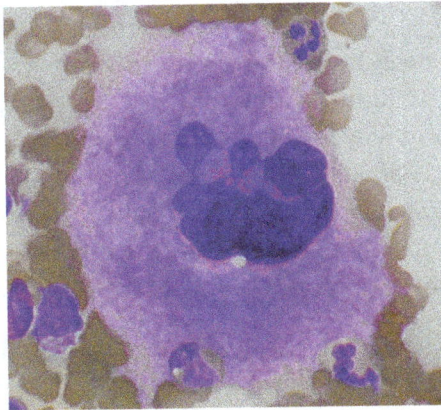

Fig. 1.8. A megakaryocyte in the bone marrow. MGG.

reduplication of chromosomes but without cell division so that the mature megakaryocyte is a giant polyploid cell (Fig. 1.8). Platelets are formed by fragmentation of the cytoplasm of megakaryocytes. In healthy subjects only the platelets and the end cells of the myeloid and erythroid lineages are released into the blood stream in significant numbers. In the case of the erythrocyte lineage, the cell that is released is a reticulocyte or polychromatic erythrocyte. It is formed from a nucleated erythroblast that squeezes through the endothelium into a bone marrow sinusoid, leaving its nucleus behind. The reticulocyte still has ribosomes (which the mature red cell does not) so it can carry on synthesising haemoglobin. It does this for 1–3 days in the circulation before it loses its ribosomes and remodels its shape to that of a hollowed out disc and becomes a mature red cell.

The differentiation of stem cells and progenitor cells to cells of specific lineages is controlled by a considerable number of cytokines, including stem cell factor, various interleukins, erythropoietin (erythrocytes), thrombopoietin (megakaryocytes) and granulocyte- and granulocyte-macrophage colony-stimulating factors (G-CSF and GM-CSF) (granulocytes and monocytes). Erythropoietin is produced mainly (about 90%) by juxtatubular cells in the kidney in response to a reduced oxygen tension (Fig. 1.9). It increases erythropoiesis and leads to earlier release of reticulocytes from the bone marrow. Thrombopoietin is produced by the liver (production being upregulated by infection, inflammation and iron deficiency) and in small amounts by bone marrow stromal cells (production being upregulated by severe thrombocytopenia). Thrombopoietin combines with a specific receptor on cell membranes. It enhances survival and expansion of haemopoietic stem cells and promotes differentiation of these cells to megakaryocytes. G-CSF is produced by fibroblasts, endothelial cells and macrophages; it increases neutrophil production, survival and functional activity and accelerates the release of neutrophils from the bone

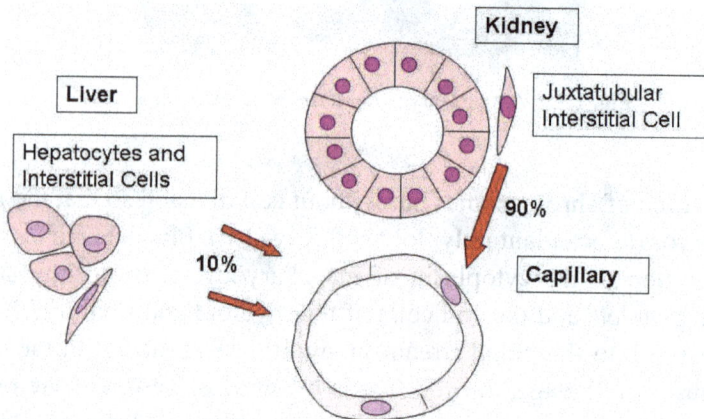

Fig. 1.9. Diagram showing production of erythropoietin by renal and, to a lesser extent, hepatic cells.

marrow. GM-CSF is produced by lymphocytes and macrophages; it increases the proliferation of progenitor cells, accelerates the production and release of neutrophils and monocytes from the bone marrow and increases the functional activity of both cell types.

In the adult the haemopoietic marrow (red marrow) is found mainly in the skull, sternum, ribs, vertebrae, upper sacrum, pelvis and proximal long bones. Marrow that is haemopoietically inactive is composed largely of fat (yellow marrow). In children the red marrow extends through a much larger proportion of the skeleton, e.g. into the distal long bones; in infants, haemopoietic marrow may be found even in the fingers and toes. In adults, under conditions of sustained need for more blood cells (particularly red cells), the red marrow can re-expand into more distal parts of the skeleton.

Normal haemopoiesis requires a supply of amino acids and various vitamins and minerals. The most important of the minerals is iron, which is an essential constituent of haemoglobin. The most important of the vitamins are vitamin B_{12} and folic acid. Both of these are needed for the synthesis of deoxyribonucleic acid (DNA), and rapidly proliferating tissues, such as the bone marrow, have a high requirement for these vitamins.

Iron

Iron is a crucial element in the human body, essential for the synthesis of haemoglobin, myoglobin, cytochromes and ribonucleotide reductase (needed for DNA synthesis). It is absorbed from the diet with foodstuffs of animal origin (e.g. red meat, offal, fish and eggs) being the richest source; some plant products, e.g. lentils, also contain a useful amount of iron. Haem iron is better absorbed than non-haem iron (about 10% can be absorbed in contrast with only 1–2%). Very little iron is normally lost from the body. The small about that is lost occurs through desquamating cells from the skin or gastrointestinal tract or in the red cells of blood. Uptake of about 1 mg a day is needed in adult men while menstruating women need about 2 mg a day. Pregnant women have a high requirement and lactation also increases need. Growing infants, children and adolescents have a greater requirement than adult men. Premature babies have increased iron needs as around half of the transfer of iron from the mother to the fetus is in the last month of intrauterine life. Blood donation increases the need for iron by 0.7 mg/day for each unit donated in a year so that men and women donating three times a year would have a daily requirement of 3 and 4 mg respectively. Since normally only about 10% of dietary iron is absorbed, the dietary iron intake needs to be considerably higher than the body's needs.

Iron is released from food in the stomach through the action of peptic enzymes and gastric acid. Iron passes into the duodenum where absorption is maximal. Some absorption also occurs in the jejunum. Any ferric (Fe^{3+}) iron is first converted to the ferrous form (Fe^{2+}) by a membrane enzyme, duodenal cytochrome B (Fig. 1.10). Ferrous iron is then able to bind to the membrane dimetal transporter 1 to enter the enterocyte. To be absorbed into the body, iron must pass right through the enterocyte, exiting by means of membrane ferroportin, so that it can be delivered to plasma transferrin. This requires re-conversion to the ferric form, achieved

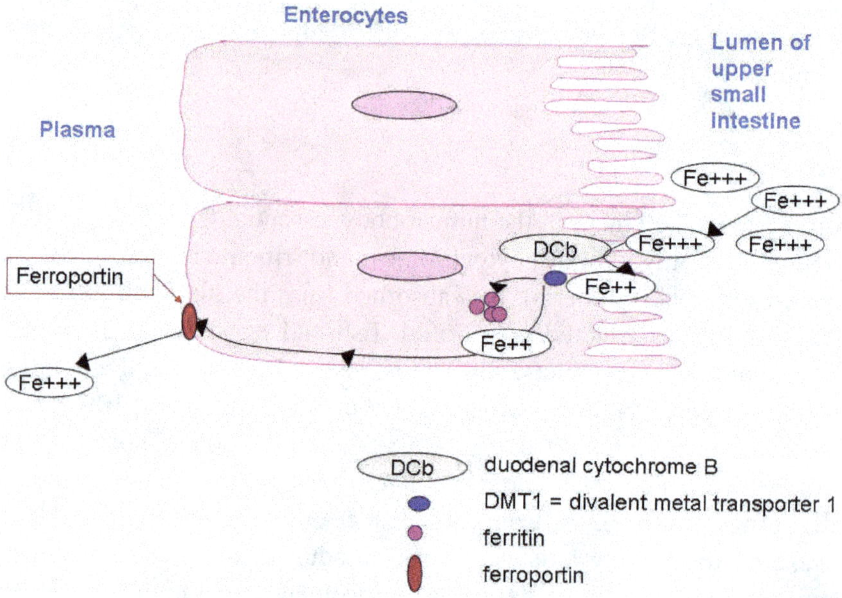

Fig. 1.10. The absorption of iron by mucosal cells of the upper intestine, particularly the duodenum.

with the help of several other co-operating proteins. If export from the cell does not happen, iron is converted to ferritin and is lost to the body when the enterocyte is shed into the gut lumen.

Since the body has no effective means of getting rid of excess iron, the rate of absorption must be carefully controlled. This is achieved by means of hepcidin, a protein synthesised by the liver. When body stores of iron are low, hepcidin synthesis is low and iron absorption is facilitated. In conditions of iron excess, hepcidin is synthesised in increased amounts and this leads to ferroportin of enterocytes being internalised and degraded (Fig. 1.11). Iron then cannot pass through the cell, so is lost to the body when the cells are shed. When there is iron deficiency, much less hepcidin is synthesised and iron absorption is promoted. Hepcidin has another role in maintaining plasma iron for delivery to erythroid precursors and other cells. The iron stored in macrophages in the form of haemosiderin can be mobilised and, by means of ferroportin, exported from the cell to the

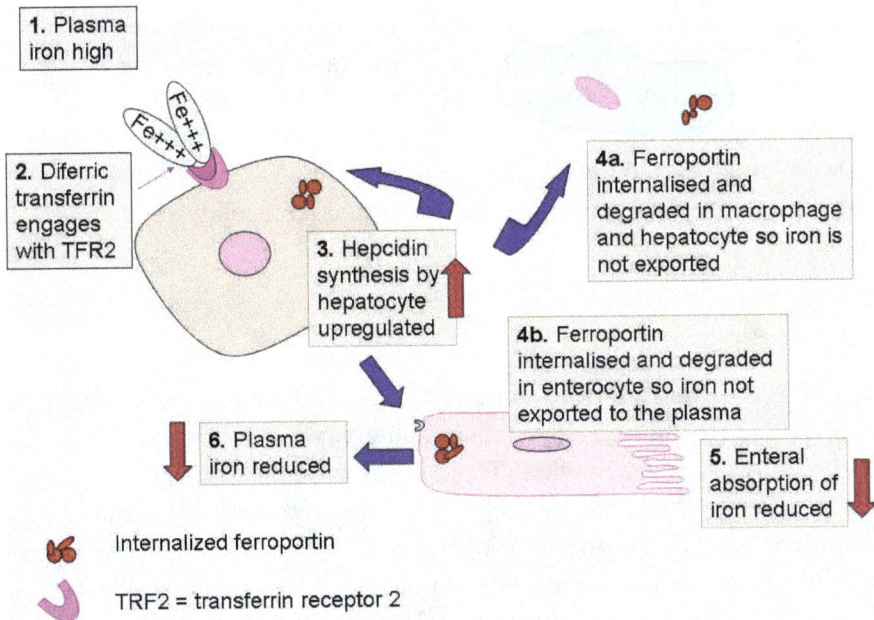

Fig. 1.11. The control of iron absorption and release from stores by hepcidin when plasma iron is high.

plasma. In the macrophage, as in the enterocyte, hepcidin leads to internalisation and degradation of ferroportin so that iron is trapped in the macrophage. In summary, in iron deficiency or depletion, when little hepcidin is synthesised, both macrophage export and intestinal absorption of iron are promoted. This maximises the iron available for erythropoiesis. Conversely, if iron is replete and more hepcidin is synthesised, iron stays in macrophages and is not absorbed by the intestine.

Another hormone links hepcidin synthesis to erythropoiesis. This is erythroferrone, which is produced by erythroblasts when erythropoiesis is stimulated by erythropoietin. Erythroferrone suppresses hepatic synthesis of hepcidin, thus leading to increased availability of iron when there is increased erythropoiesis.

The iron that is conserved in the body is in the form of haemosiderin within macrophages, referred to as the iron stores. Body iron can be viewed as belonging to three pools: (i) the functional pool, such as haemoglobin and myoglobin (about 2–3 g); (ii) the storage pool of ferritin and haemosiderin (about 1 g); and (iii) the transit pool of iron bound to transferrin in the plasma (only about 3 mg, but functionally very important).

The difference between iron deficiency and iron depletion is that in deficiency the amount of iron available to tissues is inadequate for haemoglobin synthesis whereas in depletion the iron stores are reduced or absent, but absorption is keeping up with the body's needs. The roles of some proteins important in iron transport and storage are summarised in Table 1.1.

Vitamin B_{12}

Vitamin B_{12} is derived from animal products in the diet. A vegetarian diet therefore has a reduced B_{12} content, and a vegan diet has negligible B_{12} and requires supplementation. The daily requirement is about 1 μg and, since not all is absorbed, an intake of 2.4 μg is advised. The main loss of B_{12} from the body is in the bile, where only about half of the 1.4 μg secreted each day is resorbed — and less if there is a defect in absorption. Dietary vitamin B_{12} is released from food by the action of hydrochloric acid and peptic enzymes. It binds to intrinsic factor (secreted by the stomach) in the duodenum and the B_{12}-intrinsic factor complex is then

Table 1.1. Some proteins important in iron absorption, transport and utilisation.

Protein	Nature and role
Duodenal cytochrome b	An enterocyte luminal membrane protein that converts ferric iron (Fe^{3+}) to ferrous (Fe^{2+}) so that it can be absorbed
Dimetal transporter 1	An enterocyte luminal membrane protein that transports ferrous iron into the enterocyte
Ferroportin	An enterocyte basal membrane protein and macrophage membrane protein that transports iron out of enterocytes and macrophages to the plasma
Transferrin	A plasma protein that accepts iron from ferroportin of enterocytes or macrophages and delivers it to erythroid precursors and other cells; it binds to transferrin receptors on the cell membrane and the iron–transferrin complex is then internalised with the transferrin and its receptor subsequently being recycled to the cell surface
Hepcidin	A peptide hormone synthesised by the liver that controls plasma iron by reducing iron absorption and promoting retention of iron in macrophages when iron is plentiful
Ferritin	A cytoplasmic protein, a storage form of iron, present in many cells
Erythroferrone	Produced by erythroblasts; suppresses hepatic synthesis of hepcidin thus increasing iron availability when erythropoiesis is stimulated
Haemosiderin	A cytoplasmic protein, a storage form of iron, formed from ferritin and mainly present in macrophages

internalised by ileal cells. The process is quite complex and is illustrated in Figs. 1.12 and 1.13. In the plasma, B_{12} is transported and delivered to the cells by transcobalamin. It is also bound to haptocorrin, of uncertain function, but this protein is not capable of delivering the vitamin to cells.

Vitamin B_{12} is essential for two metabolic pathways. It is a coenzyme in the conversion of 5-methyl-tetrahydrofolate to tetrahydrofolate and the simultaneous conversion of homocysteine to methionine; this pathway is essential for synthesis of DNA and RNA (ribonucleic acid). It is also a coenzyme for the synthesis of succinyl coenzyme A, a necessary step in catabolism of some fatty acids and some amino acids. Because of its role in DNA synthesis, the effects of any deficiency of vitamin B_{12} are prominent in rapidly dividing tissues, such as the bone marrow.

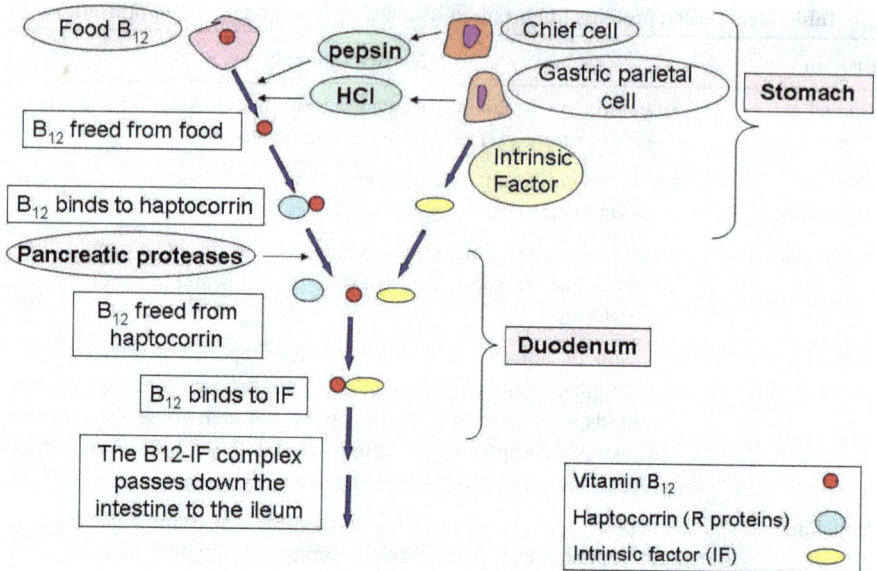

Fig. 1.12. The gastric and duodenal stages of vitamin B_{12} absorption: food containing vitamin B_{12} is digested in the stomach by means of hydrochloric acid and pepsin secreted by gastric cells; B_{12} is freed and combines with haptocorrin (of salivary gland origin); the B_{12}-haptocorrin complex passes into the duodenum where the action of pancreatic proteases and the higher pH lead to the B_{12} being released from haptocorrin and combining with intrinsic factor, also of gastric origin; the B_{12}-intrinsic factor complex passes down the intestine to the ileum where absorption occurs.

Folic acid

Rich dietary sources of folic acid include fruit and vegetables (particularly green vegetables), liver, kidney, yeast and yeast extracts. In many countries (e.g. the USA and Canada) flour is fortified with folic acid. Folic acid refers specifically to pteroylglutamic acid (a monoglutamate form), but most dietary folate is in the form of polyglutamates. The folate within body cells is also mainly in the form of polyglutamates with 3 to 7 glutamic acid residues. The term 'folate' refers to all these forms of folic acid.

Dietary folate is absorbed maximally in the upper jejunum. Polyglutamates must first be deconjugated to folic acid. This happens at the brush border, but whether in the lumen or within the cell is not clear.

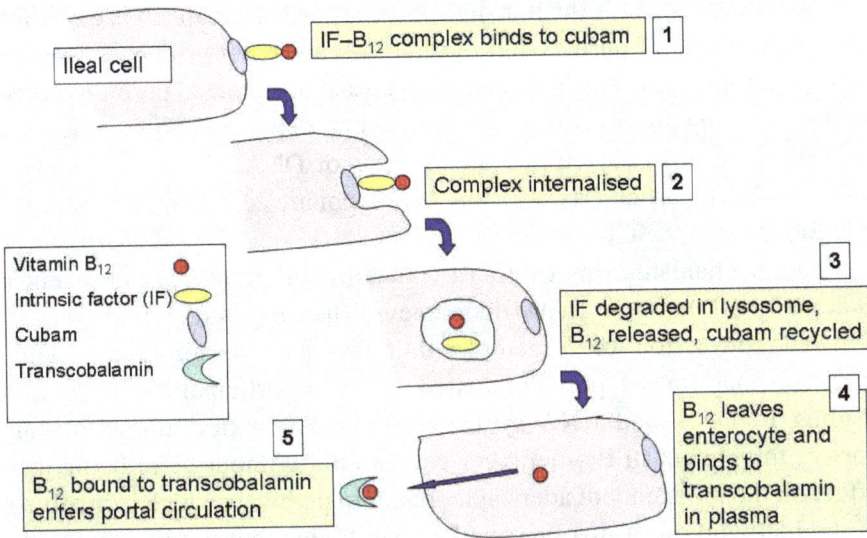

Fig. 1.13. The ileal stage of vitamin B_{12} absorption: (1) the intrinsic factor (IF)-B_{12} complex binds to cubam, an IF receptor on the surface membrane of ileal cells; (2) the IF-B_{12} complex is internalised; (3) the complex dissociates with IF being degraded and cubam being recycled to the cell surface; (4) B_{12} being exported from the cell to the plasma where it is bound to transcobalamin; (5) transcobalamin delivers B_{12} to hepatocytes for storage and to body cells that require it for DNA synthesis.

Absorption is an active process. Folic acid that is absorbed into the entero-cyte is mainly converted to methyl-tetrahydrofolate before being exported to the plasma. Methyl-tetrahydrofolate is actively taken up from the plasma by cells. Within cells it is converted to a polyglutamate form. This conversion plus the binding of folate to intracellular folate-binding pro-teins means that the folate is retained within the cell where it is required for various metabolic processes.

The daily requirement of folate is about 50–100 μg. About half of dietary folate is absorbed. To ensure the body's needs are met, the mini-mum recommended daily intake is 400 μg with the average diet containing 400–600 μg. Folate is stored in the liver and can be mobilised from there to other tissues. Body stores are 5–10 mg, sufficient to last for about four months if intake stops. Folate is lost from the body in urine, in the bile and in desquamating cells from the skin and the intestine.

The role of folate is the transfer of single carbon groups. It is essential for the synthesis of purines and pyrimidines and for interconversions of various amino acids. The body can compensate for reduced purine synthesis by reducing the rate of degradation, but if pyrimidine synthesis is reduced there is a reduced rate of synthesis of DNA with serious pathological effects, particularly affecting haemopoietic cells and other rapidly dividing cells.

The mechanism of megaloblastic anaemia in vitamin B_{12} deficiency is actually a functional folate deficiency. When B_{12} is deficient there is reduced conversion of 5-methyl-tetrahydrofolate to tetrahydrofolate, the form that can be polyglutamated and can participate in pathways leading to DNA and RNA synthesis. Providing extra folic acid can correct this defect in B_{12}-deficient patients but without there being any effect on the independent adenosylcobalamin pathway, which is involved in the methylation of myelin. The haematological but not the neurological effects of vitamin B_{12} deficiency can thus be improved by folic acid.

Folic acid is not only essential for haemopoiesis but an adequate intake during pregnancy is required to reduce the incidence of spina bifida to a minimum. Folic acid in a dose of 400 μg daily should be taken if pregnancy is possible. The prevention of neural tube defects is the reason that flour is now fortified in many countries.

Other essential requirements for haemopoiesis

Normal haemopoiesis requires a supply of amino acids and energy so that protein-calorie malnutrition leads to anaemia. Various growth factors are also essential but in general these are not rate limiting. However, erythropoietin is of critical importance for erythropoiesis and reduced synthesis in renal failure leads to anaemia. There is also a requirement for normal levels of hormones such as growth hormone, thyroxine, adrenal steroids and androgens so that anaemia is a feature of hypopituitarism, hypothyroidism, Addison disease and hypogonadism in men. In addition there is a requirement for copper, vitamin C, vitamin B_6 (pyridoxine) and vitamin B_2 (riboflavin). However, deficiency of any of these haematinics is quite uncommon as a cause of anaemia or other cytopenia.

Conclusions

Production and destruction of blood cells is finely balanced and maintained throughout life. Production is controlled by growth factors and cytokines and can be increased in response to increased needs. Normal haemopoiesis requires normal numbers of haemopoietic stem cells in an appropriate microenvironment, normal concentrations of various hormones and availability of amino acids, iron and various vitamins. The major functions of blood cells are oxygen transport and defence against infection.

2

The Blood Count and Film

Barbara J. Bain

What Do You Need To Know?

☞ The constituent parts of a blood count
☞ The meaning and clinical significance of a reticulocyte count
☞ The meaning of the words that are frequently used to describe abnormalities in the blood count and blood film and their possible clinical significance
☞ The meaning of 'normal range' and 'reference range'
☞ The approximate normal ranges for the white cell count, haemoglobin concentration, mean cell volume and platelet count in healthy adults
☞ How to interpret a blood count and develop a differential diagnosis
☞ The meaning and clinical significance of the erythrocyte sedimentation rate

---

Full Blood Count

The term 'full blood count' (FBC) refers to a group of tests performed simultaneously on a blood sample to assess whether there is any

Table 2.1. The full blood count.

Test	Abbreviation	Units	Normal range in men*	Normal range in women*
White blood cell count	WBC	$\times 10^9/l$	3.7–9.5	3.9–11.1
Red blood cell count	RBC	$\times 10^{12}/l$	4.32–5.66	3.88–4.99
Haemoglobin concentration	Hb	g/l	133–167	118–148
Haematocrit	Hct	l/l	0.39–0.50	0.36–0.44
Mean cell volume	MCV	fl	82–98	
Mean cell haemoglobin	MCH	pg	27.3–32.6	
Mean cell haemoglobin concentration	MCHC	g/l	316–349	
Platelet count		$\times 10^9/l$	168–411[†]	188–445[†]

*From BJ Bain (2022) *Blood Cells*, Sixth Edition, Wiley–Blackwell, Oxford.
[†]Reported ranges from different instruments vary.

haematological abnormality or to monitor a known abnormality. The tests that are almost always included in an FBC are shown in Table 2.1. In modern haematological practice these tests are performed on large automated analysers capable of processing many hundreds of samples in a day. Further tests are sometimes also included. The blood count is performed on a blood specimen that has been anticoagulated by being mixed with ethylene diamine tetra-acetic acid (EDTA), a chelating agent that prevents clotting by binding calcium. If you are obtaining a blood specimen from a patient for an FBC be sure to use a tube containing EDTA, add the correct volume of blood and mix the blood sample with the anticoagulant.

White blood cell count

The white blood cell count (WBC, also known as the white cell count) was initially determined by counting cells using a microscope and a glass counting chamber. Nowadays it is counted by an automated instrument that detects individual cells flowing in a stream through a sensor. Recognition is either because the cell interrupts a beam of light or because it alters the electrical current flowing between two electrodes. A WBC is performed on a sample in which the mature red cells have been lysed by solutions to which they are exposed within the instrument so that the only cells that will be counted are the white cells and any nucleated red blood cells that might be present.

Red blood cell count

The red blood cell count (RBC, also known as the red cell count) was initially determined with a counting chamber. As with the WBC, it is now determined by an instrument that counts red cells flowing through a sensor. However, the red cells are not lysed. White cells will actually also be included in the count but because they are infrequent in relation to the red cells this does not usually introduce much error.

Haemoglobin concentration

The haemoglobin concentration (Hb) is determined by lysing red cells and measuring light transmitted through a diluted sample of the blood at a specific wavelength after conversion of the haemoglobin to a stable form.

Haematocrit

It is possible to measure the proportion of red cells in an anticoagulated blood sample by centrifuging a tube of the blood and comparing the height of the column of red cells with the total height of the blood sample. This test is called a packed cell volume (PCV). It is no longer performed because it is not suitable for dealing with large numbers of blood specimens. The modern equivalent is called a haematocrit (Hct). It has the same significance as a PCV, but instruments calculate it rather than measuring it directly. This is done by multiplying the average size of a red cell, the mean cell volume (MCV), by the RBC.

Mean cell volume

The MCV was once estimated by dividing the PCV (obtained by centrifugation) by the RBC (from a counting chamber). This was a very laborious technique so it was not done very often. Modern instruments estimate the MCV from the height of the electrical impulse generated by interruption of a light beam or an electrical current. The same electrical impulse is therefore used both to count the cells and to size them.

Mean cell haemoglobin

The mean cell haemoglobin (MCH) is the average **amount** of haemoglobin in an individual red cell. Instruments calculate it by dividing the haemoglobin in a given volume of blood by the number of red cells in the same volume.

Mean cell haemoglobin concentration

The mean cell haemoglobin concentration (MCHC) is the average **concentration** of haemoglobin, rather than the absolute amount, in an individual red cell. Figure 2.1 is a visual representation of the difference between the MCH and the MCHC. Instruments calculate it by dividing the haemoglobin in a given volume of blood by the proportion of the whole blood sample that is occupied by red cells.

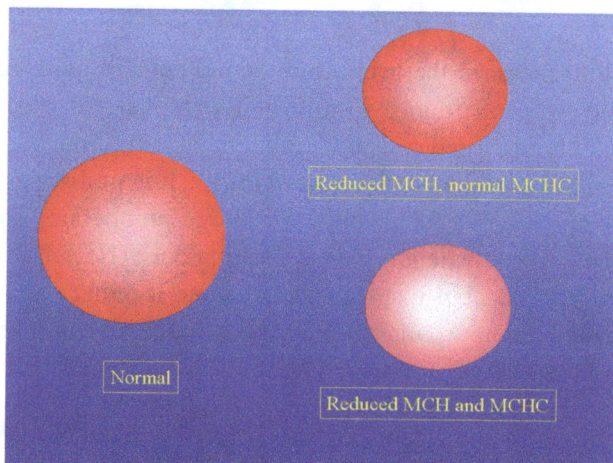

Fig. 2.1. A diagram to illustrate the difference between the mean cell haemoglobin (MCH) and the mean cell haemoglobin concentration (MCHC).

Red cell distribution width

The red cell distribution width (RDW) is a measurement of the amount of variation in the size of the red cells.

Haemoglobin distribution width

The haemoglobin distribution width (HDW), produced by some instruments, is a measurement of the amount of variation in the haemoglobinisation of red cells.

Platelet count

Platelets are counted by the same principles as red cells and white cells. They can be distinguished from red and white cells by their smaller size. Some automated instruments can also quantitate platelets with the aid of a fluorescent-labelled antibody directed at a platelet antigen.

Mean platelet volume

Platelets are sized in the same manner as red cells, yielding a mean platelet volume (MPV).

Red cell indices

The term 'red cell indices' refers to the RBC, MCV, MCH and MCHC. The formulae (which you do not need to know) for calculating the latter three values are:

$$\text{MCV (fl)} = \frac{\text{Hct (l/l)} \times 1{,}000}{\text{RBC (cells/l)} \times 10^{-12}}$$

$$\text{MCH (pg)} = \frac{\text{Hb (g/l)}}{\text{RBC (cells/l)} \times 10^{-12}}$$

$$\text{MCHC (g/l)} = \frac{\text{Hb (g/l)}}{\text{Hct (l/l)} \times 10}$$

Red cell indices are very useful for indicating the likely cause of anaemia. Note that if the RBC is, for example, $5 \times 10^{12}/l$ then the figure that is inserted in the formula is the RBC by $\times 10^{-12}/l$, which is 5. Note also that the symbol used for litre can be either 'l' or 'L'.

Reticulocyte count

A reticulocyte count is a supplement to a FBC, rather than a normal part of it. It can be performed by using a microscrope to count the percentage of erythrocytes that have developed a 'reticulum' or network of precipitated dye after incubation of the blood sample with a dye such as methylene blue (Fig. 2.2). This is a method for identifying ribonucleic acid (RNA) within red cells, thus demonstrating that these are cells newly released from the bone marrow (1–3 days old). Reticulocyte counts can also be performed by automated instruments, using either the same principle as the reticulocyte count with a microscope or, alternatively, using a fluorescent dye that binds to RNA.

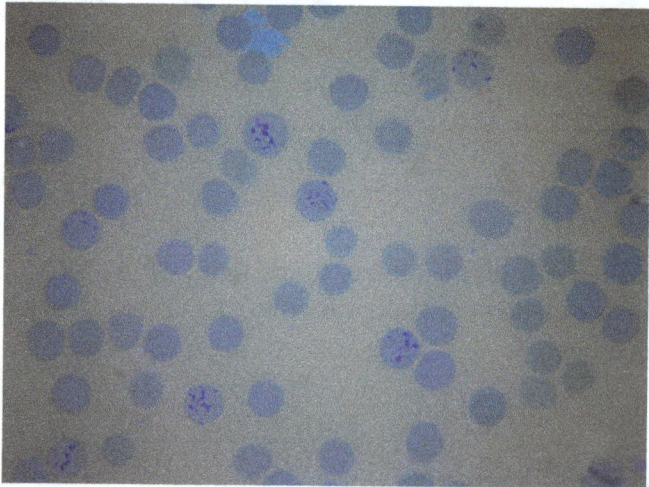

Fig. 2.2. A reticulocyte preparation, showing a reticulum of precipitated dye within some erythrocytes following incubation of blood with methylene blue.

Differential White Cell Count

The different types of white cell can be distinguished from each other by examining a stained blood film. If a hundred cells are counted and the percentages are multiplied by the WBC, the absolute number of cells of each type can be calculated. Calculating the percentage or absolute number of each cell type is referred to as a differential count. It is much more useful to calculate the absolute count than to try to make deductions from the percentages. For example, if a patient had 5% neutrophils and 95% lymphocytes this could indicate either a severe reduction of neutrophils or a marked increase in lymphocytes.

Many automated instruments can recognise the five normal types of white cell and can detect the presence of nucleated red blood cells (NRBC) and other cells that are not normally present in the circulating blood. If only normal cells are present, they are capable of performing a differential count. If abnormal cells are present, it is usually still necessary to perform a differential count on a blood film. However, many instruments are capable of counting NRBC and automated differential counts performed on a blood film are increasingly finding a role. Normal ranges for the differential white cell count are shown in Table 2.2.

Table 2.2. The differential white cell count.

Test	Units	Normal range in men[*]	Normal range in women[*]
Neutrophil count	$\times 10^9/l$	1.7–6.1	1.7–7.5
Lymphocyte count	$\times 10^9/l$	1.0–3.2	
Monocyte count	$\times 10^9/l$	0.2–0.6	
Eosinophil count	$\times 10^9/l$	0.03–0.46	
Basophil count	$\times 10^9/l$	0.09–0.29	

[*]From BJ Bain (2022) *Blood Cells,* Sixth Edition, Wiley–Blackwell, Oxford. Figures are for an automated instrument and will differ slightly between instruments. Figures for manual differential counts will have broader limits.

B. J. Bain

Haematological Terminology

Haematologists use precise terms to refer to abnormalities in the blood count and film. Since they use these terms to report abnormalities to clinical staff it is necessary for all doctors to understand them. The terms used to describe quantitative abnormalities are shown in Table 2.3; unfortunately these terms are not necessarily logical or consistent, so you just have to learn how they are used. The terms used to describe erythrocytes and their abnormalities are shown and illustrated in Table 2.4. Measurements made by automated instruments correlate with observations on a blood film. Thus MCHC correlates with hypochromia, RDW with anisocytosis and HDW with anisochromasia. MCV and MPV correlate with the observed size of red cells and platelets respectively. Polychromasia and the presence of polychromatic macrocytes are reflected in the reticulocyte count.

Table 2.3. Terminology used for describing quantitative abnormalities in blood counts.

Term	Meaning
Anaemia	Reduced Hb
Polycythaemia or erythrocytosis	Either term can be used to indicate an increase in the RBC, Hb and Hct
Leucocytosis	Increased WBC
Leucopenia	Reduced WBC
Thrombocytosis	Increased platelet count
Thrombocytopenia	Reduced platelet count
Neutrophilia	Increased neutrophil count
Neutropenia	Reduced neutrophil count
Lymphocytosis	Increased lymphocyte count
Lymphopenia* or lymphocytopenia	Reduced lymphocyte count
Monocytosis	Increased monocyte count
Eosinophilia	Increased eosinophil count
Basophilia[†]	Increased basophil count
Reticulocytosis	Increased reticulocyte count
Reticulocytopenia	Reduced reticulocyte count

*The term 'lymphopenia' is illogical because it is used to mean a reduced lymphocyte count not a reduced amount of lymph, but it is the term most often used.
[†]Basophilia has a quite different alternative meaning; it also means an increased uptake of basic dyes by the cytoplasm of a cell so that when examined with a microscope it appears blue.

Table 2.4. Terminology used for describing erythrocytes.

Term	Significance	Picture
Normocytic Normochromic	Of normal size With normal staining characteristics	
Anisocytosis	Increased variation in size	
Poikilocyte Poikilocytosis	An erythrocyte of abnormal shape Increased variation in shape	
Microcyte Microcytosis	Smaller than normal erythrocyte The presence of microcytes	
Macrocyte Macrocytosis	Larger than normal erythrocyte The presence of macrocytes	

(Continued)

Table 2.4. *(Continued)*

Term	Significance	Picture
Hypochromic	Paler than normal (more than a third of the diameter of the cell is pale)	
Hypochromia	The presence of hypochromic cells	
Anisochromasia	Variation in haemoglobinisation between cells	
Polychromasia	Having a blue tinge	
Elliptocyte	An erythrocyte that is elliptical in shape	
Ovalocyte	An erythrocyte that is oval in shape	
Macro-ovalocyte	An oval macrocyte	

Table 2.4. (*Continued*)

Term	Significance	Picture
Spherocyte	An erythrocyte that is spherical in shape and is therefore lacking central pallor	
Irregularly contracted cell	An erythrocyte that lacks central pallor and has an irregular outline	
Teardrop cell (dacrocyte)	An erythrocyte that is shaped like a tear	
Target cell	An erythrocyte that has haemoglobin concentrated at the periphery of the cell and also as a dot in the centre	
Sickle cell	An erythrocyte with a crescent or sickle shape	

(*Continued*)

Table 2.4. *(Continued)*

Term	Significance	Picture
Stomatocyte	An erythrocyte with a slit-like 'stoma'	
Schistocyte or fragment	A small piece of a red cell	
Acanthocyte	An erythrocyte that has a small number of spicules of irregular length and shape	
Echinocyte or crenated cell	An erythrocyte that has a large number of short regular spicules	
Rouleaux	Red cells stacked up like a flattened pile of pennies	

Table 2.4. (*Continued*)

Term	Significance	Picture
Agglutination	Red cells forming irregular clumps	
Howell–Jolly body	A fragment of the nucleus remaining in a mature red cell (stains purple)	
Pappenheimer body	An iron-containing granule (stains navy blue)	
Basophilic stippling	Fine or coarse dark blue-staining dots scattered through the cytoplasm	

Normal Ranges and Reference Ranges

Once we have got a laboratory result how do we know if it is normal? Laboratories issue test results with a reference range or normal range for comparison. A reference range is derived from a carefully defined

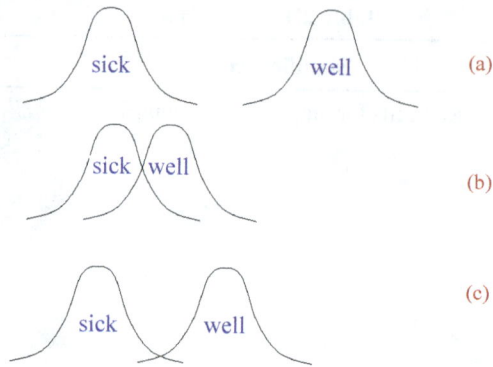

Fig. 2.3. Paired histograms showing the possible results of applying a test in sick and healthy individuals: (a) an ideal test; (b) a non-ideal test that will necessarily result in either false positive or false negative results, depending on the threshold chosen; (c) a test that shows sufficient discrimination between sick and healthy individuals to be useful in clinical practice.

population: the definition will include the age and gender of the subjects and sometimes the ethnic origin or other relevant details. If a requirement to be in good health is part of the definition then a 'reference range' becomes a 'normal range'. Conventionally reference ranges and normal ranges include the central 95% of results from the reference population. Ideally tests would give a clear separation of healthy subjects (the normal range) and an unhealthy population, as shown in Fig. 2.3(a). More often, the situation will be as shown in Fig. 2.3(c), with a small amount of overlap between sick and well people. Sometimes a test gives poor separation of sick and well (Fig. 2.3(b)). Either the laboratory or the clinician looking after the patient has to decide the threshold to accept. If the figure chosen includes all sick people, then a lot of normal people will also be included; the test becomes sensitive but at the cost of a high rate of false positives. If the threshold is moved down so that no healthy person is falsely classified as sick, there are no false positives but the test becomes very insensitive (a lot of false negative results). Fortunately the overlap between healthy and sick is not often as extreme as shown in Fig. 2.3(b).

It can be useful to have a 'health-related range', rather than a normal range that represents 95% of the apparently healthy population. For example, if the upper 20% of results for serum cholesterol in a typical Western population indicated an increased risk of myocardial infarction, an individual and his physician might aim to alter his life style and medications so that his results fell in the bottom 80% of the reference range rather than the central 95%. This bottom 80% would be the health-related range.

When laboratories collect data to establish a normal range, they perform the specified test on healthy volunteers using exactly the same instruments and methods that they are going to use for analysing patient samples. They will also analyse the data using appropriate statistical methods. If the data have a Gaussian distribution, as for the Hb (Fig. 2.4), then the arithmetic mean ±2 standard deviations (or, more strictly, 1.96 standard deviations) can be used. The WBC, however, has a logarithmic distribution (Fig. 2.5) and the data have to be converted to logarithms before they can be analysed. Other non-Gaussian distributions have to be dealt with by other statistical techniques.

It is important when interpreting laboratory tests to take account of the following: (i) the normal range may not be appropriate; (ii) the test result may be within the normal range but abnormal for that patient; and (iii) the test result might be outside the reference range but actually normal for that individual.

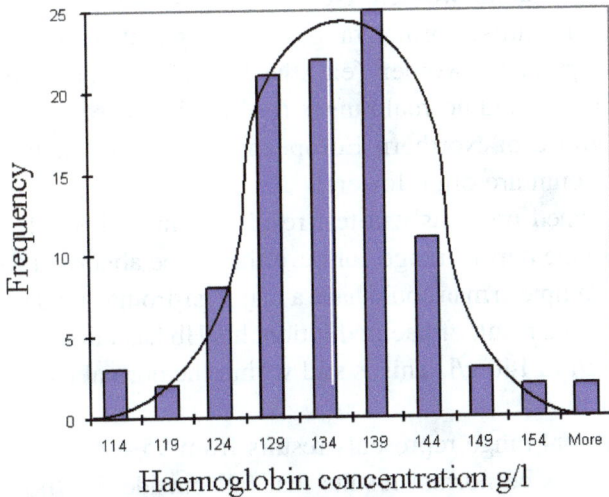

Fig. 2.4. A histogram of haemoglobin concentration (Hb) results in healthy subjects showing a Gaussian distribution.

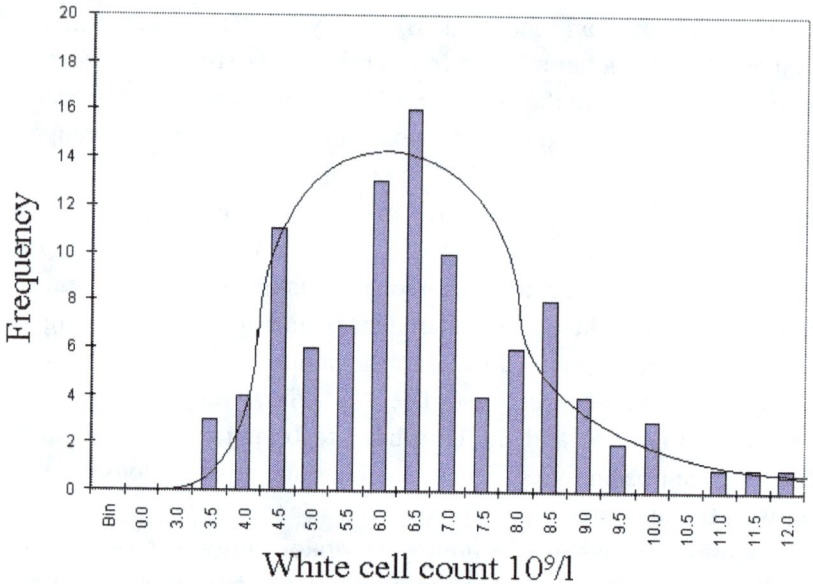

Fig. 2.5. A histogram of white cell count (WBC) results in healthy subjects showing a skewed distribution that will become Gaussian on logarithmic transformation.

Laboratories usually have only two normal ranges, one for adult men and one for adult women. Normal ranges for children often differ from those for adults, normal ranges for pregnant women differ from those of non-pregnant women (e.g. the Hb is lower and the WBC and MCV are higher), and normal ranges for individuals of African ancestry differ from those of Northern Europeans (the WBC, neutrophil count and platelet count are often lower).

As mentioned previously, a test result for an individual patient may still be within the normal range but nevertheless be abnormal for that individual. For example, a man could have a major gastrointestinal haemorrhage and next day, as a result of haemodilution, his Hb has fallen from his usual level of 165 g/l to 140 g/l. This is still within the normal range but is very abnormal for him.

If the normal range represents results from 95% of healthy subjects there will always be normal results that fall outside the 'normal' range. This will be so for 5% of results for each test. If a lot of tests are done it is very probable that at least one will be abnormal. For example, if the eight core tests that usually form part of the FBC are performed it is likely that a third of patients will have an abnormal result.

How to Interpret a Blood Count and Develop a Differential Diagnosis

When interpreting a blood count, or any other laboratory result, you should ask yourself the following questions:

- Is this result abnormal for this patient?
- If it is abnormal, is it a trivial abnormality that should be ignored or might it be important?
- If it might be important, is it so abnormal that there is a clinical urgency in dealing with the result?
- What is the likely cause of the abnormality?

To determine the likely cause of an abnormality you might need to consider the clinical history, any medications the patient is taking, any abnormalities found on physical examination and the results of any other tests that have already been done. You may then need to develop a differential diagnosis and do extra tests to find out the cause.

The differential diagnosis indicated by various blood count abnormalities will be dealt with in the chapters that follow but will be outlined here, according to which test is abnormal.

Abnormal white cell counts

If the WBC is abnormal it is necessary to go further and look at the different components of the differential count to see which parts are abnormal. The automated instrument that produces the WBC is likely to have produced an automated differential count. If the abnormality is purely quantitative, for example an increased neutrophil count, then the clinical history may reveal the cause (e.g. known bacterial infection) so that no further haematological tests are indicated. On other occasions there may be immature cells present or abnormalities of mature cells so that the automated instrument either does not produce a differential count or 'flags' the result, indicating an abnormality. In this instance a blood film is usually needed.

Neutrophil count

In deciding if a neutrophil count is elevated or reduced it is important to make a comparison with a relevant reference range (e.g. counts are higher in pregnancy and lower in some individuals of African ancestry).

A high neutrophil count is usually reactive to infection, inflammation, trauma or surgery, and is due to increased production by the bone marrow. Rarely, it is due to leukaemia.

A low neutrophil count can be due to: (i) inadequate production by the bone marrow; (ii) inability of the bone marrow to respond sufficiently to increased need, e.g. in infected neonates; (iii) peripheral destruction, e.g. drug-induced immune destruction; or (iv) abnormal pooling, e.g. in the spleen in hypersplenism.

Lymphocyte count

A high lymphocyte count can be due to increased production of lymphocytes or to altered distribution within the body. Increased production can be reactive, e.g. to viral infection, or be the result of leukaemia. A high lymphocyte count due to mobilisation of lymphocytes from tissues occurs as a transient acute response to stress, e.g. following severe trauma or a myocardial infarction. Lymphocytosis due to redistribution of lymphocytes within the body also occurs following splenectomy.

A low lymphocyte count can be due to inherited and acquired immune deficiency, e.g. human immunodeficiency virus (HIV) infection, or can be a stress response to illness, surgery or trauma, in that case being mediated by corticosteroids. A stress-induced lymphocytosis is followed by a stress-induced lymphopenia.

Monocyte count

An increased monocyte count is usually reactive, as the result of chronic infection, inflammation or malignancy and is the result of increased production by the bone marrow. Less often it represents leukaemia.

A reduced monocyte count is usually due to inadequate production by the bone marrow. It is uncommon but when it does occur it renders the patient susceptible to infection.

Eosinophil count

An increased eosinophil count is usually reactive, as a result of allergy (including some adverse drug reactions) or parasitic infection, and is due to increased bone marrow production.

A low eosinophil count occurs as a stress reaction, mediated by corticosteroids.

Basophil count

An increased basophil count is often a feature of a haematological neoplasm and results from increased bone marrow production. It is diagnostically useful since reactive basophilia (e.g. due to hypothyroidism or ulcerative colitis) is uncommon.

A reduced basophil count is rarely noted and is even more rarely of diagnostic importance.

Anaemia

The cause of the anaemia may be apparent from the clinical history. If not, a differential diagnosis can be developed by considering the size of the cells or by trying to work out the mechanism of the anaemia. A classification of anaemia based on cell size is shown in Table 2.5. This approach is very useful and often indicates a likely diagnosis and the tests that are needed to confirm it. If consideration of clinical features and erythrocyte size does not suggest a diagnosis, it can be useful to seek evidence of a mechanism of the anaemia, as shown in Table 2.6.

Polycythaemia

Polycythaemia refers to an increase of RBC, Hb and Hct. These laboratory abnormalities can be the result of a true polycythaemia, in which the total volume of red cells circulating in the blood stream is increased. They can also be the result of an acute or chronic reduction of plasma volume, referred to as pseudopolycythaemia. The cause of an acute reduction in plasma volume, such as shock, burns or dehydration, will be apparent from the clinical history, but a chronic pseudopolycythaemia requires

Table 2.5.   Causes of anaemias according to cell size.

Cell size	Microcytic	Macrocytic	Normocytic
Causes	Iron deficiency (common) Anaemia of chronic disease (common) Thalassaemia (common in some ethnic groups)	Liver disease Alcohol excess Megaloblastic anaemia (vitamin B_{12} or folate deficiency or exposure to certain drugs) Myelodysplastic syndromes Hypothyroidism Aplastic anaemia Haemolysis	Early stages or iron deficiency and anaemia of chronic disease Blood loss Renal failure Bone marrow suppression (e.g. by chemotherapy)

Table 2.6.   Supporting evidence for mechanisms of anaemia.

Mechanism	Possible supporting evidence
Failure of bone marrow production	Low reticulocyte count, lack of polychromasia
Blood loss	Clinical evidence and later increased reticulocyte count
Increased destruction (i.e. haemolysis)	Increased reticulocyte count, polychromasia, increased bilirubin concentration, increased lactate dehydrogenase, cells of abnormal shape (spherocytes, elliptocytes, fragments)
Red cell pooling in the spleen plus increased plasma volume	Clinical evidence — presence of splenomegaly

laboratory tests to distinguish it from true polycythaemia. The differential diagnosis of polycythaemia will be discussed in Chapter 9.

Thrombocytosis

A high platelet count is almost always due to increased production by the bone marrow. The exception is following a splenectomy, when it is due to redistribution. Thrombocytosis is usually reactive, due to infection, inflammation, blood loss or malignancy. Less often it is the result of a chronic haematological neoplasm known as a myeloproliferative neoplasm.

Thrombocytopenia can be the result of: (i) failure of bone marrow production; (ii) increased destruction by antibodies; (iii) increased consumption during coagulation; (iv) acute blood loss with failure to replace platelets that are lost; or (v) pooling in an enlarged spleen. The causes of thrombocytopenia will be discussed in more detail in Chapter 11.

Erythrocyte Sedimentation Rate

This test involves mixing blood with the correct amount of citrate anticoagulant, allowing it to sediment in a tube of precise dimensions and measuring the number of mm of sedimented red cells at the end of one hour. The normal range is 1–10 mm in an hour for a man and 0–20 mm in an hour for a woman. The erythrocyte sedimentation rate (ESR) is increased by anaemia and decreased by polycythaemia. It is increased by an increase in large plasma proteins (such as fibrinogen, $\alpha 2$ macroglobulin and immunoglobulins, particularly immunoglobulin M) and by a reduction in albumin concentration. The ESR is increased by pregnancy and by infection, inflammation, tissue infarction and malignancy. Although this test is very non-specific, it remains useful for monitoring chronic inflammatory conditions, such as rheumatoid arthritis, and in the follow up of Hodgkin lymphoma.

Conclusions

In order to interpret a full blood count and blood film you need to be familiar with the terminology and the abbreviations that are often used. You also need to know the approximate normal range for common measurements. By the time you get to the end of this book, or your haematology course, you should also be able to interpret a blood count and film, develop a differential diagnosis and explain what tests you would do next.

3

Microcytic Anaemias
and the Thalassaemias

Vishal Jayakar

What Do You Need To Know?

☞ How to diagnose, investigate and treat iron deficiency anaemia
☞ When to suspect and how to diagnose anaemia of chronic disease
☞ The nature of thalassaemia, how it is diagnosed, why diagnosis is important and how the condition is managed
☞ That there are other causes of microcytic anaemia

Introduction

A microcytic anaemia is one in which the erythrocytes are smaller than normal (i.e. microcytic). Often they are also hypochromic (i.e. they appear paler than normal in a stained blood film). The anaemia may thus be referred to as a hypochromic microcytic anaemia. The blood count shows a reduced haemoglobin concentration (Hb), haematocrit (Hct) and mean cell volume (MCV). Cells of reduced size have a reduced haemoglobin content so the mean cell haemoglobin (MCH) is also reduced. In addition, the concentration of haemoglobin in the erythrocytes may be reduced; this is reflected in a low normal value or a reduction in the mean cell haemo-globin concentration (MCHC).

Microcytic anaemias result from a reduced rate of synthesis of haemoglobin. This, in turn, results from a reduced rate of synthesis of either **haem** or **globin**. A reduced rate of synthesis of haem occurs in iron deficiency and also in a type of anaemia that occurs in patients with chronic infection or inflammation, known as 'anaemia of chronic disease'. Unlike iron deficiency, in the anaemia of chronic disease body stores of iron are normal or increased; however, the availability of iron to the developing red cell is reduced. A reduced rate of synthesis of either α or β globin chains also leads to a reduced rate of synthesis of haemoglobin and thus to microcytosis. A reduced rate of synthesis of one or other of the globin chain types is usually an inherited condition, known as α thalassaemia (reduced rate of synthesis of α globin chains) or β thalassaemia (reduced rate of synthesis of β globin chains). A rare cause of a microcytic anaemia is an inherited defect in the synthesis of haem in which iron accumulates within the mitochondria of erythroblasts rather than being incorporated into haem: this is known as sideroblastic anaemia. Rarely, acquired defects in haem synthesis occur, for example in lead poisoning.

The various mechanisms of microcytosis are summarised in Fig. 3.1.

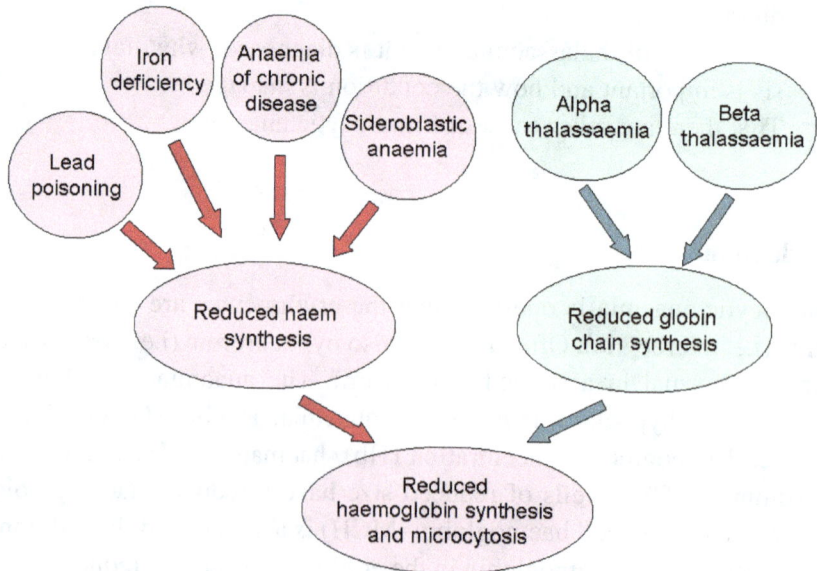

Fig. 3.1.   Diagrammatic representation of the causes of microcytosis.

Iron Deficiency Anaemia

Iron, which is essential for the synthesis of haemoglobin, is obtained from the diet and recycled and conserved in the body. Dietary sources and absorption are discussed on pages 11–12. To maintain a normal Hb, iron absorption needs to keep up with any physiological or pathological loss and cope with any increased demands. Iron deficiency therefore results from: (i) inadequate intake; (ii) malabsorption; (iii) increased need; (iv) increased or abnormal loss; or (v) any combination of these factors (Fig. 3.2, Table 3.1). In developed countries iron deficiency is the most common cause of anaemia, accounting for almost a third of cases. This proportion is even higher in developing countries. Common causes of iron deficiency are poor dietary intake of iron, increased requirements (in infancy or during pregnancy) and abnormal blood loss. In developing countries blood loss from intestinal parasites is a major factor. Low socio-economic status and poverty correlate with an increased rate of iron deficiency. In infants, early replacement of breast feeding with cow's milk and late introduction of solid foods can contribute to iron deficiency.

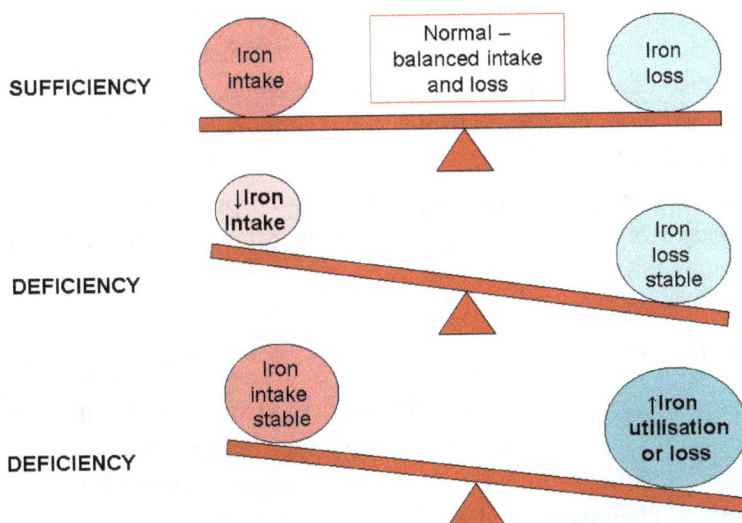

Fig. 3.2. Diagrammatic representation of the causes of iron deficiency: (a) balanced intake and loss, normal iron status; (b) decreased iron intake that does not balance iron loss and iron deficiency occurs; and (c) increased iron utilisation in excess of what is provided by normal intake and iron deficiency occurs.

Table 3.1. Factors that can cause or contribute to iron deficiency anaemia.

Increased utilisation
  Growth spurts, e.g. in infants, children and adolescents
  Repeated pregnancies and lactation

Inadequate intake
  Weaning babies onto iron-poor milk or substitutes (e.g. 'goat's milk anaemia')
  Vegetarian diet

Malabsorption
  Coeliac disease
  Autoimmune gastric atrophy
  Helicobacter pylori infection

Increased loss
  Menorrhagia
  Gastrointestinal bleeding (e.g. induced by aspirin or non-steroidal anti-inflammatory
    drugs, other ulceration, inflammatory bowel disease, carcinoma and (in some
    countries) intestinal parasites)
  Haemoglobinuria
  Frequently repeated blood donation

Sequestration of iron
  Pulmonary haemosiderosis

Paterson–Brown–Kelly syndrome (or Plummer–Vinson syndrome) is a rare cause of iron deficiency anaemia, accompanied by dysphagia and oesophageal webs with a predisposition to squamous cell carcinoma of the pharynx and oesophagus.

Iron deficiency anaemia is preceded by a period of iron depletion, when body stores of iron are greatly reduced but the patient has not yet become anaemic.

Clinical features

Patients with iron deficiency anaemia demonstrate the usual signs and symptoms of anaemia such as fatigue, tachycardia and poor exercise tolerance. Specific clinical features suggestive of iron deficiency are uncommon. They include pica (the ingestion of unusual substances such as ice or soil), glossitis (flattening and soreness of the tongue), angular cheilosis (cracking at the angle of the mouth), dysphagia and koilonychia (spoon-shaped nails). In children there can also be impaired intellectual performance, which may not be reversible.

Laboratory features

Iron deficiency anaemia is initially normocytic and normochromic. As it becomes more severe, it becomes hypochromic and microcytic. The red cell count (RBC), Hb, Hct, MCV and MCH are all reduced. When the anaemia is severe, the MCHC is also reduced. The platelet count may be increased. When iron deficiency is the result of intestinal parasites such as hookworms (Fig. 3.3), the blood count may show eosinophilia.

The blood film shows hypochromia and microcytosis (Fig. 3.4). When anaemia is more severe there is anisocytosis and poikilocytosis, with thin elliptocytes, known as pencil cells, being particularly characteristic. There may be small numbers of target cells.

Serum ferritin is usually low and as other causes of a low ferritin are very rare a reduced ferritin, less than 15 μg/l (normal range 15–300), confirms that anaemia is the result of iron deficiency. Serum iron level is

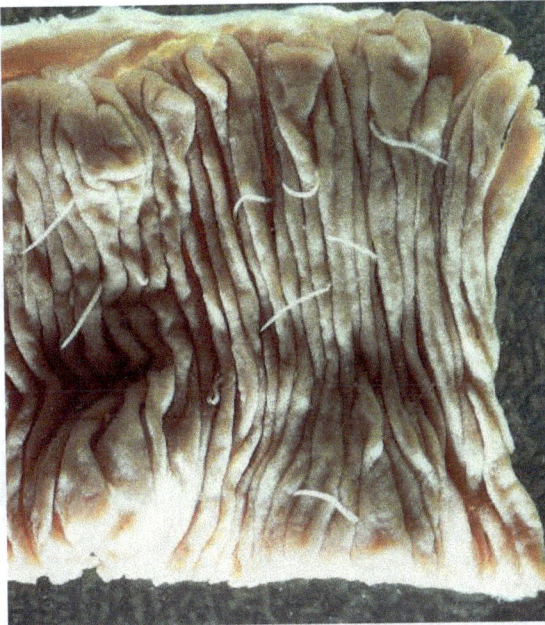

Fig. 3.3. Adult hookworms attached by their buccal capsule to the villi of the small intestine. Hookworm is an significant worldwide cause of iron deficiency anaemia. Eosinophilia is maximal at the stage of larval migration through the lung. Reproduced with permission from W Peters and G Pasvol, *Atlas of Tropical Medicine and Parasitology*, 6th Edn, Elsevier, 2007.

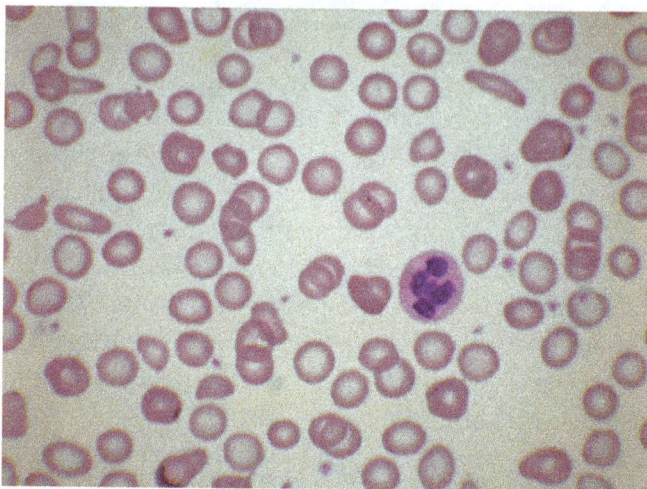

Fig. 3.4. Peripheral blood (PB) film in iron deficiency anaemia showing hypochromia, anisochromasia, microcytosis and several elliptocytes. May–Grünwald–Giemsa stain (MGG).

low, with elevated transferrin concentration and iron-binding capacity, but these measurements are not necessary if the ferritin level is low.

In patients with chronic inflammation the diagnosis of iron deficiency is more difficult since serum ferritin is elevated by infection, acute and chronic inflammation and many tumours. In patients known to have these conditions, a ferritin of up to 50 μg/l or even higher is consistent with iron deficiency. If the results of blood tests do not clearly distinguish between these two types of anaemia, a bone marrow aspirate will provide the answer, though this is not routinely required in clinical practice. In patients with iron deficiency there is no stainable iron in the macrophages of the bone marrow particles, whereas in anaemia of chronic disease storage iron is present and may be increased.

Diagnosis

A blood count, blood film and serum ferritin assay are usually all that is required for diagnosis. In uncomplicated iron deficiency there is a hypochromic microcytic anaemia and a low serum ferritin. When diagnosis is difficult, it may be necessary to examine the bone marrow and perform a Prussian blue stain on a bone marrow film. In a normal bone marrow, iron

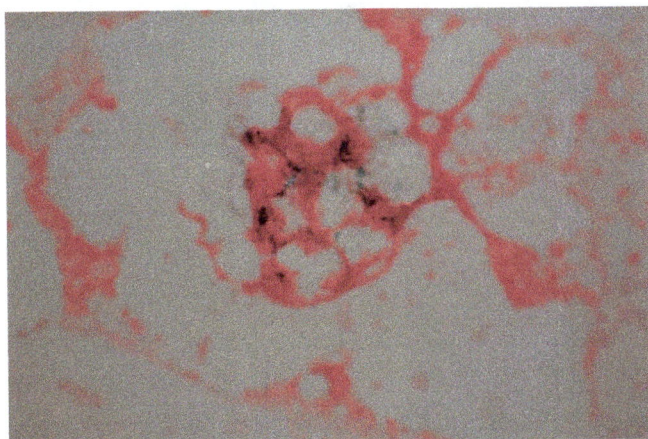

Fig. 3.5. Bone marrow (BM) fragment stained with a Perls stain for iron showing that storage iron (haemosiderin in macrophages) is present (blue-staining material).

is present in macrophages within bone marrow fragments and stains deep blue (Fig. 3.5); it is also seen as small blue-staining particles within erythroblasts, referred to as siderotic granules. In iron deficiency no blue-staining material is apparent in the fragments (Fig. 3.6) and siderotic granules are reduced or absent.

Management

Having established a diagnosis of iron deficiency it is necessary both to find the cause and deal with it and also to treat the deficiency. Dietary history, travel history and, for women of childbearing age, the number and frequency of pregnancies must be assessed. The possibility of menorrhagia or other abnormal bleeding must be considered. In young women, low dietary iron intake, menstruation and pregnancy are the likely causes. In middle-aged or elderly people of either gender, gastrointestinal tract bleeding (which may be occult) is likely and further investigations including gastroscopy and colonoscopy may be needed. Other potential causes to consider are malabsorption of iron due to achlorhydria or coeliac disease (serology for anti-tissue transglutaminase antibodies should be performed). Patients with pernicious anaemia (see page 73) have achlorhydria and are prone to iron deficiency. In middle-aged and elderly patients (i.e. above 50 years) investigations to exclude

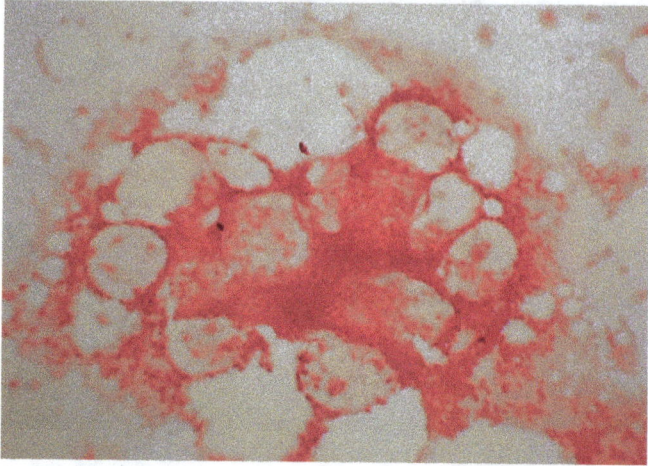

Fig. 3.6. BM stained with a Perls stain for iron in a patient with iron deficiency anaemia showing that storage iron (haemosiderin in macrophages) is absent (no blue-staining material).

gastrointestinal carcinoma or other tumour must be carried out, even in the absence of relevant symptoms.

Iron deficiency is usually treated with oral ferrous salts, which will cause the Hb to rise by about 10 g/l/week. Available ferrous salts include ferrous fumarate, ferrous sulphate and ferrous gluconate. What is important is the amount of elemental iron, which varies by preparation. For example, the usual dose of ferrous sulphate (containing 65 mg of elemental iron) is 200 mg three times a day. The patient should be warned that the stools will become black and that there may be gastrointestinal side effects (nausea, diarrhoea, constipation, abdominal pain). Mothers of children should also be specifically warned to keep the iron preparation in a safe place away from children. Accidental iron poisoning in children can be fatal. Oral iron is better absorbed early in the morning (when hepcidin levels are lowest, enabling more iron absorption) on an empty stomach; however, if the patient cannot tolerate it, then it can be taken with food. If it is taken with a source of vitamin C, such as orange juice, absorption is increased. Other medications, multivitamins and antacids should not be taken at the same time. Repeat Hb testing is desirable 3–4 weeks after commencing treatment to assess compliance, correct administration and response to treatment. Once Hb is in the normal range, replacement should continue for 3–6 months to replenish iron stores. If the patient cannot tolerate oral iron, various parenteral preparations are available; these are most conveniently administered as a total-dose intravenous infusion. Single-dose preparations of iron carboxymaltose and iron isomaltoside are popular alternatives. Genuine hypersensitivity and anaphylaxis are rare; hypophosphataemia can occur, particularly after a dose of ferric carboxymaltose.

Anaemia of Chronic Disease

Anaemia of chronic disease, also known as anaemia of inflammation, characteristically occurs in patients with chronic infection or inflammation. It also occurs in some patients with malignant disease. Typical causes include tuberculosis, rheumatoid arthritis, ulcerative colitis, Crohn disease, carcinoma of the ovary and Hodgkin lymphoma. Anaemia of

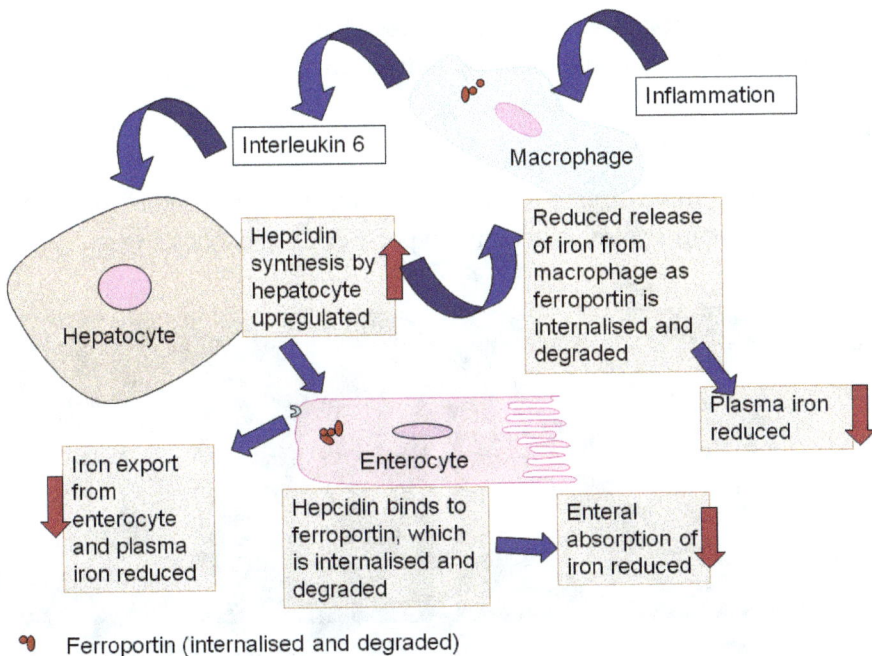

Fig. 3.7. Diagram showing how hepcidin regulates iron absorption and release from macrophages and how increases in interleukin 6 (synthesised by macrophages when there is inflammation) leads to increased hepcidin synthesis and contributes to the anaemia of chronic disease.

chronic disease is characterised by iron-deficient erythropoiesis but body stores of iron are normal or increased. The mechanism is synthesis of an inflammatory cytokine, interleukin 6, by macrophages. This stimulates hepcidin synthesis by the liver. The result of a high plasma hepcidin level is that iron is retained in macrophages rather than being released to transferrin for delivery to erythroblasts (Fig. 3.7). Hepcidin also reduces export of iron from enterocytes to the plasma, again reducing availability of iron. Other mechanisms can contribute to the anaemia of chronic disease, including a blunted erythropoietin response to anaemia and some reduction in red cell life span.

Clinical features

There are no specific clinical features. Usually the primary disease responsible for anaemia of chronic disease is clinically apparent, but sometimes the cause is an occult infection or tumour. Anaemia of chronic disease is the second most common cause of anaemia in developed countries, not far behind iron deficiency in frequency.

Laboratory features

Anaemia of chronic disease is initially normocytic and normochromic. As it becomes more severe, it become hypochromic and microcytic. At this

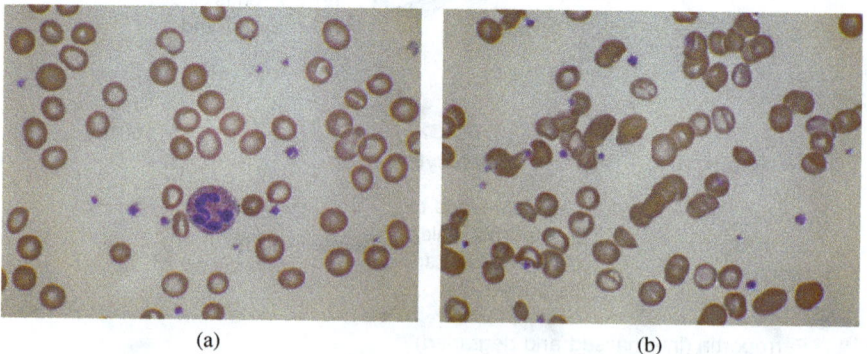

(a)   (b)

Fig. 3.8. PB in anaemia of chronic disease in a patient with rheumatoid arthritis showing (a) hypochromia, anisochromasia, microcytosis and (b) some increase in rouleaux formation. MGG.

stage the RBC, Hb, Hct, MCV and MCH are all reduced. The white blood cell count (WBC) and platelet count may be increased. The blood film initially shows normocytic normochromic and later hypochromic microcytic red cells. There may be increased rouleaux formation and increased background staining (giving a bluish tinge to the blood film), both resulting from increased plasma proteins (Fig. 3.8).

Serum ferritin is elevated. Serum iron is reduced but, in contrast to iron deficiency anaemia, serum transferrin and iron-binding capacity are also reduced. There may be an increased erythrocyte sedimentation rate (ESR) and increased C-reactive protein, $\alpha2$ macroglobulin, fibrinogen and immunoglobulins. The usual test results in comparison with those in iron deficiency are shown in Table 3.2. In most patients with anaemia of chronic disease, examination of the bone marrow shows normal or increased iron stores but siderotic granules are reduced as iron is not being delivered to the developing erythroblasts.

Table 3.2. Blood tests in iron deficiency anaemia and the anaemia of chronic disease.

Blood test	Iron deficiency anaemia	Anaemia of chronic disease	Normal range Men	Normal range Women
Serum ferritin	↓	Normal or ↑	15–300 μg/l	15–200 μg/l
Serum iron	↓	↓	12–24 μmol/l	9–23 μmol/l
Serum transferrin	↑	Normal or ↓	1.7–3.4 g/l	
Iron-binding capacity			54–72 μmol/l	55–81 μmol/l
Transferrin saturation	↓	↓	18–40%	13–37%
Soluble transferrin receptor*	↑	Normal	0.85–3.06 mg/l*	
Soluble transferrin receptor* / Log ferritin	>1.36 (or >1.5)	<1.36 (or <1.5)	≤1.36 (or ≤1.5)*	
C-reactive protein	Normal	↑	<10 mg/l	
Erythrocyte sedimentation rate	Normal or near normal	↑	1–10 mm in 1 hour	1–20 mm in 1 hour
Bone marrow storage iron	Absent	Normal or ↑	Present	Usually present

*Very dependent on method of measurement of soluble transferrin receptor.

However, many of the conditions that can cause anaemia of chronic disease can also lead, directly or indirectly, to iron deficiency. Inflammatory bowel disease can lead to gastrointestinal blood loss, as can the drugs used for treatment of rheumatoid arthritis (aspirin and non-steroidal anti-inflammatory drugs). When anaemia of chronic disease co-exists with iron deficiency, results of laboratory tests may be equivocal and sometimes a bone marrow aspirate is necessary to demonstrate that there is absent bone marrow iron.

Management

Effective management of the primary disease will lead to improvement of the anaemia. Other types of therapy that are sometimes used include recombinant erythropoietin injections and blood transfusion.

The Thalassaemias

To understand the thalassaemias, it is necessary to know which haemoglobins are normally present in a fetus, baby and adult (Table 3.3), and

Table 3.3. Haemoglobins present at various stages of life.

Haemoglobin	Constituent globin chains	When present	Genes needed	Proportion in adult
F (fetal haemoglobin)	$\alpha_2\gamma_2$	Fetal life and early neonatal period; minor component in child and adult	α $^G\gamma$, $^A\gamma$ or both	Less than 1%
A (adult haemoglobin)	$\alpha_2\beta_2$	Late fetal life and increasingly major proportion in neonate, infant, child and adult	α β	95.5–97.5%
A_2	$\alpha_2\delta_2$	Increases from neonatal period onwards but always very minor component	α δ	3.0–3.5%

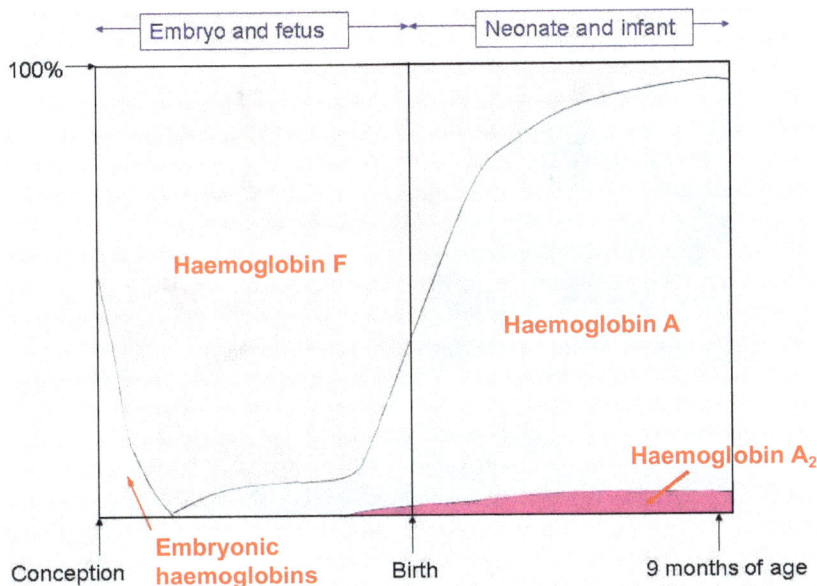

Fig. 3.9. The proportions of various haemoglobins present in intrauterine life and in neonates and young infants.

to understand the basics of the genetic control of globin chain synthesis. A normal fetus has mainly fetal haemoglobin (haemoglobin F) but before birth synthesis of adult haemoglobin (haemoglobin A) commences and steadily increases as haemoglobin F synthesis decreases (Fig. 3.9). Haemoglobin A_2 synthesis starts later than synthesis of haemoglobin A; it is always a minor component but is diagnostically important. The α globin chains are encoded by a pair of α genes ($\alpha2$ and $\alpha1$) in the α gene cluster on each chromosome 16. The γ, β and δ chains are encoded by γ, β and δ genes in the β cluster on each chromosome 11.

The thalassaemias are a group of inherited disorders in which a mutation or deletion of a gene encoding one of the globin chains results in absent or a reduced rate of synthesis of the equivalent chain. This leads to a reduced rate of synthesis of haemoglobin and therefore microcytosis. In milder forms of thalassaemia (often referred to as thalassaemia trait), the bone marrow can compensate by producing more red cells so that there is microcytosis without anaemia. In more severe forms of thalassaemia there

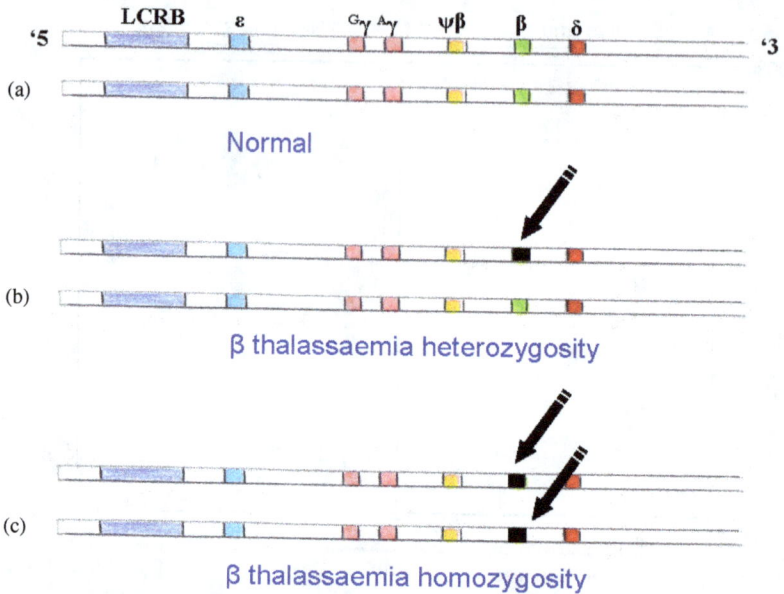

Fig. 3.10. Diagram of the β globin gene cluster showing the γ, β and δ genes. ε is a gene that operates only in embryonic life and $\psi\beta$ is a pseudogene (i.e. it is non-functional). LCRB indicates a master control of these genes, the locus control region beta. (a) normal β globin gene cluster; (b) a mutation (indicated by a black arrow) has occurred in one β gene, leading to heterozygosity for β thalassaemia, also known as β thalassaemia trait; (c) a mutation has occurred in both β globin genes, leading to homozygosity for β thalassaemia or, if the two mutations are different, to compound heterozygosity for β thalassaemia, both of these generally leading to β thalassaemia major.

is anaemia and, in the most severe forms, either this is fatal or life is sustained only by regular blood transfusion.

β Thalassaemias

Normal cells have two β globin genes. β thalassaemia is a condition resulting from mutation in one or both of the β globin genes (Fig. 3.10), which leads to a reduced rate, or even a total absence, of synthesis of β globin. Mutations in β thalassaemia genes are highly prevalent in many parts of the world: about 15% in Cyprus; up to 20% in some parts of Italy, Greece and Turkey; 5–10% in Southeast Asia; about 5% in the Indian subcontinent; about 1% in Afro-Caribbeans.

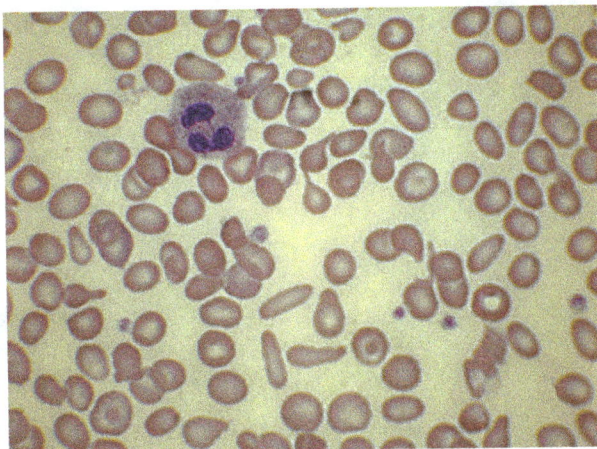

Fig. 3.11. PB film in β thalassaemia heterozygosity showing microcytosis, occasional hypochromic cells, elliptocytes, target cells and other poikilocytes. MGG.

β thalassaemia heterozygosity

If there is a mutation in only one of the two β globin genes there is a reduced rate of synthesis of β globin and therefore microcytosis. However, the bone marrow compensates by producing more red cells so that the blood count usually shows an increased RBC, normal Hb and Hct and reduced MCV and MCH. These red cell indices are quite different from those of iron deficiency, in which a fall of Hb precedes the development of microcytosis (low MCV and MCH). The MCHC, which can be low in iron deficiency, is typically normal. The blood film may show only microcytosis or there may also be poikilocytes including target cells (Fig. 3.11).

β thalassaemia trait is an asymptomatic condition. Only occasionally, e.g. during pregnancy or intercurrent infection, does anaemia occur. However, genetics are important. If a child inherits a β thalassaemia gene from both parents, the result is usually a clinically severe condition known as β thalassaemia major (Fig. 3.12). For this reason, doctors should test for β thalassaemia heterozygosity in pregnancy (or preconceptually), and if this is found to be present the partner should also be tested so that, if a fetus is found to be homozygous for β thalassaemia, termination of pregnancy can be offered.

Diagnosis of β thalassaemia heterozygosity is based on the presence of microcytosis plus an elevated proportion of haemoglobin A_2 (measured

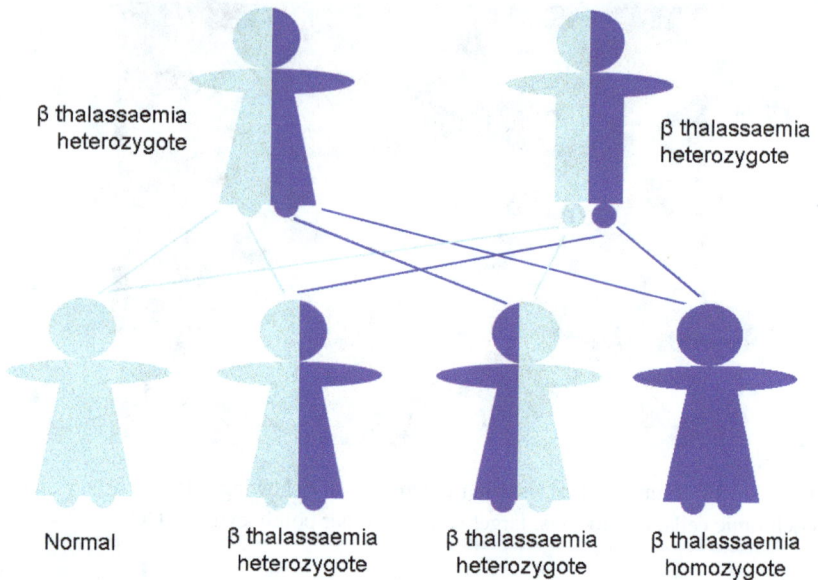

Fig. 3.12. The inheritance of β thalassaemia. Both parents have β thalassaemia heterozygosity. For each pregnancy that occurs, there is a 1 in 2 chance of β thalassaemia heterozygosity, a 1 in 4 chance of normal globin genes and a 1 in 4 chance of β thalassaemia major.

by high performance liquid chromatography or capillary electrophoresis). The elevated percentage of this usually minor haemoglobin occurs because its synthesis requires δ chain rather than the deficient β chain. For similar reasons there is often an increase in the percentage of haemoglobin F since this requires γ chains rather than the deficient β chains.

β thalassaemia homozygosity or compound heterozygosity

If there is a mutation in both β genes the situation is much more serious than when only one is mutated. Synthesis of β globin is totally absent (β^0 thalassaemia) or severely reduced ($\beta^0\beta^+$ thalassaemia or $\beta^+\beta^+$ thalassaemia). This leads to β thalassaemia major, a condition in which survival for more than a few years is dependent on blood transfusion. Failure to thrive is noted between 3 and 6 months of age as haemoglobin F synthesis declines but haemoglobin A synthesis does not take over. The mechanism of the severe anaemia is threefold: (i) inadequate synthesis of globin and therefore of haemoglobin leading to a microcytic anaemia; (ii) ineffective haemopoiesis – death

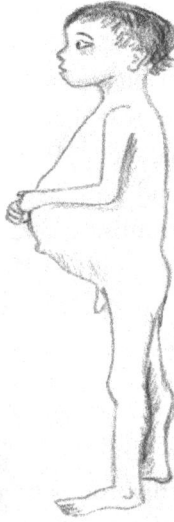

Fig. 3.13. A drawing of a child with β thalassaemia major who has been receiving inadequate transfusion support. He has skull expansion with frontal bossing, expanded maxillae and mandible, gross hepatosplenomegaly (note eversion of the umbilicus) and wasting of his limbs.

of red cell precursors in the bone marrow when they are damaged by excess α chains; (iii) shortened red cell survival. The severe anaemia leads to increased erythropoietin synthesis, which stimulates a further increase in largely ineffective erythropoiesis. This occurs within an expanded bone marrow space (leading to bony deformity) and at extramedullary sites (leading to gross hepatosplenomegaly) (Fig. 3.13). The splenomegaly further aggravates the anaemia as red cells are pooled in the spleen.

In countries in which economic circumstances permit, β thalassaemia major is treated by regular blood transfusion. This prevents death from thalassaemia but instead leads to iron overload, with deposition of iron in tissues including the heart, pancreas, pituitary and liver. Tissue damage from iron overload leads to death (usually in early adult life from cardiac failure) if iron is not removed by chelation. Chelation therapy can be administered through daily oral deferasirox or deferiprone, or subcutaneous infusion of desferrioxamine (also known as deferoxamine), usually over-night for five nights a week.

Bone marrow transplantation should be considered in younger patients who do not yet have serious organ damage from iron overload. While this is considered a curative treatment, its applicability is hampered by the requirement of a fully matched, HLA-identical donor, the risk of immunological complications, and the need for long-term immunosup-pression. Gene therapy offers promise as transformative treatment, and both gene addition and gene editing with CRISPR-cas9 have shown prom-ising success with transfusion independence in initial trials of beta thalassaemia patients aged 12–35.

β thalassaemia intermedia

The term 'β thalassaemia intermedia' refers to a genetically heterogeneous group of conditions that range from mildly to severely symptomatic. By definition, survival without blood transfusion is possible although, in the more severe forms, quality of life may be poor in the absence of transfusion. Iron absorption is increased, and iron overload can occur in the absence of regular transfusion with resultant organ dysfunction. β thalassaemia inter-media can result from heterozygosity for β thalassaemia with aggravating factors or from inheritance of two β thalassaemia genes but with ameliorat-ing factors. In Southeast Asia, co-inheritance of β thalassaemia and haemoglobin E is a common cause of the clinical picture of β thalassaemia intermedia, the β^E chain being synthesised at a reduced rate.

α Thalassaemias

Normal cells have two alpha genes on each chromosome 16. Various α thalassaemia syndromes occur when there is deletion or loss of function of 1, 2, 3 or 4 α genes (Fig. 3.14). Usually α thalassaemia results from α gene deletion rather than mutation. The consequences of α gene loss are shown in Table 3.4. The only important things to know are:

1. Loss of one or two α genes (Fig. 3.14(b)–(d)) can cause microcytosis but is harmless to the individual. It is very common in some ethnic

groups (e.g. 25% of Afro-Caribbeans have loss of a single α gene, known as α^+ thalassaemia heterozygosity). Although loss of two α genes from a single chromosome (Fig 3.14(d)), known as α^0 thalassaemia, is harmless to the individual, it is of genetic significance since this condition in both parents leads to a 1 in 4 chance of haemoglobin Bart's hydrops fetalis (see below). Diagnosis is by DNA analysis in individuals with microcytosis who are of relevant ethnic origin (Southeast Asian, Greek, Cypriot, Turkish or Sardinian).

2. Loss of three α genes (Fig. 3.14(e)) causes haemoglobin H disease, a condition in which there is a moderately severe microcytic anaemia with haemolysis and splenomegaly. Haemoglobin H is a non-functional haemoglobin with four β chains, formed because of a lack of α chains. Haemolysis results from erythrocyte damage from haemoglobin H.

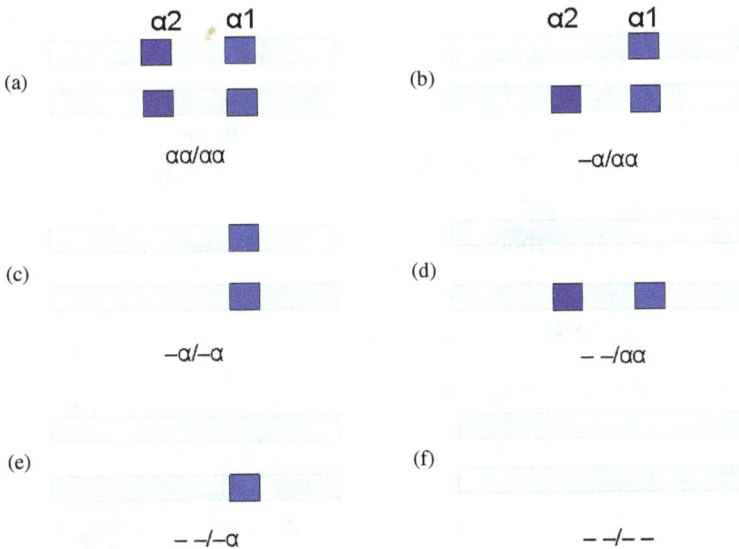

Fig. 3.14. Diagram of normal and abnormal α globin genes: (a) normal, two α genes on each chromosome 16; (b) deletion of a single α gene (α^+ thalassaemia heterozygosity); (c) deletion of a single α gene from each chromosome (α^+ thalassaemia homozygosity); (d) deletion of both α genes from a single chromosome (α^0 thalassaemia heterozygosity); (e) deletion of one α gene from one chromosome 16 and both α genes from the other (haemoglobin H disease); (f) loss of all four α genes (haemoglobin Bart's hydrops fetalis).

Table 3.4.   Consequences of loss of one or more α genes.

Alpha genes	Consequences
$\alpha\,\alpha/\alpha\,\alpha$	Normal
$-\alpha/\alpha\,\alpha$	Haematologically normal or mild microcytosis
$-\alpha/-\alpha$	Microcytosis, no clinical or genetic significance
$--/\alpha\,\alpha$	Microcytosis, no clinical significance but is genetically significant
$-\alpha/--$	Haemoglobin H disease
$--/--$	Haemoglobin Bart's hydrops fetalis

This condition is not generally regarded as being sufficiently severe to justify prenatal prediction and termination of pregnancy.

3.   A total absence of α genes (Fig. 3.14(f)), homozygosity for α^0 thalassaemia, leads to haemoglobin Bart's hydrops fetalis. When no α chain can be produced there can be no production of haemoglobins F, A or A_2. Instead there is production of haemoglobin Bart's, a nonfunctional haemoglobin with four γ chains. This condition leads to death of the severely anaemic and oedematous fetus *in utero* or death shortly after birth. In addition, women carrying a hydropic fetus have an increased rate of complications of pregnancy. Modern medical practice aims to prevent this condition by its prediction leading to termination of pregnancy.

Other Causes of Microcytic Anaemia

Congenital sideroblastic anaemia

Congenital sideroblastic anaemia is a rare X-linked condition, in which an inherited defect in haem synthesis causes a microcytic anaemia. The distinctive feature is that the blood film is dimorphic, i.e. there is a population of hypochromic microcytic cells and a population of normal cells (Fig. 3.15).

Lead poisoning

Lead poisoning can cause an acquired defect in haem synthesis leading to a microcytic anaemia and can also lead to haemolysis with an

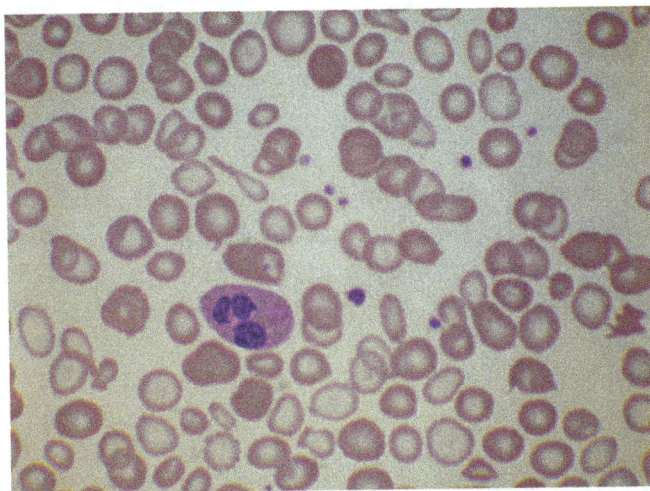

Fig. 3.15. PB film in congenital sideroblastic anaemia showing a dimorphic film: hypochromic microcytic cells and normocytic normochromic cells. There is also anisocytosis and poikilocytosis. MGG.

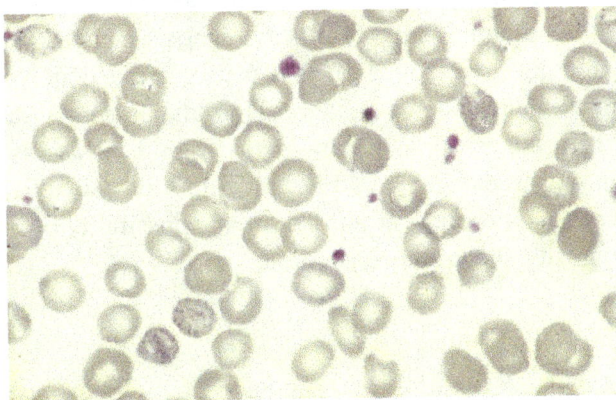

Fig. 3.16. PB film in lead poisoning showing hypochromia and basophilic stippling. MGG.

increased reticulocyte count. The most distinctive blood film feature is basophilic stippling (Fig. 3.16). Lead poisoning is very rare in developed countries.

Haemoglobinopathies

The presence of a structural variant of haemoglobin is known as a haemo-globinopathy. Often this term is used to also encompass the thalassaemias. Some haemoglobinopathies are associated with microcytosis.

Haemoglobin E heterozygosity (common in Southeast Asia) is usually associated with microcytosis whereas haemoglobin E homozygosity is usually associated with a microcytic anaemia. Haemoglobin C homozygosity (found in those of West African ancestry) is also associated with a microcytic anaemia.

Haemoglobinopathies are discussed in Chapter 5.

Conclusions

When a microcytic anaemia is identified, the age, gender, ethnic origin and geographic origin of the patient should be considered. It is also necessary to assess the diet, and whether or not there are clinical features to suggest blood loss or chronic infection or inflammation. This information permits a differential diagnosis and indicates the necessary tests to identify iron deficiency, anaemia of chronic disease and other causes of microcytosis can then be requested. If a diagnosis of iron deficiency has been made, it is important to identify the cause. In a patient found to have microcytosis without anaemia, a diagnosis of 'thalassaemia trait' is likely. In these circumstances their ethnic origin should be assessed and the haemoglobin A_2 percentage should be measured; in individuals of child-bearing age of an appropriate ethnic origin, the possibility of α^0 thalassae-mia heterozygosity should be considered.

Test Case 3.1

A 63-year-old retired truck driver presents to his general practitioner complaining of fatigue. He has a past history of hypertension and a myocardial infarction and is now taking a β blocker and aspirin, 75 mg daily. A year previously he had suffered from an ill-defined arthritis, which is not currently troubling him. Other than pallor, no abnormality is found on physical examination, so some blood tests are done. These show Hb 90 g/l (normal range [NR] 133–167) and MCV 75 fl (NR 82–98). The WBC and platelet count are normal. The erythrocyte sedimentation rate is 12 mm in 1 hour (NR <10) and C-reactive protein is 5.5 mg/l (NR 0–5). Liver and renal function are normal.

Questions

1. What is the most likely cause of the anaemia?
2. What should be done next?
3. How would you manage the patient?

Write down your answers before checking the correct answer (page 403) and re-reading any relevant part of the chapter.

4

Macrocytic Anaemias

Barbara J. Bain

What Do You Need To Know?

☞ The causes of macrocytosis and macrocytic anaemia
☞ How to diagnose, investigate and treat vitamin B_{12} and folate deficiency
☞ When to suspect other causes of macrocytosis

Introduction

A macrocytic anaemia is one in which the average red cell size is greater than normal. The blood count shows an increased mean cell volume (MCV). Macrocytosis can also occur without anaemia. To decide if erythrocytes are larger than normal, it is necessary to compare their size with what is normal for an individual of that age and to compare the MCV of the patient with an appropriate normal range. For example, healthy newborn babies have much larger red cells than children or adults and their erythrocytes would only be considered macrocytic if the MCV was above a normal range for neonates.

Macrocytosis occurs for many reasons (Table 4.1). If there is a deficiency of vitamin B_{12} or folic acid there will be an interference with

Table 4.1. Some causes of macrocytosis and macrocytic anaemia.

Classification	Causes
Megaloblastic anaemia	Deficiency of vitamin B_{12} or folic acid
	Drugs interfering with the action of vitamin B_{12} or folic acid and inactivation of vitamin B_{12} by repeated exposure to nitrous oxide (N_2O)*
	Other defects in DNA synthesis, e.g. drug-induced and rare congenital defects in pyrimidine synthesis or metabolism of vitamin B_{12} or folic acid
	Some congenital dyserythropoietic anaemias
	Some erythroid leukaemias and myelodysplastic syndromes
Macrocytic anaemia with macronormoblastic erythropoiesis	Liver disease
	Ethanol toxicity
	Hypothyroidism
	Some myelodysplastic syndromes
	Some congenital dyserythropoietic anaemias
	Some cases of aplastic anaemia
	Some cases of multiple myeloma
	Chronic hypoxic lung disease
Stress erythropoiesis[†]	Haemolytic anaemia
	Recovery from anaemia or blood loss

*N_2O exposure, including repeated recreational use, can also cause dominant neurological abnormalities typical of vitamin B_{12} deficiency, with only minor haematological abnormities.
[†]This term indicates very active, erythropoietin-driven erythropoiesis.

synthesis of deoxyribonucleic acid (DNA) so that the development of the nucleus is retarded in relation to the maturation of the cytoplasm. The erythroblast continues to grow but cell division is delayed. These large erythroblasts with nucleocytoplasmic dissociation are referred to as megaloblasts (in contrast to erythroblasts without these features, which are known as normoblasts). This type of erythropoiesis is called megaloblastic. In megaloblastic anaemia due to deficiency of vitamin B_{12} or folic acid, the red cell lifespan is reduced by 30–50%. However, the major cause of the anaemia is ineffective haemopoiesis; this term means that the bone marrow is very cellular but many haemopoietic cells are dying rather than maturing in the bone marrow. Drugs that act as antagonists to vitamin B_{12} (nitrous oxide) or folic acid (methotrexate) also cause a megaloblastic anaemia. Other drugs interfere with DNA synthesis and can cause megaloblastic anaemia; important among these are: (i) the antiretro-viral drug, zidovudine; (ii) the immunosuppressive agent, azathioprine; and (iii) a number of anti-cancer chemotherapeutic agents. There can also be retarded DNA synthesis when the erythroblasts are neoplastic cells, arising from a haemopoietic stem cell that has undergone mutation. This occurs sometimes in acute leukaemias, particularly erythroleukaemias where a large proportion of the leukaemic cells are of erythroid lineage, and also in the myelodysplastic syndromes, which are neoplastic preleu-kaemic conditions.

In a second major group of macrocytic anaemias the normal relation-ship between the development of the nucleus and of the cytoplasm is retained but the erythroblasts are larger than normal, as are the resulting red cells. This can be referred to as macronormoblastic erythropoiesis. It occurs in liver disease, as a toxic effect of alcohol and, less often, in hypothyroidism. It also occurs in some myelodysplastic syndromes.

Macrocytosis and macrocytic anaemia can also result from reticulocy-tosis due to a markedly shortened red cell life span or during the recovery phase after rapid blood loss. A high level of erythropoietin leads to expanded and accelerated erythropoiesis, which is macronormoblastic, and is sometimes called 'stress erythropoiesis'. The circulating red cells include an increased proportion of reticulocytes and other young red cells, which are larger than older red cells. The blood film shows polychromatic macrocytes, representing reticulocytes; some of these have skipped a cell division during erythropoiesis, meaning that they can be very large.

Vitamin B_{12} Deficiency

Dietary sources, absorption and function of vitamin B_{12} are discussed on pages 14–16. The causes of vitamin B_{12} deficiency are summarised in Table 4.2. Anaemia due to vitamin B_{12} (cobalamin) deficiency is much less common than that due to iron deficiency or the anaemia of chronic disease. The most prominent cause in clinical practice is pernicious anae-mia (see pages 71–72). Malabsorption of food-B_{12} (attributed to declining levels of gastric HCl and pepsin with increasing age, possibly aggravated by intake of proton-pump inhibitors) with preserved absorption of crystal-line B_{12} is actually more common than pernicious anaemia, but it usually causes milder, often subclinical, deficiency.

Table 4.2. Some of the causes of vitamin B_{12} deficiency.

Nature of cause	Examples
Dietary deficiency	Veganism; a vegetarian diet can contribute to deficiency but does not alone cause tissue deficiency
Gastric causes	Pernicious anaemia, food-B_{12} malabsorption, gastric atrophy associated with *Helicobacter pylori* infection, total or partial gastrectomy, bariatric surgery
Pancreatic causes	Pancreatic insufficiency
Small bowel causes	Coeliac disease, Crohn disease (particularly after ileal resection), blind loop syndrome, tropical sprue

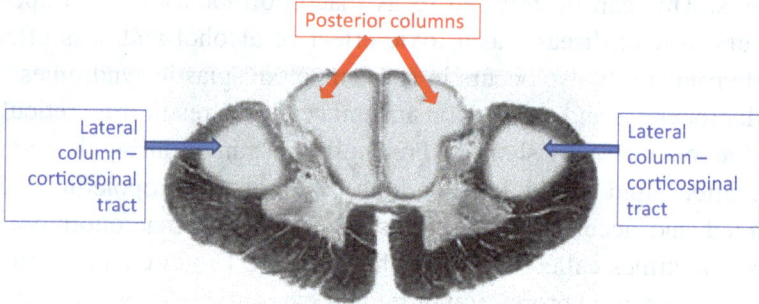

Fig. 4.1. Diagram of the spinal cord in cross section showing the areas of degeneration in subacute combined degeneration: posterior columns (vibration sense and proprioception) and lateral columns (upper motor neurons).

Clinical features

Patients with vitamin B_{12} deficiency may be discovered to have macrocytosis without anaemia or may present with clinical features of anaemia or with neurological complications. There may also be mild jaundice and glossitis. Recognised neurological features include peripheral neuropathy, subacute combined degeneration of the spinal cord, dementia, psychiatric manifestations and optic atrophy. Subacute combined degeneration of the spinal cord involves the dorsal and the corticospinal tracts of the lateral columns resulting in spastic paresis, a Babinski response and reduced proprioception and vibration sense (Fig. 4.1). It should be noted that

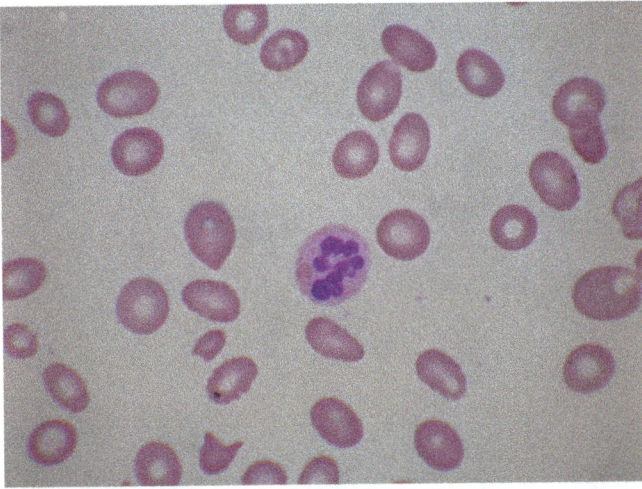

Fig. 4.2. Peripheral blood (PB) film in megaloblastic anaemia showing anisocytosis, macrocytosis, oval macrocytes, a teardrop poikilocyte and a hypersegmented neutrophil. May–Grünwald–Giemsa (MGG) stain.

patients who present with neurological manifestations of vitamin B_{12} deficiency sometime have only a mild macrocytosis and no anaemia.

Laboratory features

Early in the development of vitamin B_{12} deficiency there is usually macrocytosis without anaemia. Later there is a macrocytic anaemia and, when deficiency is very severe, neutropenia and thrombocytopenia. A blood film shows anisocytosis and poikilocytosis with macrocytes, oval macrocytes, teardrop poikilocytes and hypersegmented neutrophils (six or more nuclear lobes) (Fig. 4.2). The absolute reticulocyte count can be reduced, normal or slightly elevated, but is inappropriately low for the degree of anaemia. Biochemical tests show increased bilirubin and lactate dehydrogenase and usually increased iron and ferritin. Serum B_{12} is reduced. A bone marrow aspirate shows megaloblastic erythropoiesis and giant metamyelocytes (Figs. 4.3 and 4.4).

Haematological abnormalities can be very mild in those who present with neurological features.

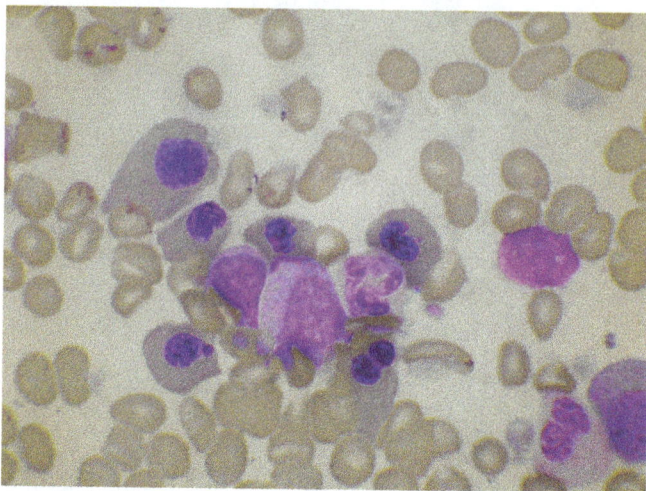

Fig. 4.3. Bone marrow film in severe megaloblastic anaemia. The late erythroblasts show marked megaloblastosis with abundant mature cytoplasm but immature nuclei. Dyserythropoiesis, which is a feature of the megaloblastosis, is present (nuclear lobulation in erythroblasts). MGG.

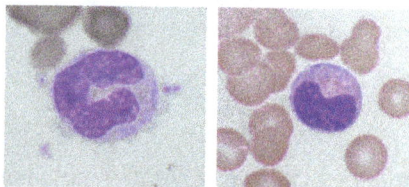

Fig. 4.4. A giant metamyelocyte in the bone marrow in megaloblastic anaemia (left) in comparison with a normal sized metamyelocyte (right). MGG.

Diagnosis

Diagnosis is based on a blood count, blood film and serum vitamin B_{12} assay. However it should be noted that many elderly people have a low serum B_{12} without any evidence of tissue deficiency. Conversely, the B_{12} assay is normal in a small minority of patients with confirmed deficiency (less than 5% of patients). If the B_{12} assay is normal when B_{12} deficiency appears otherwise likely, the patient should be further investigated, for example by a bone marrow aspirate and by tests relevant to pernicious anaemia (see below). The red cell folate is reduced in about 60% of patients with vitamin B_{12} deficiency.

Management

Treatment is usually with parenteral vitamin B_{12}, in the United Kingdom in the form of hydroxocobalamin. Initially 1,000 μg can be given at fairly short intervals, for example three times a week for 2 weeks, to build up body stores. The maintenance dose is then 1,000 μg each 3 months. It is customary to give a higher dose in patients with neurological abnormalities, but there is no evidence that this is of more benefit than a standard dose. It is also possible to treat vitamin B_{12} deficiency with oral vitamin B_{12}, but a dose of 1,000 μg a day is needed; absorption is better if not taken with food. Unless a patient has had an allergic reaction to parenteral B_{12} there is no clear advantage to oral therapy.

If vitamin B_{12} deficiency is due to veganism, supplementation of the diet with physiological doses of oral B_{12} is sufficient for maintenance of normality once body stores have been built up.

Management of the patient also requires investigation to establish the cause of the B_{12} deficiency, with treatment of the underlying disease if necessary. The patient's clinical history may indicate a likely diagnosis. Otherwise investigations are directed mainly at identifying pernicious anaemia, food-B_{12} malabsorption and diseases of the small intestine.

Pernicious anaemia

Pernicious anaemia is an autoimmune disease in which gastric atrophy leads to loss of secretion of pepsin, hydrochloric acid and intrinsic factor with resultant vitamin B_{12} deficiency. There is an association with other autoimmune diseases, such as Addison disease, hypothyroidism and vitiligo, and there may also be a family history of pernicious anaemia. Autoantibodies directed at gastric parietal cells are present in about 95% of patients and autoantibodies against intrinsic factor in about 60%.

The clinical, haematological and biochemical features are as for any patient with B_{12} deficiency. The diagnosis is most simply made by investigation for intrinsic factor antibodies which, if present, are sufficient to confirm the diagnosis. Investigation for parietal cell antibodies is much less specific since such antibodies are common in elderly people. If intrinsic factor antibodies are not detected (about 30–40% of patients) confirmation of the diagnosis is more difficult. A Schilling test, in which oral radiolabelled vitamin B_{12} is administered and urinary radioactivity is then measured, is no longer possible as reagents are not now available.

Management is as for other patients with B_{12} deficiency. Because gastric atrophy also reduces iron absorption, some patients with pernicious anaemia have co-existing iron deficiency at presentation and in others the inadequacy of iron stores is revealed by the development of iron deficiency once a haematological response to B_{12} occurs. Oral iron therapy may then be needed.

It is important to try to establish a definite diagnosis in pernicious anaemia since patients require life-long therapy.

Folic Acid Deficiency

Dietary sources, absorption and function of folic acid are discussed on page 16. The causes of folic acid deficiency are summarised in Table 4.3. The most common causes are decreased intake and increased requirements.

Clinical features

Patients with folic deficiency have clinical features resulting from anaemia and ineffective erythropoiesis (fatigue, pallor, dyspnoea, mild jaundice).

Laboratory features

The haematological features are usually the same as those of vitamin B_{12} deficiency. However one of the possible causes of folate deficiency is an increased need for the vitamin so that occasionally the features of a haemolytic anaemia (e.g. hereditary spherocytosis, autoimmune haemolytic anaemia or sickle cell anaemia) are combined with the features of

Table 4.3. Some causes of folic acid deficiency.

Increased need	Pregnancy and lactation Prematurity Growth spurts Alcoholism Increased cell turnover (e.g. haemolytic anaemia, psoriasis, chronic exfoliative dermatitis, leukaemia)
Decreased availability	Reduced dietary intake (poverty, old age, alcoholism, ill-advised diets, e.g. 'goat's milk anaemia') Decreased absorption (coeliac disease, jejunal resection, tropical sprue, malabsorption induced by drugs — sulfasalazine, cholestyramine, triamterene)
Interference with metabolism	Inborn errors of metabolism Anti-folate drugs (methotrexate, pyrimethamine, trimethoprim)[*]
Increased loss	Increased urinary loss (congestive cardiac failure, active liver damage) or other loss (haemodialysis or peritoneal dialysis)

[*]In addition, folate deficiency appears to sometimes be the result of use of other drugs including phenytoin, primidone and barbiturates.

a megaloblastic anaemia. The serum folate and red cell folate are usually low. Serum B_{12} is reduced in up to a third of patients. Serum bilirubin and lactate dehydrogenase (LDH) are increased. Although not widely available, assays of serum methylmalonic acid and homocysteine can help to distinguish between deficiency of vitamin B_{12} and of folic acid (Table 4.4).

Diagnosis

Assay of serum folate is the test now most often used for the diagnosis of folic acid deficiency. It is more sensitive than assay of red cell folate although it is much less specific since serum folate falls within days of a reduction in intake. It is also essential to measure serum vitamin B_{12} since the red cell folate is low in 50% of patients with B_{12} deficiency. Treating B_{12}-deficient patients with pharmacological doses of folic acid will correct the megaloblastic anaemia but permits the neurological abnormalities to progress.

Table 4.4. Methylmalonic acid and homocysteine assays in deficiency of Vitamin B_{12} and folic acid.

	Methylmalonic acid*	Homocysteine*
Vitamin B_{12} deficiency	↑	↑
Folic acid deficiency	Normal	↑

*Also increased in renal insufficiency.

It should be noted that red cell folate may not be low if megaloblastic anaemia develops very acutely. It is therefore important to interpret the laboratory tests in light of the clinical features.

Management

Treatment is with oral folic acid in a dose of 1–5 mg daily. Management also includes ascertaining the cause of the folic acid deficiency so that the patient can be given dietary advice and conditions such as coeliac disease can be treated.

In patients prone to develop folic acid deficiency, such as those with a chronic haemolytic anaemia, folic acid supplementation (e.g. 5 mg a day) is usually given. It is also important to prevent subclinical folate deficiency in women who are, or who might become, pregnant since even sub-clinical deficiency can cause defects in neural tube closure in the fetus leading to spinal bifida, anencephaly and related developmental abnormalities. In many countries (e.g. Canada and the United States) this is achieved by supplementing flour that is used for bread making. The proposed UK policy is for fortification of non-wholemeal wheat flour. In countries where this is not the practice, it is desirable to supplement the normal dietary intake with a further 400 μg of folic acid daily, preferably starting before conception.

Other Causes of Macrocytosis

Macrocytosis is common in the myelodysplastic syndromes, as a result of the dysplastic erythropoiesis (Fig. 4.5). These syndromes will be discussed further in Chapter 6.

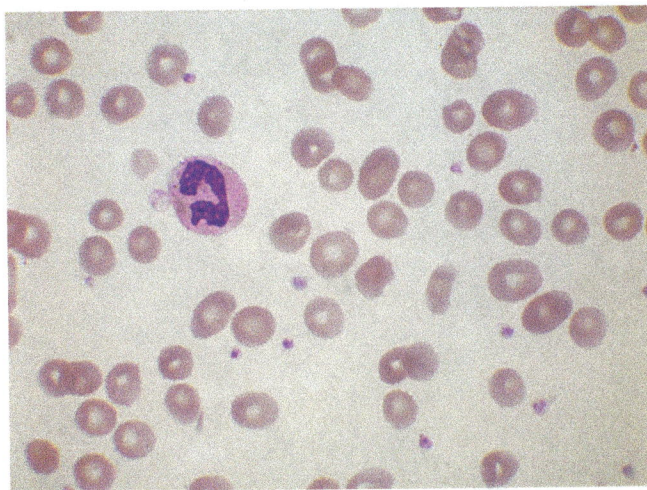

Fig. 4.5. PB film of a patient with a myelodysplastic syndrome, showing mild anisocytosis and the presence of some macrocytes. MGG.

In Western countries excess alcohol intake is probably the most frequent cause of macrocytosis, often accompanied by mild anaemia and thrombocytopenia (Fig. 4.6). The mechanism is complex. There may be poor dietary intake of folate and alcohol has a weak antifolate effect, leading to megaloblastosis in some cases. In other patients macronormoblastic erythropoiesis occurs without any biochemical evidence of folate deficiency. When excess alcohol intake is the cause of macrocytosis, the blood film may also show stomatocytosis (Fig. 4.7).

Macrocytosis is also common in liver disease that is not caused by alcohol. In these patients there may also be target cells. When there is obstructive jaundice, target cells can be very numerous (Fig. 4.8).

Erythrocytes become smaller as they age. Therefore, when there is a chronic haemolytic anaemia the younger red cell population is composed, on average, of larger red cells than when the red cell population shows a normal spread of cell ages. This is most marked when the reticulocyte count is high as reticulocytes are considerably larger than other erythrocytes. The presence of polychromatic macrocytes is a clue to reticulocytosis as a cause of macrocytosis (Fig. 4.9).

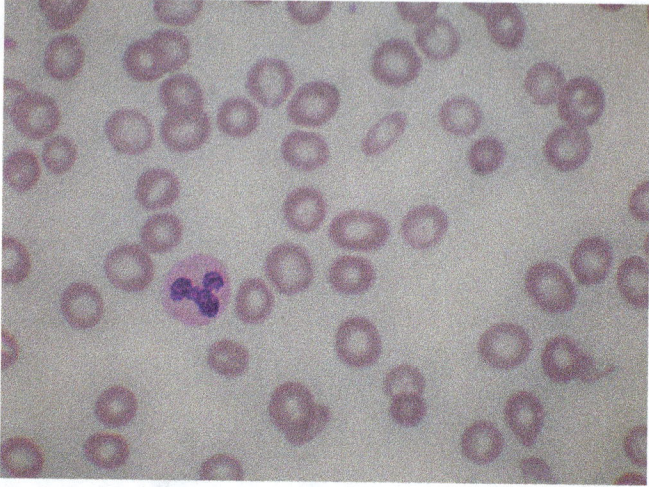

Fig. 4.6. PB film from a patient taking excess alcohol showing anaemia, anisocytosis and macrocytosis. Note that, in contrast to megaloblastic anaemia, the neutrophil is normally segmented. MGG.

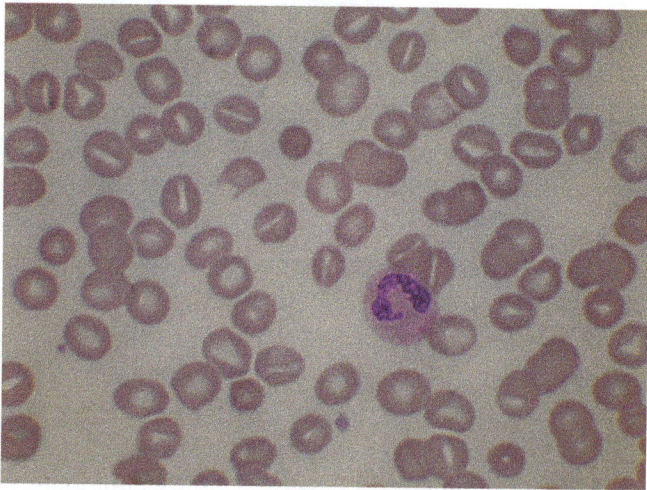

Fig. 4.7. PB film from a patient taking excess alcohol showing anaemia, marked macrocytosis and numerous stomatocytes. Note that, in contrast to megaloblastic anaemia, the neutrophil is normally segmented. MGG.

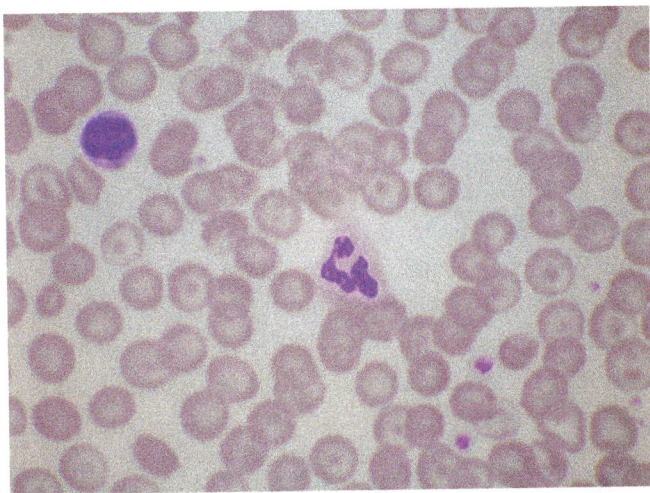

Fig. 4.8. PB film from a patient with obstructive jaundice showing macrocytosis and target cells. MGG.

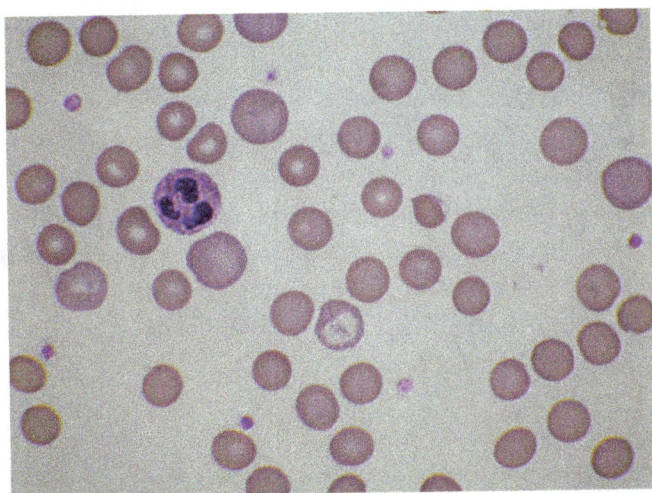

Fig. 4.9. PB film from a patient with glucose-6-phosphate dehydrogenase deficiency and recent acute haemolysis showing macrocytosis as a result of marked reticulocytosis. It is clear that the polychromatic cells are larger than other erythrocytes. There is also an irregularly contracted cell and an erythrocyte showing basophilic stippling. MGG.

Conclusions

The correct diagnosis in patients with macrocytic anaemia is important since missing a deficiency state can lead to a patient becoming severely pancytopenic and, in the case of vitamin B_{12} deficiency, can permit the progression of neurological damage that may not be fully reversible. The correct diagnosis can usually be made on the basis of clinical history including drug history, vitamin B_{12} and folate assays and liver and thyroid function tests. If the diagnosis is still not clear a bone marrow aspirate is indicated. If the diagnosis still proves difficult, a trial of vitamin B_{12} and folic acid therapy is indicated. Assays of methylmalonic acid and homocysteine can also be useful in diagnostically difficult cases.

Test Case 4.1

A 55-year-old Caucasian school teacher presents to her general practitioner with a four-month history of numbness and tingling in her hands and feet and a two-week history of weakness in her legs. She is on no medications, has a normal diet, takes 1–2 units of alcohol each night and does not smoke. On examination, she has reduced power and brisk tendon reflexes in her legs, an extensor plantar response, reduced proprioception and vibration sense to the ankles and a normal appreciation of light touch and heat. Laboratory tests show normal liver and renal function, Hb 110 g/l (normal range 118–148) and MCV 103 fl (normal range 82–98). The WBC and platelet count are normal.

Questions

1. What is the most likely diagnosis and why?
2. What other tests would you do next and what would you expect?
3. If your suspicions are correct, what treatment would be needed?

Write down your answers before checking the correct answer (page 404) or re-reading any relevant parts of the chapter.

5

Haemoglobinopathies and Haemolytic Anaemias

Vishal Jayakar

What Do You Need To Know?

☞ The structure and function of the red cell membrane (outline)
☞ The role of the glycolytic pathway and the pentose shunt in maintaining the integrity of the red cell
☞ The inheritance, clinicopathological features, diagnosis and management of sickle cell anaemia
☞ That there are other forms of sickle cell disease
☞ The clinicopathological effects of other significant haemoglobinopathies (outline)
☞ How haemolysis and haemolytic anaemia are defined
☞ The mechanisms and causes of haemolytic anaemia
☞ How haemolytic anaemia is diagnosed
☞ The clinicopathological effects, diagnosis and management of representative hereditary and acquired haemolytic anaemias
☞ The function of the spleen and the consequences of hyposplenism

Introduction

An erythrocyte (or red cell) passes through the heart half a million times and travels 300 miles during its 120-day lifespan. It is subject to deformation as it squeezes through capillaries, which are only a third of its own diameter. In addition to physical trauma, the red cell is exposed to endogenous and exogenous oxidants that can oxidise both membrane and intracellular constituents, including haemoglobin. It is particularly vulnerable to damage when passing from the splenic cords to the splenic sinuses. To survive the vicissitudes of its life, the red cell needs to generate energy, protect itself against oxidative damage, maintain its haemoglobin in its reduced form, enhance oxygen delivery from haemoglobin and maintain a flexible semipermeable membrane. In addition to the capabilities of mature red cells, reticulocytes can synthesise proteins; they are thus able to synthesise haemoglobin. Conversely, mature red cells lack ribosomes and therefore do not have the capacity for protein synthesis.

The disciform erythrocyte has 40% more membrane than a spherical one of the same size. This is very important for its flexibility. It is also important that the concentration of haemoglobin is not abnormally high within the red cell; otherwise, there is an increase in internal viscosity, which again reduces deformability.

The red cell membrane

The red cell membrane is a lipid bilayer with integral membrane proteins supported by a cytoskeleton composed of spectrin, actin and other proteins (Fig. 5.1). It serves to maintain the shape and flexibility of the red cell and to pump ions and water across the membrane.

The glycolytic pathway

The erythrocyte derives energy from glycolysis, also known as the Embden–Meyerhof pathway (Fig. 5.2). Energy is necessary for the ion pumps, which maintain an ion gradient across the red cell membrane and prevent swelling or shrinking of the cell. In addition, the glycolytic

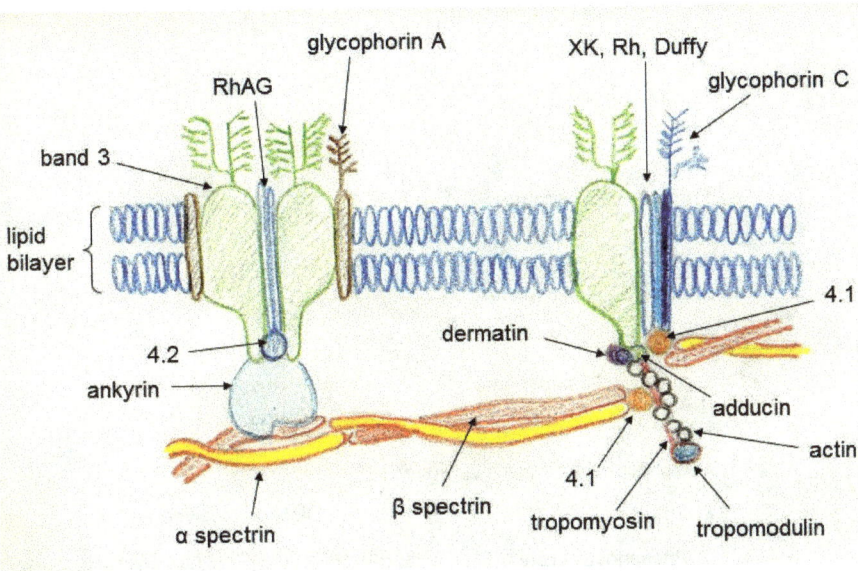

Fig. 5.1. Diagram of the red cell membrane and cytoskeleton. The red cell membrane is composed of a lipid bilayer composed of similar amounts of cholesterol and phospholipids; cholesterol is disposed equally between the two layers, whereas phospholipids are asymmetrically disposed. Phosphatidyl choline and sphingomyelin are mainly in the outer leaflet, while phosphatidylethanolamine and phosphatidyl serine are mainly in the inner leaflet. There are more than 100 integral membrane proteins; some having a transport function and some connecting the lipid bilayer to the underlying cytoskeleton. The cytoskeleton is composed of the dimers of α and β spectrin, which are assembled into a network of tetramers. The transmembrane band 3 and RhAG proteins bind to protein 4.2 and ankyrin; ankyrin binds to spectrin. The cytoskeleton is also tethered to the lipid bilayer by glycophorin C, XK, Rh and Duffy, which bind to protein 4.1 and thus to spectrin. Band 3 also binds to adducin and dermatin. In addition to these vertical interactions, spectrin binds to protein 4.1 and thus to actin microfilaments, creating horizontal interactions. It is these highly complex interactions that maintain the shape and flexibility of the red cell.

pathway leads to the synthesis of 2,3-diphosphoglycerate (2,3-DPG), also known as 2,3-biphosphoglycerate (2,3-BPG), which enhances oxygen delivery from a haemoglobin molecule that has already given up one oxygen; it does this by binding with greater affinity to deoxyhaemoglobin

V. Jayakar

Glucose
ATP
ADP
hexokinase

Glucose-6-phosphate

glucose phosphate isomerase

Fructose-6-phosphate
ATP
ADP
phosphofructokinase

Fructose-1,6-bisphosphate

aldolase

Dihydroxyacetone
phosphate

Glyceraldehyde-3-phosphate
NAD
NADH
triosephosphate isomerase

glyceraldehyde phosphate dehydrogenase

1,3-Bisphosphoglycerate
ADP
ATP
bisphosphoglycerate mutase

phosphoglycerate kinase

2,3-Disphosphoglycerate

3-Phosphoglycerate
bisphosphoglycerate kinase

phosphoglycerate mutase

2-Phosphoglycerate

enolase

Phosphoenolpyruvate
ADP
ATP
pyruvate kinase

Pyruvate
NADH
NAD
lactate dehydrogenase

Lactate

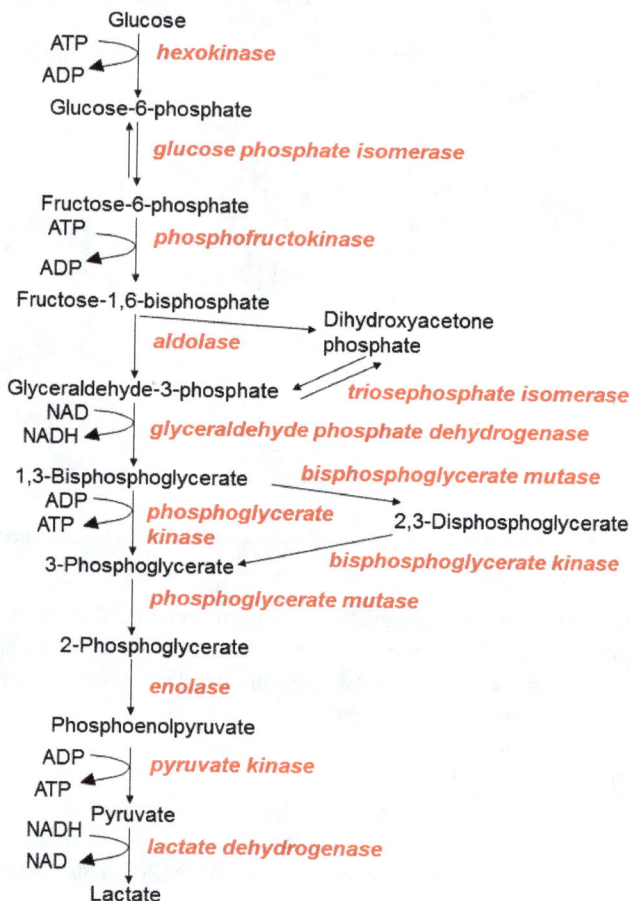

Fig. 5.2. Diagram of the glycolytic pathway. Enzymes are shown in red and metabolites in black. Glycolysis provides adenosine triphosphate (ATP), needed for red cell ion pumps whilst some ATP is converted to adenosine diphosphate (ADP) in the early steps of glycolysis, overall there is net production of ATP.

and allosterically favouring the release of further oxygen molecules. 2,3-DPG thus contributes to cooperativity (see page 2). Increased synthesis of 2,3-DPG in circumstances of increased need helps the body adapt to anaemia, living at high altitude and chronic hypoxia due to disease.

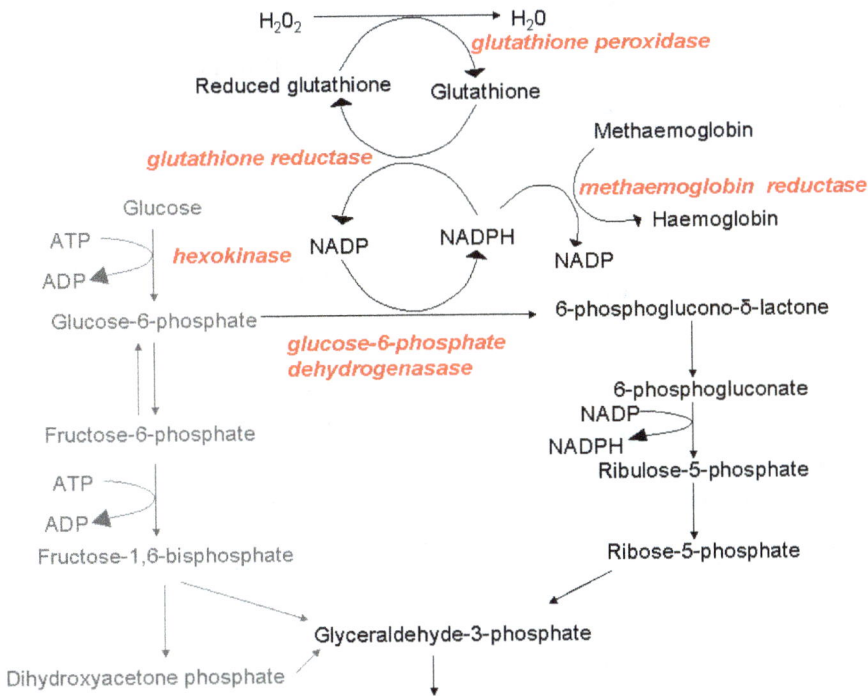

Fig. 5.3. The pentose shunt showing how nicotinamide–adenine dinucleotide phosphate (NADP) is converted to its reduced form, NADPH, thus permitting the reduction of oxidised proteins, including methaemoglobin, and the protection of the red cell from peroxides, particularly hydrogen peroxide. The glycolytic pathway is shown in grey and the pentose shunt and related pathways in black. Some key enzymes are in red.

The pentose shunt

The pentose shunt, also known as the hexose monophosphate shunt, is very important in the erythrocyte since it generates the reduced form of nicotinamide–adenine dinucleotide phosphate (NADPH) and reduced glutathione, and thus protects the cell from oxidant damage (Fig. 5.3). It is also essential for the synthesis of 5-carbon sugars and, thus, nucleic acids.

Table 5.1.   Some causes of haemolysis.

Haemolysis type	Example
Congenital haemolytic anaemia	
Defect in glycolytic pathway	Pyruvate kinase deficiency
Defect in pentose shunt	Glucose-6-phosphate dehydrogenase deficiency
Defect in haemoglobin	Sickle cell anaemia, unstable haemoglobin
Defect in membrane	Hereditary spherocytosis
Acquired haemolytic anaemia	
Mechanical damage	Microangiopathic haemolytic anaemia, malfunctioning prosthetic heart valve
Antibody damage	Autoimmune haemolytic anaemia
Oxidant damage	Exposure to oxidant drugs or chemicals
Enzymatic damage	Envenomation by certain snakes
Heat damage	Severe burns

Mechanisms of Haemolysis

Haemolysis means shortened red cell survival. This is compensated for by an erythropoietin-driven increase in erythropoiesis. The bone marrow can increase its output of red cells five- to six-fold to compensate for a red cell lifespan as short as 20–30 days. If the bone marrow cannot compensate fully, haemolytic anaemia occurs. There are inherited and acquired causes of haemolysis. Some of these are summarised, with examples, in Table 5.1. Congenital and acquired factors can interact. Thus, an inherited deficiency of glucose-6-phosphate dehydrogenase (G6PD) may only become apparent after the cell is exposed to some unusual oxidant stress.

Diagnosis of Haemolysis

It is possible to measure the red cell lifespan by labelling red cells with a radioactive isotope and thus definitively identify haemolysis. However, in practice, the conclusion that there is haemolysis is made by indirect means using: (i) evidence that there is increased red cell breakdown (e.g. increased bilirubin — particularly unconjugated bilirubin — and lactate dehydrogenase (LDH), free haemoglobin in the plasma or urine, reduced serum haptoglobin, haemosiderin in the urine or increased urinary urobilinogen); (ii) evidence of increased bone marrow activity (e.g. increased reticulocyte count and the presence of polychromatic macrocytes and nucleated red cells in the blood film); (iii) abnormal red cells of a type that is found in haemolytic anaemia (e.g. spherocytes, elliptocytes, irregularly contracted cells, sickle cells and red cell fragments); or (iv) evidence for a specific type of haemolytic anaemia (e.g. a positive direct antiglobulin test or a reduced concentration of red cell G6PD). A low haptoglobin concentration provides evidence of haemolysis because, when there is intravascular haemolysis, the haemoglobin released from red cells forms a complex with haptoglobin, and the complex is removed by the liver. Other clinical features can also suggest haemolysis, although they are not specific to it, for example splenomegaly or gallstones at a young age. The gallstones in haemolytic anaemia are bile pigment stones, formed because of the increased load of bilirubin that is excreted; they may lead to acute cholecystitis and biliary obstruction.

Examples of some of the blood film abnormalities that might indicate a haemolytic anaemia are shown in Table 5.2.

Table 5.2. Some of the blood film abnormalities that might suggest haemolytic anaemia.

Abnormality	What is it and what might it mean?	Abnormality	What is it and what might it mean?
	Sickle cell: sickle cell disease		Haemoglobin C crystal: haemoglobin C disease
	Spherocyte: hereditary spherocytosis or autoimmune haemolytic anaemia		Elliptocyte: hereditary elliptocytosis
	Stomatocyte: hereditary stomatocytosis		Crenation: renal failure or pyruvate kinase deficiency (particularly post-splenectomy)

(*Continued*)

Table 5.2. (*Continued*)

Abnormality	What is it and what might it mean?	Abnormality	What is it and what might it mean?
	Acanthocyte: inherited membrane defect; liver failure		Irregularly contracted cell: glucose-6-phosphate dehydrogenase deficiency or oxidant damage
	Red cell fragment (schistocyte): microangiopathic haemolytic anaemia or mechanical haemolysis		Keratocyte: oxidant damage or mechanical or microangiopathic haemolysis

The Haemoglobinopathies

The haemoglobinopathies are a group of inherited disorders in which a mutation of a globin gene leads to the synthesis of a structurally abnormal haemoglobin, known as a variant haemoglobin. Such mutations can affect any globin gene; however, those of clinical significance mainly affect either the α or β globin gene. The thalassaemias, which have been discussed in Chapter 3, can be regarded as a specific type of haemoglobinopathy. The possible results of a mutation in a globin gene are as follows:

- The same amino acid is encoded, no phenotypic effect.
- A similar amino acid is encoded, no clinical effect.
- Haemoglobin is prone to polymerise, e.g. haemoglobin S.
- Haemoglobin is prone to crystallise, causing haemolysis, e.g. haemoglobin C.
- Haemoglobin is unstable, causing haemolysis.
- High-affinity haemoglobin, polycythaemia occurs.
- Low-affinity haemoglobin, anaemia occurs (but there is no functional effect as tissue delivery of oxygen is normal).
- Haemoglobin is prone to oxidise, causing methaemoglobinaemia and cyanosis.
- Haemoglobin is synthesised at a reduced rate, e.g. haemoglobin E and the thalassaemias.

The great majority of mutations in globin genes are harmless. However, a small number of mutations that are potentially harmful are very common in certain ethnic groups, specifically haemoglobin S and haemoglobin C (in those of African ancestry) and haemoglobin E (in those of Southeast Asian descent).

Sickle cell trait

The sickle cell trait, or heterozygosity for haemoglobin S, is not a disease. It is the carrier state for haemoglobin S. It is of genetic significance but rarely of clinical significance.

Haemoglobin S has an uncharged valine instead of a charged glutamic acid at position 6 of the β globin chain, which makes its deoxy form far less soluble than normal. The point mutation in the β globin gene that gives rise to haemoglobin S has arisen independently at least three times in different parts of Africa as well as at certain locations in an area extending from the Arabian Peninsula to India. The mutation can thus be found in people of African ancestry and from the Indian subcontinent but is also present in a significant proportion of Arabs, Greeks and Sicilians.

Clinical features

Most individuals with the sickle cell trait have no relevant clinical abnormalities. Occasionally, they suffer from haematuria or reduced renal concentrating ability, and rarely from renal papillary necrosis. Very rarely, an individual is exposed to hypoxia of sufficient severity to lead to signs and symptoms due to sickling. This can happen with vigorous, prolonged exercise, as in athletes; at high altitudes, when flying in an unpressurised aircraft; and if hypoxia is allowed to occur during anaesthesia.

A rare form of cancer (renal medullary carcinoma) has been associated with the trait.

Laboratory features

The blood count is normal. Haemoglobin electrophoresis, high-performance liquid chromatography (HPLC) or capillary electrophoresis shows that about 45% of the total haemoglobin is haemoglobin S, the rest being haemoglobin A and a small amount of haemoglobin A_2 (Fig. 5.4, lane d). The red cells can be induced to sickle in the laboratory by adding a sample of the patient's blood to a phosphate buffer acting as a reducing

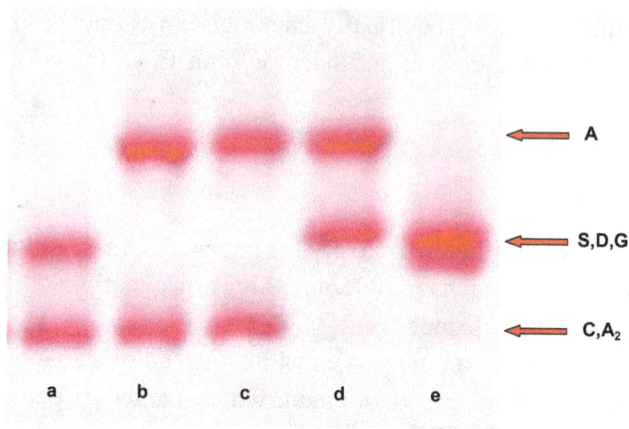

Fig. 5.4. Haemoglobin electrophoresis on a cellulose acetate membrane at an alkaline pH showing: (a) haemoglobin S + haemoglobin C; (b) haemoglobin A + haemoglobin C; (c) haemoglobin A + haemoglobin C; (d) haemoglobin A + haemoglobin S + haemoglobin A_2; (e) haemoglobin S + haemoglobin A_2.

agent, leading to a visible cloudiness. This is called a sickle solubility test and is necessary because not all haemoglobins that look like haemoglobin S on haemoglobin electrophoresis or HPLC are actually haemoglobin S.

Management

It is important to avoid hypoxia during anaesthesia. Testing is therefore performed before surgery in patients from ethnic groups in which this mutation is prevalent. When emergency surgery is needed, time permits only a blood count and a sickle solubility test, but this should be followed by definitive testing. Individuals undertaking vigorous exercise, particularly at high altitudes and in hot climates, should avoid dehydration and, when the environmental temperature is high, need to acclimatise.

Testing for haemoglobin S must also be considered for individuals who are planning to become pregnant or are already pregnant since there is a one in four chance of the child of two carriers of haemoglobin S having sickle cell anaemia (Fig. 5.5).

Sickle cell anaemia

Sickle cell anaemia results from homozygosity for the β^S gene and occurs when the gene is inherited from both parents. Since there are no normal β

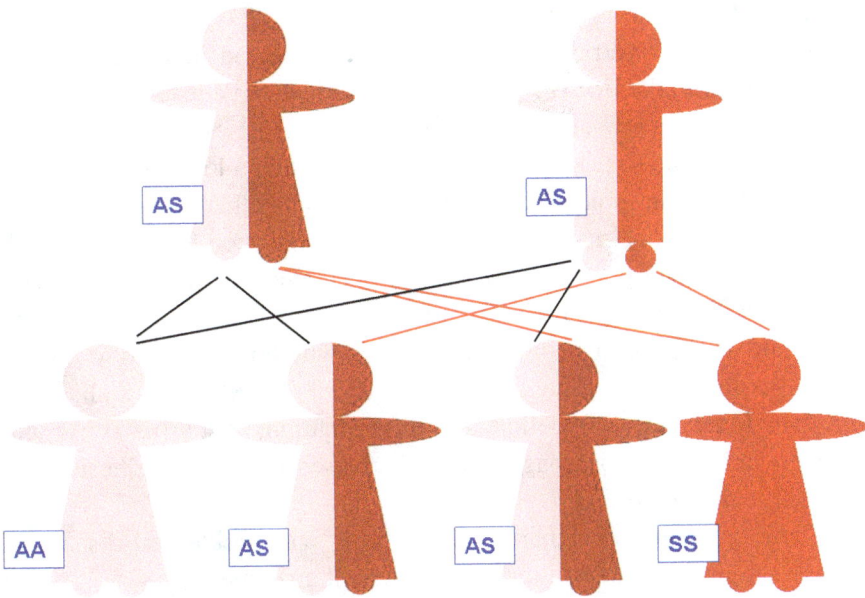

Fig. 5.5. Diagram showing the possible outcomes of a pregnancy when both parents have sickle cell trait. The β^S gene is represented in deep red and the normal β^A gene in pink. On average, a quarter of offspring will have no inherited haemoglobinopathy, a quarter will have sickle cell anaemia and a half will have sickle cell trait.

genes, haemoglobin A is completely absent (Fig. 5.4(e)). Sickle cell anaemia is one form of sickle cell disease. Haemoglobin S is prone to polymerise at low oxygen tension, leading to the formation of long, twisted polymers that deform the cell into the shape of a sickle. This process is reversible when the cell is again exposed to high oxygen tension; however, after several cycles of sickling, secondary changes in the cell membrane make the shape change irreversible. Sickle cell formation leads to obstruction of blood vessels and resultant tissue infarction. Vascular obstruction is due not only to the abnormal shape and rigidity of the sickled red cell but also to secondary changes in the erythrocyte membrane: dehydration of the cell that increases internal viscosity and the interaction of the sickled cell with neutrophils and endothelial cells. Intravascular haemolysis also leads to the destruction of nitric oxide (NO), an important physiological vasodilator. Over time, recurrent infarction can lead to permanent tissue damage in multiple organs.

Red cell lifespan is reduced from the normal 120 days to 10–20 days, which results in hyperbilirubinaemia and an increased incidence of gall-stones. However, the low Hb level in sickle cell anaemia is largely because haemoglobin S is a low-affinity haemoglobin that releases oxygen to tissues very readily. Since tissue oxygen delivery is normal, a lower Hb level suffices, and the erythropoietic drive is less than would otherwise be expected. The hyperactive bone marrow leads to an increased need for folic acid.

Haemoglobin S polymerisation, vaso-occlusion, and haemolytic anaemia are central to the pathophysiology of sickle cell disease. They precipitate a cascade of pathological events, which in turn lead to a wide range of complications. These processes include vascular endothelial dysfunction, functional NO deficiency, inflammation, oxidative stress and reperfusion injury, hypercoagulability, increased neutrophil adhesiveness and platelet activation.

There are now more than 17,000 people with sickle cell disease in Britain, the majority of whom have sickle cell anaemia.

Clinical features

Sickle cell anaemia is a multisystem disorder, with nearly every organ in the body being affected. Patients suffer recurrent painful crises as a result of tissue infarction in the chest, abdomen, spine and limbs; the infarction may involve bones, soft tissues or both. Pulmonary infarction can lead to hypoxia, which can be fatal. Infarction of the kidneys can cause haematuria. In children, infarction of small bones of the hands and feet can lead to painful swelling, referred to as dactylitis or the 'hand-foot syndrome' (Fig. 5.6). Young children can suffer from splenic sequestration, in which there is a rapid increase in spleen size due to pooling of red cells in the spleen resulting in severe acute anaemia; it can lead to hypovolaemic shock and, if not treated rapidly and appropriately, can be fatal. In older children, splenic sequestration no longer occurs because splenic fibrosis, following recurrent episodes of infarction, causes the spleen to no longer be distensible. In children, and to a lesser extent in adults, thrombosis in cerebral vessels leads to stroke. From adolescence onwards, males may suffer from priapism as a result of obstruction of venous drainage from the penis (Box 5.1).

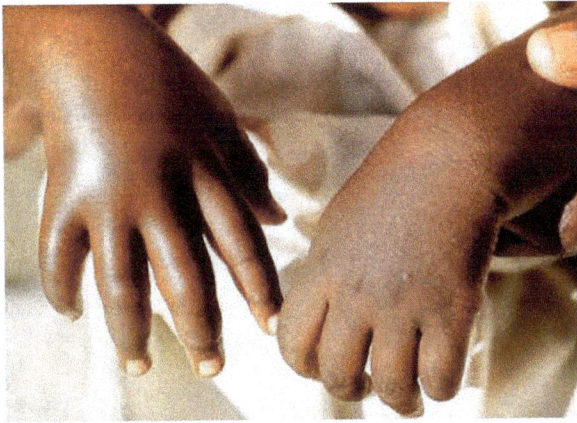

Fig. 5.6. Dactylitis in a child with sickle cell anaemia.

Box 5.1
Sickle cell emergencies (crises)

Crisis	Clinical features	Management
Acute chest syndrome	Chest pain, cough, fever, respiratory distress with pulmonary infiltrates and hypoxia	Treat infection, bronchodilators, incentive spirometry, O_2 supplementation May need exchange transfusion to get haemoglobin S <30% and/or non-invasive/invasive ventilation Hydroxycarbamide to prevent further chest crises
Acute stroke/ transient ischaemic attack (TIA)	Ischaemic stroke is more common than haemorrhagic stroke in children/ adolescents	Exchange transfusion Neurology review Primary prevention through regular exchange transfusions to keep haemoglobin S <30% if middle cerebral artery velocity >200 cm/s on transcranial Doppler

(Continued)

Box 5.1   *(Continued)*

Aplastic crisis	Acute drop in Hb with severe reticulocytopenia, commonly associated with parvovirus B19 infection in children	Top-up transfusion Consider intravenous immunoglobulin (IvIg) for parvovirus infection
Splenic sequestration	Acute drop in Hb with red cells captured and pooled in spleen, leading to its rapid enlargement	Restoration of blood volume with red cell transfusions
Painful vaso-occlusive crisis	Most common crisis with severe pain in bones needing hospital review/admission	Potent analgesia as per individual patient protocol, often involving opioids, plus hydration and rest
Priapism	Persistent painful erection not related to sexual desire	Urology intervention with corporal aspiration/irrigation Sympathomimetics

Hb: haemoglobin concentration.

Box 5.2
The function of the spleen

Removal of senescent or damaged red cells.
Antibody synthesis.
Removal of encapsulated microorganisms.
Removal of antibody- or complement-coated microorganisms.
Removal of red cell inclusions, such as malaria parasites and babesia.

Infarction due to sickling may have medium- and long-term sequelae. Recurrent splenic infarction leads to a clinically significant loss of splenic function. In considering the significance of this, it is useful to think about the function of the spleen (Box 5.2). Infarction of the soft tissues of the legs can lead to chronic ulceration (Fig. 5.7). There is an increased incidence of osteomyelitis, as infarcted bone is prone to secondary infection, with salmonella osteomyelitis being common. Rarely, infarction of the

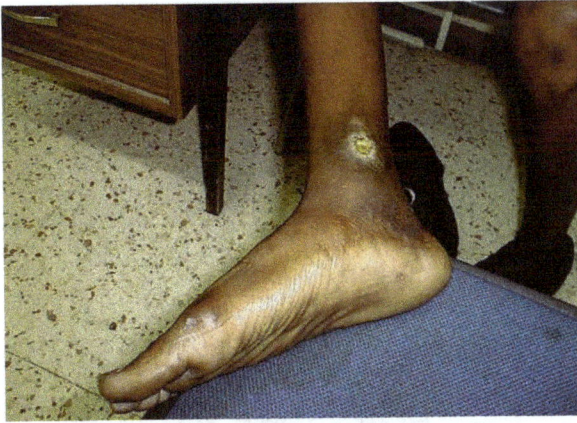

Fig. 5.7. A leg ulcer in a patient with sickle cell anaemia.

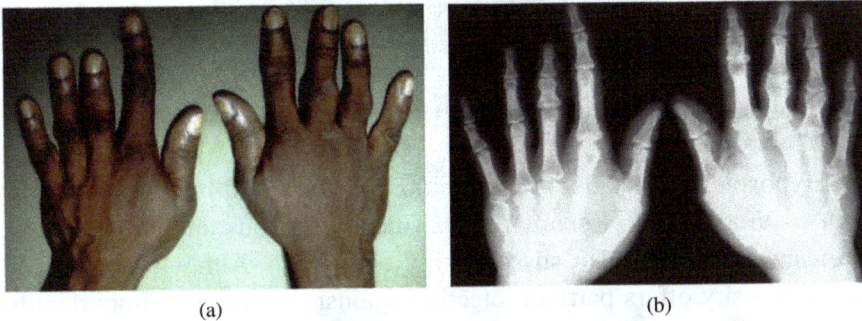

(a) (b)

Fig. 5.8. Clinical (a) photograph and (b) radiograph showing possible sequelae of bone infarction in young children with sickle cell anaemia; the third and fourth fingers of the left hand are abnormally short due to shortening of the metacarpals.

growth plate prevents bone growth so that there is shortening of one or more fingers or toes (Fig. 5.8). Infarction of the femoral heads can lead to osteonecrosis and osteoarthritis (Fig. 5.9). Recurrent renal infarction can lead to renal failure in early middle age.

Because of the short red cell lifespan, infection by parvovirus B19 (which infects red cell precursors and causes a temporary arrest in erythroblast maturation) can cause a rapid fall of Hb, leading to symptomatic anaemia.

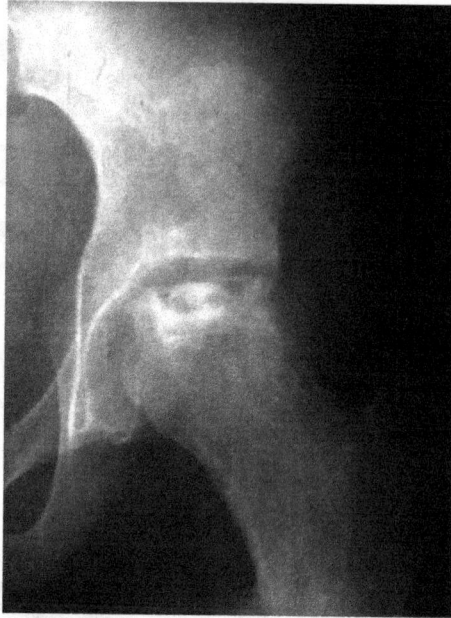

Fig. 5.9.   Radiograph showing osteoarthritis of the hip as a result of previous osteonecrosis.

Hyposplenism leads to susceptibility to blood-borne infections, such as those due to pneumococcus, meningococcus and *Haemophilus influenzae*. There is also susceptibility to malaria. Although sickle cell heterozygosity offers partial protection against malaria, it is important to realise that sickle cell anaemia definitely does not (Box 5.3).

Chronic complications fall into two main groups: those related to large vessel vasculopathy (cerebrovascular disease, pulmonary hypertension, priapism and retinopathy) and those caused by progressive ischemic organ damage (hyposplenism, renal failure, bone disease and liver damage).

Laboratory features and diagnosis

The Hb level is usually around 60–80 g/l, with an increased reticulocyte count. The blood film shows sickle cells, target cells, polychromasia, nucleated red blood cells and the features of hyposplenism (Howell–Jolly

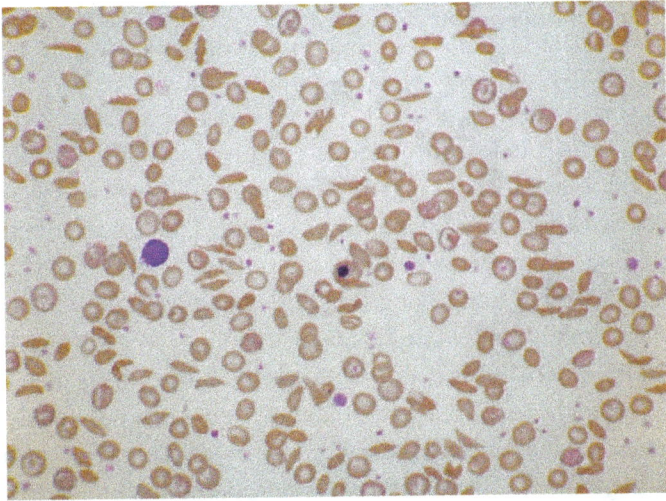

Fig. 5.10. Blood film of a patient with sickle cell anaemia showing numerous sickle cells, target cells, one lymphocyte and one nucleated red cell. There are some Howell–Jolly bodies and large platelets as an effect of hyposplenism (May–Grünwald–Giemsa (MGG) stain).

bodies, Pappenheimer bodies and an increased platelet count) (Fig. 5.10). A sudden fall in Hb to lower levels can be the result of splenic sequestration, folic acid deficiency (leading to megaloblastic anaemia) or infection by parvovirus B19. Parvovirus causes a temporary arrest of erythropoiesis, which remains unnoticed in people with a normal red cell lifespan, but in patients with a shortened red cell lifespan, it can cause symptomatic worsening of the anaemia; a very low reticulocyte count is a clue to this complication.

A sickle solubility test is positive when haemoglobin S is above 20%. False positives can occur in patients with a paraprotein or with numerous Heinz bodies because of an unstable haemoglobin imparting turbidity in the test tube.

Haemoglobin electrophoresis or HPLC shows haemoglobins S, A_2 and F, with a complete absence of haemoglobin A.

Biochemical tests show increased bilirubin (particularly unconjugated) and LDH, both as a result of haemolysis.

Prevention and management

Premarital, antenatal and neonatal screening programmes have been established in several countries, including the UK, as a preventative measure.

Children with sickle cell anaemia require vaccination against pneumococcus, meningococcus and *Haemophilus influenzae*. Vaccination against hepatitis B is also advised. They should also be prescribed prophylactic penicillin, which ideally should continue for life. Prophylactic folic acid is also advised. Parents should be instructed as to how to palpate the abdomen to recognise an enlarged spleen due to splenic sequestration and seek urgent medical advice if this is suspected.

During a sickle cell crisis, the patient needs adequate analgesia and the avoidance of dehydration, hypoxia and cold. If there is an infection, antibiotics are required. Splenic sequestration requires urgent transfusion, and parvovirus infection can also necessitate transfusion. Patients with hypoxia due to a severe chest crisis require exchange transfusions to lower the haemoglobin S percentage rapidly without increasing the blood viscosity. Transfusions should not be used to treat the chronic anaemia of sickle cell anaemia. However, patients who suffer recurrent crises can benefit from regular transfusions, either top-up or exchange, to keep the haemoglobin S percentage below 30%. Red cells for transfusion must have extended Rh and Kell typing, and if regular transfusion is instituted, monitoring for iron overload will become necessary. Exchange red cell transfusions are iron neutral.

Patients suffering from recurrent crises can benefit from regular hydroxycarbamide (previously known as hydroxyurea), which increases the haemoglobin F percentage and reduces sickling. Children who have suffered or are at high risk of a stroke benefit from regular blood transfusions to lower the percentage of haemoglobin S. A high risk of stroke is recognised by Doppler measurements of blood flow in cerebral vessels, with an accelerated flow rate indicating that the vessel is already narrowed. Regular Doppler monitoring should commence at two years of age and continue up to the age of 16.

Clinical outcomes have gradually improved over the years, mostly as a result of developments in supportive care and treatment with hydroxycarbamide. This is a licensed drug worldwide for sickle cell anaemia. Its mode of action is based on its ability to increase haemoglobin F levels and reduce intercellular adhesion, and hence improve blood flow.

Relatively few interventions have a strong evidence base. However, those that do include penicillin prophylaxis in children, primary stroke prevention with the use of transcranial Doppler screening and blood transfusions, and hydroxycarbamide to prevent acute pain and the acute chest syndrome as well as primary stroke.

New drugs such as L-glutamine (which reduces the oxidative stress of red cells, thus reducing endothelial adhesion) is under evaluation.

Allogenic haematopoietic stem cell transplantation (HSCT) involves the administration of a healthy donor's haematopoeitic stem cells (a matched sibling transplant is currently licensed in the UK) to modify sickle cell disease genotypes, and remains a curative treatment for patients. However, HSCT can result in graft rejection, graft versus host disease and infertility — some of the reasons why the use and uptake of this has been relatively low and traditionally reserved for patients with severe sickle cell complications.

Gene therapy, involving gene addition (such as lentiglobin vector to deliver normal haemoglobin to stem cells) or gene editing with CRISPR-Cas9 (to induce pan-cellular increase in haemoglobin F by modifying the *BCL11A* gene), offers huge promise as a disease-transforming treatment. Early approvals for these products are already underway.

Other forms of sickle cell disease

Sickle cell disease can also result from the coinheritance of haemoglobin S from one parent, and either β thalassaemia or a haemoglobin that interacts with haemoglobin S from the other parent. The most frequent are sickle cell/β thalassaemia and sickle cell/haemoglobin C disease. In sickle cell/β thalassaemia, there may be a small amount of haemoglobin A (if the thalassaemia gene is a β^+ gene) or absent haemoglobin A (if the thalassaemia gene is a β^0 gene). In either instance, there is microcytosis.

In sickle cell/haemoglobin C disease, there are equal amounts of haemo-globin S and haemoglobin C (Fig. 5.4(a)); haemoglobin C does not have a reduced oxygen affinity, so the Hb level is higher than in sickle cell anaemia, even being normal in some patients.

Red Cell Membrane Defects

A defect in the cytoskeleton that supports the red cell membrane can cause haemolytic anaemia. Inherited abnormalities can lead to haemolysis in many of the proteins shown in Fig. 5.1, including band 3, RhAG, pro-tein 4.2, α spectrin, β spectrin and actin. Hereditary spherocytosis and hereditary elliptocytosis are discussed as examples of red cell membrane defects.

Hereditary spherocytosis

Hereditary spherocytosis results from an inherited defect in the red cell membrane that leads to either compensated haemolysis or haemolytic anaemia. Estimates of frequency among Caucasians vary between 1 in 1,000 and 1 in 3,000. In three-quarters of instances, there is autosomal dominant inheritance, while in the others there is either autosomal reces-sive inheritance or a new mutation occurs. Causative mutations may be in the genes encoding band 3, actin, protein 4.2, α spectrin or β spectrin. As seen in Fig. 5.1, these proteins are involved in vertical interactions between the red cell membrane lipid bilayer and the supporting cytoskeleton. Defects in the proteins therefore leave part of the membrane unsupported so that it is lost by vesiculation. The cell therefore becomes progressively more spherocytic as it ages, along with the formation of spherocytes and microspherocytes. This leads to increased rigidity so that the cell is likely to become trapped and prematurely destroyed in the spleen.

Clinical features

Patients may present with symptomatic anaemia or recurrent jaundice. There is an increased incidence of pigment gallstones. Many patients are asymptomatic.

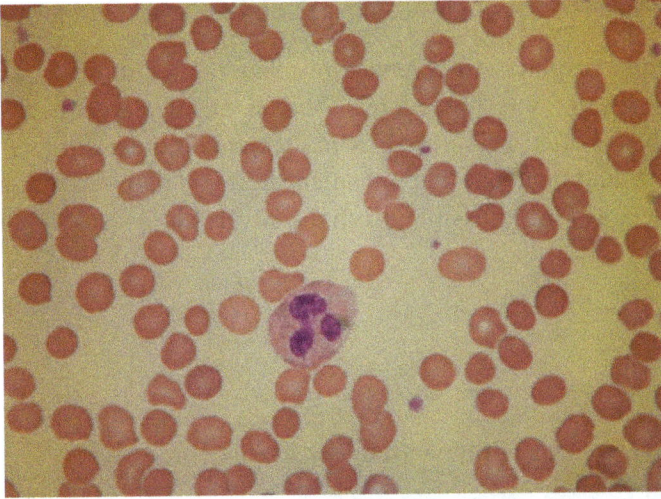

Fig. 5.11. Blood film of a patient with hereditary spherocytosis showing a neutrophil and numerous spherocytes — small dark red cells that lack central pallor (MGG stain).

Laboratory features and diagnosis

The blood count may or may not show anaemia. The mean cell haemoglobin concentration (MCHC) is often increased. The reticulocyte count is increased. The blood film (Fig. 5.11) shows spherocytosis and polychromasia. Hb may be at a reduced or normal level, but the reticulocyte count is increased. Bilirubin and LDH are increased.

Diagnosis is based on the observation of a haemolytic anaemia or compensated haemolysis with spherocytosis. If there is a family history of spherocytosis, no further tests are needed unless the anaemia is more severe than expected from the family history. In the absence of a family history, it is necessary to exclude the possibility of autoimmune haemolytic anaemia, an alternative cause of spherocytosis, by demonstrating a negative direct antiglobulin test. The diagnosis of hereditary spherocytosis can be confirmed by showing reduced binding of a dye, eosin-5-maleimide, to red cells (EMA binding, detected by measuring fluorescence in flow cytometry). An osmotic fragility test may aso be abnormal, although the test is now rarely performed. Red cell next-generation DNA sequencing (NGS) panels, inclusive of the common incriminated genes, are increasingly used for precise genetic diagnosis.

Management

The anaemia responds to splenectomy, but if it is mild, it is better to avoid the risks of this procedure. There is an increased need for folic acid, so this is often prescribed. Some patients require surgery for gall-stones. It should be noted that if a splenectomy is required, patients must be protected, as far as possible, from the adverse effects of hyposplenism (Box 5.3).

Box 5.3
Splenectomy/hyposplenism

Clinical issues

- Patients with absent or impaired splenic function are at risk of overwhelming fatal infection
- Encapsulated organisms: *S. pneumoniae, H. influenzae* and *N. meningitidis*
- Blood-borne parasites: malaria and babesia
- Dog and cat bites: *Capnocytophaga canimorsis*

Who is at risk?

- Anatomical loss: post-surgery
- Functional loss: sickle cell disease, thalassaemia, coeliac disease and other conditions
- Howell–Jolly bodies in red cells indicate hyposplenism

Management

- Essential that all clinicians, patients and carers are aware of risks
- Management evolves, so access up-to-date national or society guidelines

Prevention and treatment of infection

- Vaccinations: pneumococcal, meningococcal, Hib vaccines and seasonal flu

Box 5.3   *(Continued)*

- Prophylactic antibiotics: penicillin V daily
- Emergency antibiotics: amoxicillin-clavulanate (patients should have a supply)
- Fever in an asplenic patient is a medical emergency
- Travel advice: tick avoidance and malaria prevention

Hereditary elliptocytosis

Hereditary elliptocytosis usually causes only mild compensated haemolysis, but a few patients have haemolytic anaemia. Its prevalence is highest in West Africa, where it occurs in around 2% of individuals, although it is not infrequent among Caucasians. Inheritance is autosomal dominant. Hereditary elliptocytosis can result from mutation in genes encoding protein 4.2, α spectrin and β spectrin. Figure 5.1 shows that these proteins are concerned with horizontal interactions and the stability of the cytoskeleton. Mutations lead to mechanical instability, and erythrocytes become elliptocytic with a reduced surface-to-volume ratio as they age.

Clinical features

Most individuals with hereditary elliptocytosis are asymptomatic, and their diagnosis is incidental. Occasionally, there is symptomatic anaemia.

Laboratory features and diagnosis

Diagnosis is based on the distinctive blood film (Fig. 5.12), usually with compensated haemolysis, but sometimes with haemolytic anaemia.

Management

Usually, no treatment is necessary, but rarely, when haemolysis is severe, a splenectomy is required.

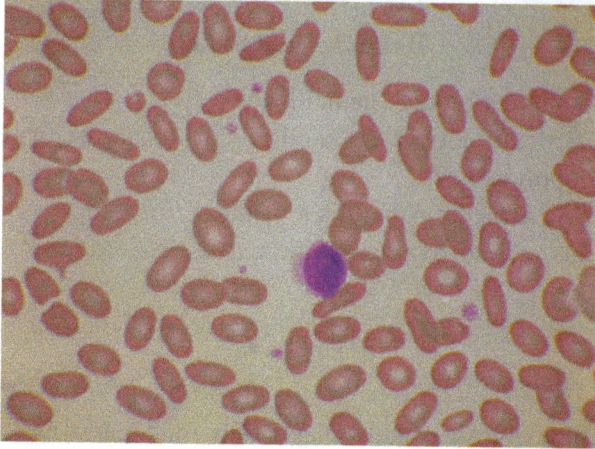

Fig. 5.12. Blood film of a patient with hereditary elliptocytosis showing a lymphocyte and numerous elliptocytes (MGG stain).

Defects in the Glycolytic Pathway

An intact glycolytic pathway leads to a net gain in adenosine triphosphate (ATP), which meets the energy needs of the red cell (Fig. 5.2). Defects in this pathway therefore lead to shortened red cell survival. All defects of the glycolytic pathway are rare.

Pyruvate kinase deficiency

Pyruvate kinase deficiency is the most common form of the rare defects in the glycolytic pathway. Although deficiency is infrequent, it occurs in many ethnic groups. The blood count, reticulocyte count and biochemical tests indicate a chronic haemolytic anaemia. The blood film shows no specific abnormality. Diagnosis is by an assay of enzyme activity. When haemolysis is severe, a splenectomy may be needed. Oral allosteric activators of the pyruvate kinase enzyme (such as mitapivat) increase the Hb level significantly in some patients.

Defects in the Pentose Shunt

Deficiency of G6PD is common in many populations worldwide. Other defects in the pentose shunt are rare. The pentose shunt maintains oxygen in its normal functionally reduced form. When it is defective and the red cells are exposed to oxidative stress, haemoglobin is oxidised to the non-functional methaemoglobin, which is incapable of oxygen transport.

Glucose-6-phosphate dehydrogenase deficiency

The gene encoding G6PD is on the X chromosome, so most affected individuals are males. However, symptomatic deficiency can also occur in homozygous females and, occasionally, in heterozygous females. G6PD deficiency is common in populations from around the Mediterranean Sea (Italians, Greeks, Cypriots and Arabs) and also in Afro-Caribbeans and others of African ancestry. In the great majority of cases, presentation is with neonatal jaundice or acute intermittent haemolysis. Rarely, when deficiency is severe, there is chronic haemolysis.

Clinical features

Most individuals with G6PD deficiency are asymptomatic until oxidative stress on the red cells leads to acute haemolysis. Such stress may involve the generation of reactive oxygen species by neutrophils during an infection or may be attributable to the ingestion of broad beans or a drug (such as primaquine or dapsone) or exposure to a chemical (such as naphthalene, a chemical once popular for mothballs but now no longer legally available in many countries). The previously healthy individual develops haemoglobinuria, jaundice and acute anaemia.

Babies with G6PD deficiency have an increased incidence of neonatal jaundice, not necessarily accompanied by anaemia since it is in part due to the effect of G6PD deficiency on hepatic cells.

Laboratory features and diagnosis

The blood film during a haemolytic episode confirms the anaemia and shows irregularly contracted cells (Fig. 5.13). Sometimes, the haemoglobin is precipitated in half of the cell, leaving the rest of the red cell membrane empty — a 'hemi-ghost'. On other occasions, the red cell loses all its haemoglobin during intravascular lysis and becomes an empty membrane — a 'ghost cell' (Fig. 5.13). A Heinz body preparation

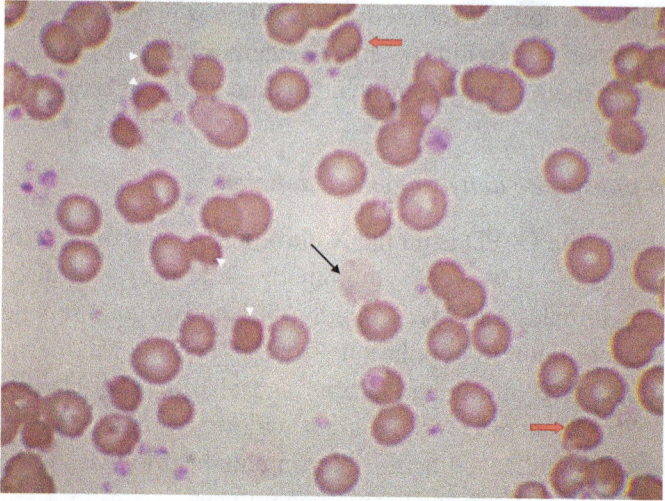

Fig. 5.13. Blood film of a patient with acute haemolysis as the result of exposure to an oxidant drug in a patient with G6PD deficiency (MGG stain). There are irregularly contracted cells (red arrows), ghost cells (black arrows) and hemi-ghost cells (white arrows). The haemolysis is very recent so that, although the anaemia is severe, there is not yet any polychromasia.

is positive, indicating that methaemoglobin is present and has precipitated (Fig. 5.14). There is rapid development of polychromasia, and the reticulocyte count rises.

The blood film is very important in diagnosis. A G6PD assay confirms the diagnosis; however, sometimes, the results appear to be normal during acute haemolysis due to the high reticulocyte count (reticulocytes have a higher concentration of the enzyme). It is then necessary to repeat the assay after the acute haemolytic episode is over.

Management

Following acute haemolysis, the anaemia may be severe enough to require transfusions. Otherwise, prevention is important. The patient must be given an accurate list of drugs that can cause haemolysis, and doctors caring for such patients should refer to a reliable list (e.g. the British National Formulary) before prescribing.

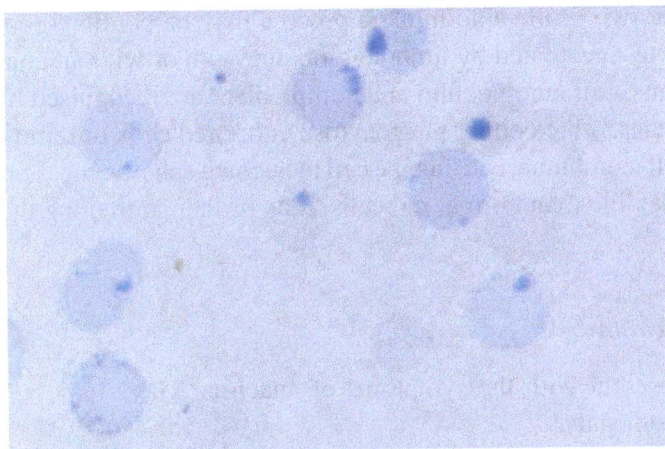

Fig. 5.14. A Heinz body preparation in a patient with G6PD deficiency and acute haemolysis showing numerous Heinz bodies. The erythrocytes have stained pale blue; the Heinz bodies are the large brilliant cresyl blue inclusions within the erythrocytes.

Neonatal jaundice should be managed by keeping the bilirubin at a safe level using phototherapy. Occasionally, exchange transfusions may be needed.

Immune Haemolytic Anaemias

Immune haemolytic anaemia is an antibody-mediated haemolytic anaemia. The antibody may be an autoantibody (as in autoimmune haemolytic anaemia), an alloantibody (as in haemolytic transfusion reactions or when maternal antibodies cross the placenta and cause haemolysis in a fetus or neonate) or a drug-dependent antibody (causing haemolysis in the presence of the drug).

Autoimmune haemolytic anaemia

Autoimmune haemolytic anaemia results from the development of an antibody directed at autologous erythrocyte antigens. This may occur as part of a recognised autoimmune disease, such as systemic lupus erythematosus, or the autoimmune process may be confined to red cells. Erythrocytes are coated by immunoglobulin, with or without complement components. Immunoglobulin and complement are recognised by splenic macrophages, which either phagocytose entire red cells or remove part of the red cell membrane, causing the cell to become spherocytic. Spherocytes are less flexible than normal red cells, thus further shortening the red cell lifespan.

Clinical features

Patients present with the symptoms of anaemia. There may be jaundice and splenomegaly.

Laboratory features and diagnosis

There is anaemia with reticulocytosis. The blood film shows sphero-cytes and polychromasia. Biochemical evidence of haemolysis is present. The diagnosis is confirmed by a positive direct antiglobulin test (also known as a Coombs test, see Fig. 13.10). This is a test for the iden-tification of immunoglobulin and complement on the red cell membrane. In contrast to hereditary spherocytosis, the binding of eosin-5-maleimide is normal.

Management

Treatment is initially with corticosteroids, which may be combined with rituximab, a monoclonal antibody directed at B lymphocytes. If the dis-ease is not easily controlled, other immunosuppressive agents may be added. In severe cases, a splenectomy may be needed.

Microangiopathic Haemolytic Anaemia

This is a type of haemolytic anaemia resulting from a pathological process in small blood vessels that causes fragmentation of red cells. The capillaries may have abnormal endothelial cells and contain fibrin strands that trap and damage red cells. There are many causes, including haemolytic uraemic syndrome, thrombotic thrombocytopenic purpura (see Chapter 11) and metastatic tumours. The blood film detection of red cell fragments is important in making a diagnosis.

Haemolytic uraemic syndrome

This syndrome typically occurs in young children and usually results from infection by a specific strain of *Escherichia coli, E. coli* O157:H7. This pathogenic *E. coli* secretes verocytotoxin, which damages endothelial cells, particularly in the kidney, leading to both fragmentation of adherent red cells and renal failure. There is diarrhoea, followed by the onset of jaundice and clinical features of anaemia. Laboratory tests show anaemia, reticulocytosis, red cell fragments, increased bilirubin and LDH and increased creatinine. The haemolysis is reversible once the acute phase of the illness is over. The renal failure is also reversible in most cases, but may require temporary renal support by haemodialysis.

Conclusions

Haemolytic anaemia can be suspected when there is evidence of increased breakdown of red cells, increased bone marrow response and the presence of red cells with an abnormal appearance. The diagnosis depends on an initial blood count and blood film, with further specific tests being indicated by the blood film abnormalities. Sickle cell anaemia has many clinicopathological manifestations, of which haemolytic anaemia is one; other features are related directly or indirectly to vascular obstruction and tissue infarction. Other haemolytic anaemias can also be a feature of a serious systemic disease, such as haemolytic uraemic syndrome or autoimmune haemolytic anaemia secondary to systemic lupus erythematosus.

Test Case 5.1

A 25-year-old woman presents with right upper quadrant pain, nausea and vomiting. On examination, she has tenderness in the right upper quadrant and scleral icterus. Ultrasonography of the abdomen shows a number of gallstones in the gall bladder. On specific questioning, she admits that occasionally in the past, she has noticed yellowness of her eyes. A blood count shows: WBC $13 \times 10^9/l$, neutrophil count $10.8 \times 10^9/l$, Hb 100 g/l (normal range (NR): 118–148), MCV 101 fl (NR: 82–98) and platelet count $407 \times 10^9/l$. A blood film shows spherocytes and polychromatic macrocytes, so further tests are done. The reticulocyte count is $250 \times 10^9/l$, and the direct antiglobulin test is negative. Bilirubin is increased and is mainly unconjugated.

Questions

1. Are you surprised that a 25-year-old has gallstones?
2. What is the most likely diagnosis and why?
3. Why was a direct antiglobulin test done, and what does it tell us?
4. What test would confirm your suspicion?

Write down your answers before checking the correct answer (page 404) or re-reading any relevant parts of the chapter.

Test Case 5.2

A 5-year-old Afro-Caribbean girl has been known to have sickle cell anaemia since birth, when the diagnosis was made after neonatal screening. She had an episode of dactylitis at the age of 18 months and suffers from painful crises several times a year. She takes penicillin and folic acid regularly. Her mother brings her to the Paediatric Accident and Emergency Department because she appears quite listless and is thought to be paler than normal. On examination, there is no jaundice and the spleen is not palpable. A blood count shows: WBC $9.6 \times 10^9/l$, Hb 35 g/l (NR for a 5-year-old girl: 100–140), MCV 87 fl (NR: 75–90) and platelet count $313 \times 10^9/l$. A blood film shows sickle cells, target cells and Howell–Jolly bodies, but polychromasia is noted to be absent. A reticulocyte count is $2 \times 10^9/l$ (NR: 50 –100 $\times 10^9/l$).

Questions

1. What does the reticulocyte count tell us?
2. What is the most likely diagnosis and why?
3. How should the child be managed?

Write down your answers before checking the correct answer (page 405) or re-reading any relevant parts of the chapter.

6

Miscellaneous Anaemias, Pancytopenia and the Myelodysplastic Syndromes

Vishal Jayakar

What Do You Need To Know?

☞ The causes, diagnosis and management of normocytic normochromic anaemias (including renal failure and aplastic anaemia)
☞ The possible causes of pancytopenia and how they are recognised
☞ The nature, diagnosis and management of aplastic anaemia
☞ The nature, clinicopathological features, diagnosis and principles of management of the myelodysplastic syndromes

Normocytic Normochromic Anaemia and Other Anaemias

Some of the causes of normocytic normochromic anaemia and associated diagnostic features are shown in Table 6.1. The clinical history and physical examination are of considerable importance in making a specific diagnosis. If no specific diagnosis is suggested from the history and examination, it can be useful to examine a blood film and measure serum ferritin, serum vitamin B_{12}, serum folate, serum creatinine and the erythrocyte sedimentation rate as the first step.

V. Jayakar

Table 6.1. Some causes of normocytic normochromic anaemia.

Causative conditions	Diagnostic features
Early iron deficiency*	Low serum ferritin
Early anaemia of chronic disease*	Increased rouleaux and erythrocyte sedimentation rate, low serum iron, normal or high serum ferritin
Double deficiency of iron and vitamin B_{12} or folic acid	Hypersegmented neutrophils, low ferritin and either low serum vitamin B_{12} or low serum folate
Blood loss	If blood loss is severe and acute, anaemia is leucoerythroblastic; polychromasia and reticulocytosis develop within a few days
Some haemolytic anaemias[†]	Polychromasia, increased reticulocyte count, increased serum bilirubin and lactate dehydrogenase, possibly specific poikilocytes
Some myelodysplastic syndromes[†]	Other features of myelodysplastic syndromes
Renal failure	Sometimes crenation or schistocytes, creatinine elevated
Liver failure[†]	Target cells, stomatocytes, acanthocytes, other cytopenias, abnormal liver function tests
Multiple myeloma[†]	Increased rouleaux and erythrocyte sedimentation rate when serum paraprotein is present
Hypothyroidism[†]	Low thyroxine and high thyroid stimulating hormone
Addison disease and hypopituitarism	Lymphocytosis, eosinophilia, neutropenia, monocytopenia
Anorexia nervosa	Small numbers of acanthocytes, sometimes other cytopenias
Pure red cell aplasia[†]	Reticulocyte count very low or reticulocytes absent; may have a thymoma, lymphoproliferative disorder or autoimmune disease

*Can also be microcytic.
[†]Can also be macrocytic.

Renal disease

Renal disease may be complicated by microangiopathic haemolytic anaemia, which is a feature of severe hypertension, haemolytic uraemic syndrome (see page 109) and thrombotic thrombocytopenic purpura (see below and page 262). Renal failure has haematological manifestations, causing both anaemia and impaired platelet function. Renal failure can result from haematological diseases, such as sickle cell disease and multiple myeloma (also known as plasma cell myeloma). All adults who present with renal failure should be tested urgently for myeloma as renal damage may be reversible if treated quickly.

Renal failure

Anaemia in renal failure is multifactorial. An important mechanism is inadequate erythropoietin synthesis but there may also be shortening of red cell survival. In acute renal failure there may be a more pronounced haemolytic element. When renal failure results from multiple myeloma, bone marrow infiltration contributes to anaemia.

Anaemia of chronic renal failure may benefit from recombinant erythropoietin therapy. For maximum effectiveness, iron stores must be adequate so that maintaining the serum ferritin above 100 μg/l is recommended. The aim of therapy should be a haemoglobin concentration (Hb) of 100–110 g/l since higher levels are not associated with a better quality of life or other outcome and may have adverse cardiovascular effects. A rapid rise of Hb should also be avoided, since this may cause hypertension.

Thrombotic thrombocytopenic purpura (TTP)

This is a rare condition characterised by some or all of five clinical features: (i) fever; (ii) neurological abnormalities; (iii) renal impairment; (iv) microangiopathic haemolytic anaemia; and (v) thrombocytopenia. It is caused by an autoantibody to Von Willebrand factor-cleaving protease (ADAMTS13). Although this condition is rare, recognising it rapidly is important because there is a high mortality without specific treatment. A detailed explanation of TTP is provided on page 262.

Liver disease

Anaemia in liver disease may be normocytic normochromic or macrocytic and may be accompanied by other cytopenias. Haematological abnormalities are multifactorial. The effects of excess alcohol consumption and folic acid deficiency may be superimposed on those of liver disease, and patients with cirrhosis can develop portal hypertension leading to hypersplenism with associated pancytopenia. The blood film may show macrocytes, stomatocytes (Fig. 6.1) or target cells. There are two specific types of haemolytic anaemia associated with liver disease. Zieve syndrome refers to acute haemolysis and hyperlipidaemia associated with an alcoholic fatty liver (Fig. 6.2). Spur cell haemolytic anaemia refers to haemolytic anaemia associated with a severe acanthocytic change, occurring in liver failure of any aetiology (Fig. 6.3).

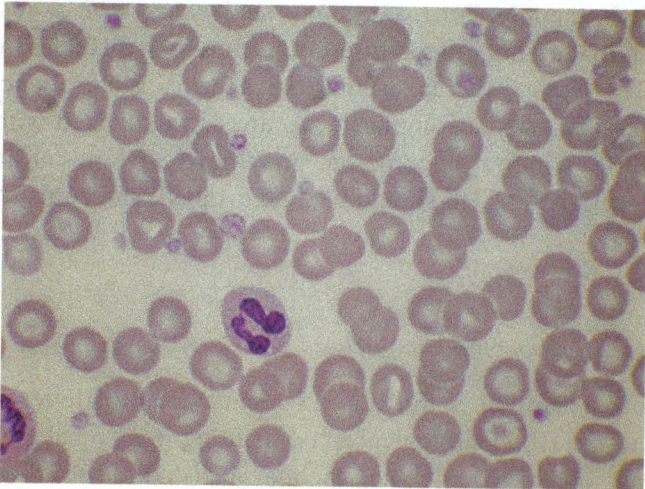

Fig. 6.1. Peripheral blood (PB) film showing macrocytes, stomatocytes and target cells in a patient with portal cirrhosis. May–Grünwald–Giemsa stain (MGG).

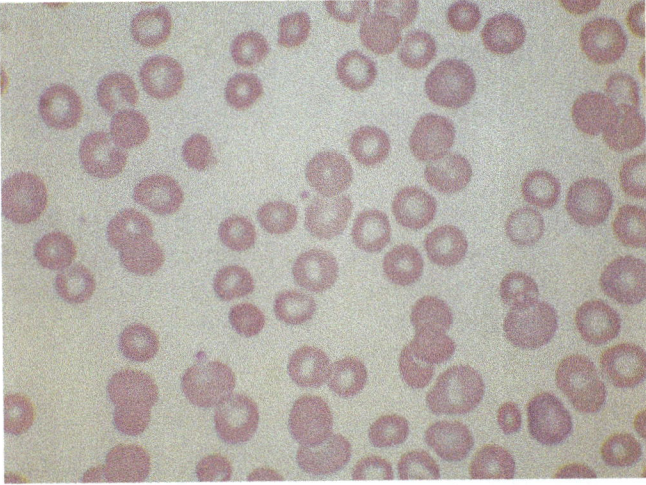

Fig. 6.2. PB film showing several irregularly contracted cells and some polychromatic macrocytes in a patient with Zieve syndrome. MGG.

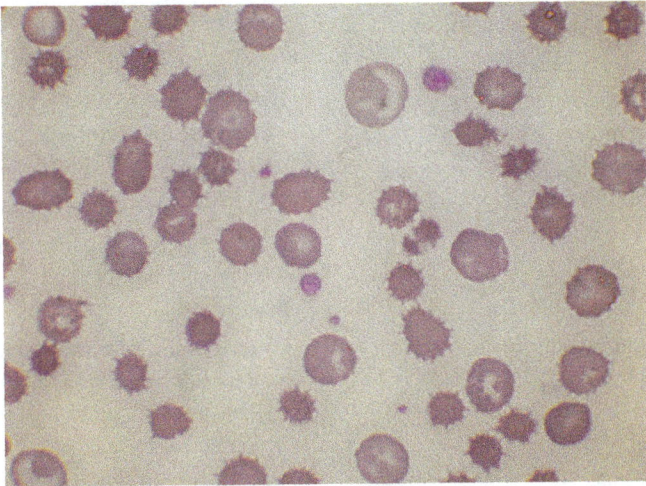

Fig. 6.3. PB film showing polychromatic macrocytes and a severe acanthocytic change in a patient with terminal liver failure and spur cell haemolytic anaemia. MGG.

Liver disease is often associated with prolongation of the prothrombin time and activated partial thromboplastin time.

Pancytopenia

Pancytopenia refers to a reduction in the total white cell count (WBC), neutrophil count, Hb and platelet count. There are many possible causes, which will often be apparent from the clinical history or suggested by blood film features (Table 6.2).

Table 6.2. Some causes of pancytopenia.

Cause	Possible diagnostic clues
Bone marrow suppression by drugs (e.g. anti-cancer drugs or immunosuppressive agents) or irradiation	Clinical history
Severe megaloblastic anaemia (including the effects of methotrexate therapy)	Macrocytes, hypersegmented neutrophils
Bone marrow replacement by leukaemic blast cells	Clinical features (splenomegaly ± lymphadenopathy), some blast cells often present in peripheral blood
Bone marrow infiltration by metastatic carcinoma	Clinical features, leucoerythroblastic blood film with teardrop poikilocytes
Primary myelofibrosis	Splenomegaly (which is often marked), leucoerythroblastic blood film with teardrop poikilocytes
Myelodysplastic syndromes	Red cell anisocytosis and poikilocytosis or a dimorphic population, dysplastic changes in neutrophils, large or hypogranular platelets
Aplastic anaemia	None
Human immunodeficiency virus (HIV) infection	Clinical history, opportunistic infections, lymphopenia
Osteopetrosis	Leucoerythroblastic blood film
Hypersplenism	Clinical or blood film features of liver disease, splenomegaly

In current medical practice, pancytopenia is often the effect of administration of anti-cancer or immunosuppressive drugs and is an expected side effect of the treatment. Much less often, it results from radiotherapy.

Patients with acute leukaemia usually present with a high WBC but sometimes with pancytopenia. Particularly in children, pancytopenia may be the result of infiltration of the bone marrow by the lymphoblasts of acute lymphoblastic leukaemia. There may be clinical features such as splenomegaly and lymphadenopathy and the blood film usually shows at least a small number of lymphoblasts. Replacement of the normal marrow by myeloid blast cells can similarly cause pancytopenia in patients of any age with acute myeloid leukaemia (AML). The blood film is likely to show at least some blast cells or other abnormal myeloid cells.

Pancytopenia can result from replacement of the bone marrow by non-haematological cells, such as metastatic carcinoma cells. There is often associated fibrosis, which contributes to the cytopenia. The patient may have a history of previous cancer or may have systemic features such as weight loss. The blood film often shows the presence of nucleated red blood cells and myelocytes, which is known as a leucoerythroblastic anaemia.

Pancytopenia can result from a marked reduction in the number of haemopoietic stem cells in the bone marrow (aplastic anaemia, see below) or from defective differentiation and maturation of cells derived from a defective stem cell (myelodysplastic syndromes, see page 121).

Pancytopenia can occur despite normal bone marrow function if the spleen is very large and blood cells are being pooled there. This is a feature of portal hypertension in patients with cirrhosis. It also occurs in Gaucher disease when the spleen contains many Gaucher cells; in this condition partial replacement of the bone marrow by Gaucher cells also contributes to the pancytopenia. In primary myelofibrosis (see page 204), pancytopenia is due both to hypersplenism and to progressive fibrosis of the bone marrow.

Aplastic anaemia

Despite its name, aplastic anaemia is characterised by pancytopenia rather than just anaemia. The reticulocyte count is low and the blood film shows

V. Jayakar

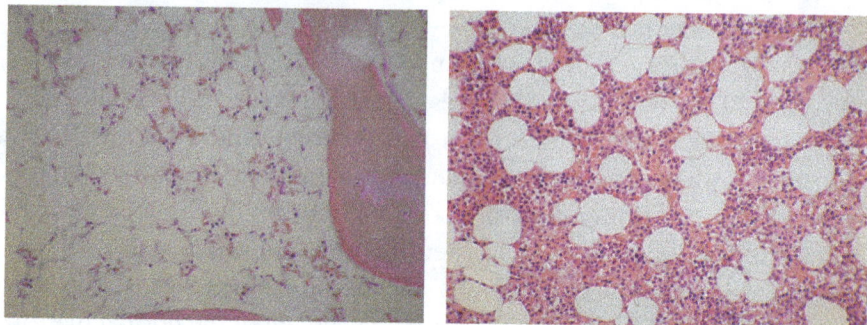

Fig. 6.4. Trephine biopsy section from a patient with aplastic anaemia (left) showing that most of the bone marrow cavity between the bones is occupied by fat cells. In comparison, a normal marrow (right) shows active haemopoiesis with the fat cells occupying a much smaller proportion of the intertrabecular space. Haematoxylin and eosin stain.

no specific morphological abnormality. Bone marrow biopsy shows that haemopoietic marrow is largely replaced by fat cells (Fig. 6.4). Aplastic anaemia may be due to an inherited genetic abnormality (such as Fanconi anaemia or dyskeratosis congenita). It can be the result of drug exposure, either from excessive doses of a drug that regularly causes bone marrow suppression (such as a cytotoxic agent) or to normal doses of a drug to which the patient suffers an idiosyncratic reaction. Drugs that can cause permanent bone marrow damage as an idiosyncratic reaction include chloramphenicol, phenylbutazone (no longer approved for human use), phenytoin, chlorpropamide and tolbutamide. The Epstein–Barr virus can lead to aplastic anaemia but mainly in individuals with a defective immune response to the virus. Aplastic anaemia may occur 2–3 months after an episode of hepatitis. This accounts for 5–10% of all cases and often affects young males. It is postulated that a viral infection may cause either T-cell activation and cytokine release or the development of a cytotoxic T-cell clone cross reacting with bone marrow cells. Hepatitis viruses A, B and C are not involved. Currently the responsible virus is unidentified. Some cases of aplastic anaemia are idiopathic (i.e. no cause is discovered).

Treatment available includes immunosuppressive treatment and allogeneic haemopoietic stem cell transplantation. Immunosuppressive treatment is usually anti-lymphocyte globulin (produced by immunising horses or rabbits, though horse is the preferred source) plus ciclosporin. The basis of its success is that in many cases of aplastic anaemia there is damage to haemopoietic cells by suppressor T lymphocytes. The addition of eltrombopag which is a thrombopoietin receptor agonist increases the rate of response and shortens the median response time. In patients with less severe aplastic anaemia, an anabolic steroid may be of benefit. Acute myeloid leukaemia sometimes develops in patients with aplastic anaemia who have responded to immunosuppressive treatment.

Pure red cell aplasia

Aplasia may affect only the erythroid lineage. The earliest morphologically recognisable red cell precursors, proerythroblasts, are present but maturing cells are markedly reduced or virtually absent. Known causes include infection by parvovirus B19 and an autoimmune process, the latter being sometimes associated with thymoma. Parvovirus-induced pure red cell aplasia is transient in people with normal immunity but may be clinically manifest in patients with haemolytic anaemia. In those with severe immune deficiency, who are unable to clear the virus, it can cause prolonged red cell aplasia.

Myelodysplastic Syndromes

Myelodysplastic syndromes (MDS), also known as myelodysplastic neoplasms, are a heterogeneous group of disorders that are characterised by a cellular bone marrow but, paradoxically, peripheral cytopenia. They are related to the myeloid leukaemias in that normal bone marrow cells are replaced by a clonal population of cells derived from a single mutated haemopoietic stem cell. The progeny of this stem cell retain the ability to proliferate, but their maturation is abnormal in two ways. Firstly, there is an increased rate of death of haemopoietic precursors in the marrow; this is known as ineffective haemopoiesis which explains the coexistence of a hypercellular marrow and peripheral cytopenia. Secondly, the maturation appears abnormal when cells are viewed down the microscope; this is referred to as 'dysplasia', hence the term myelodysplastic syndrome. Cells may also be functionally abnormal. In addition to ineffective and

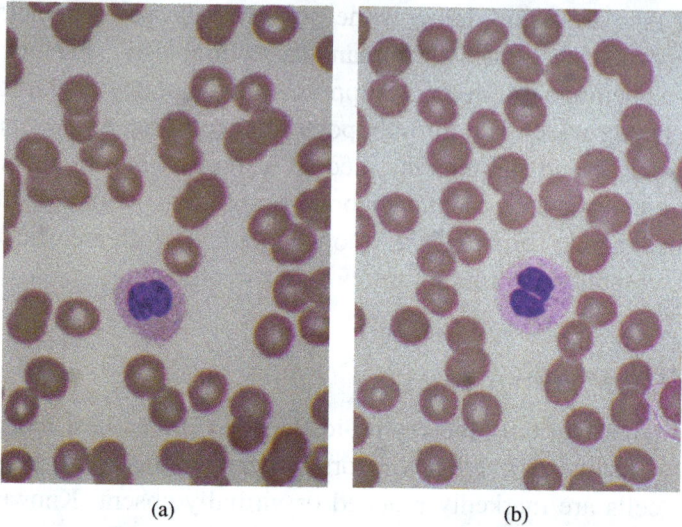

(a)   (b)

Fig. 6.5. PB film showing two hypolobulated neutrophils from the same patient (a and b); (b) the neutrophil has a nucleus shaped like a pince-nez, or a pair of spectacles. This is referred to as a pseudo- or acquired Pelger–Huët anomaly since the neutrophils resemble those of an inherited condition with the same name. Note that there are no platelets in either photograph, so the patient clearly has severe thrombocytopenia as well.

dysplastic haemopoiesis, there is a third characteristic of the abnormal clone of cells. They are genetically unstable. As a result of further muta-tion, a sub-clone of more malignant cells may emerge, leading to disease progression and transformation to AML.

Among the dysplastic features most typical of these syndromes are hypogranularity and hypolobulation of neutrophils (Figs. 6.5 and 6.6) and the presence of either small or hypolobulated megakaryocytes in the bone marrow (Figs. 6.7 and 6.8). Among red cell changes, one of the most characteristic is macrocytosis (Fig. 6.9). Bone marrow erythro-blasts may show abnormalities such as bi- or multi-nuclearity, nuclear lobulation, nuclear fragmentation and megaloblastosis. Sideroblastic erythropoiesis can also occur (Fig. 6.10); this means that there is a defect in haem synthesis and some of the erythroblasts in the bone marrow have a prominent ring of haemosiderin granules around the nucleus, rather than the small scattered iron-containing granules that are seen in normal erythroblasts.

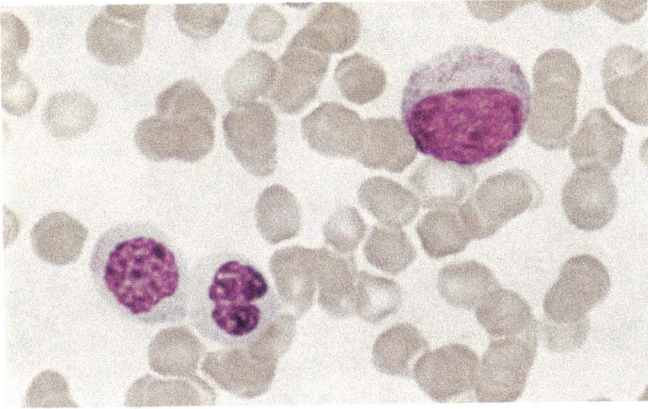

Fig. 6.6. PB film showing two neutrophils that are hypolobated and almost totally agranular. The other cell is a myelocyte. No platelets are seen. MGG.

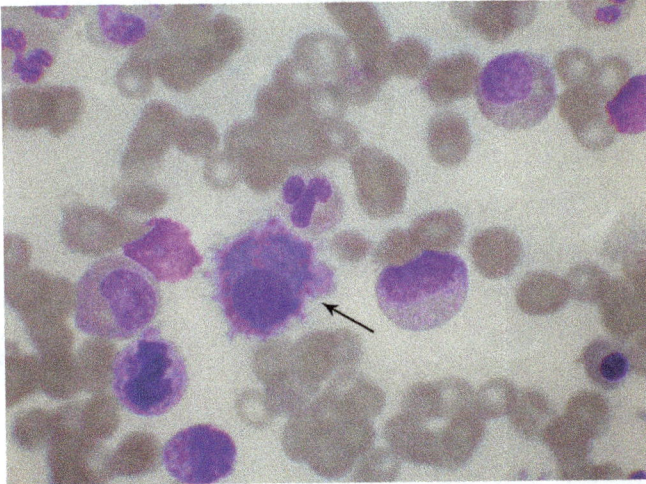

Fig. 6.7. Bone marrow (BM) aspirate film. The arrow identifies a very small megakaryocyte, referred to as a micromegakaryocyte. MGG.

In a minority of patients the bone marrow is hypocellular rather than hypercellular and such cases can be difficult to distinguish from aplastic anaemia.

MDS is mainly a disease of the middle-aged and elderly. It can arise *de novo* but some cases follow damage to stem cells by cytotoxic

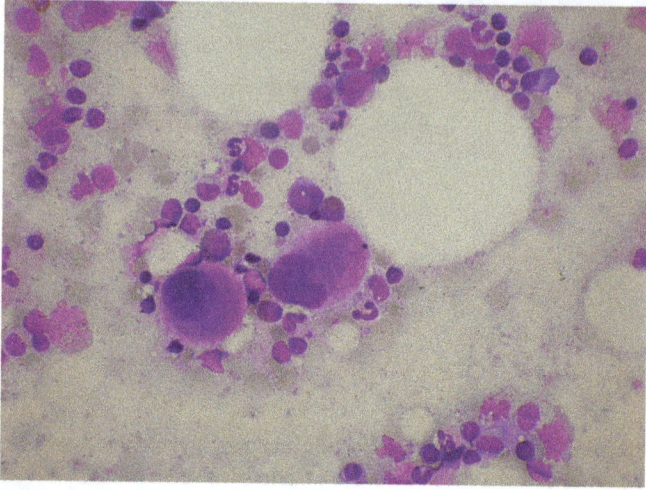

Fig. 6.8. BM aspirate film showing two megakaryocytes that are of normal size but have hypolobated nuclei. This bone marrow is from a patient with the 5q– syndrome, which is characterised by macrocytic anaemia and non-lobulated or hypolobulated megakaryocyte nuclei. MGG.

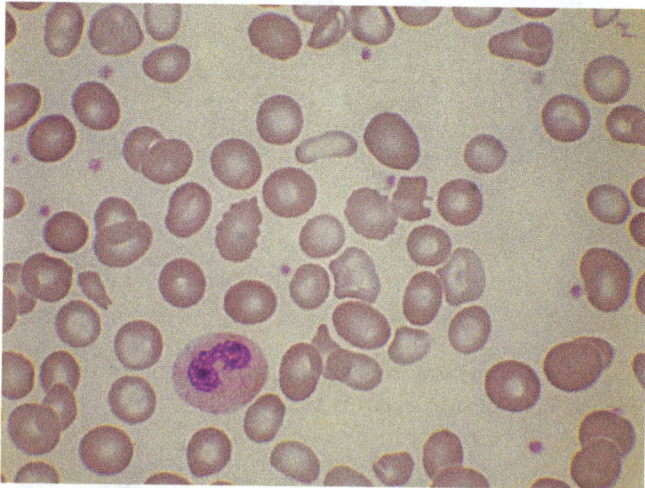

Fig. 6.9. PB film in myelodysplastic syndrome with multilineage dysplasia showing macrocytosis and mild poikilocytosis. Platelet numbers appear to be normal. MGG.

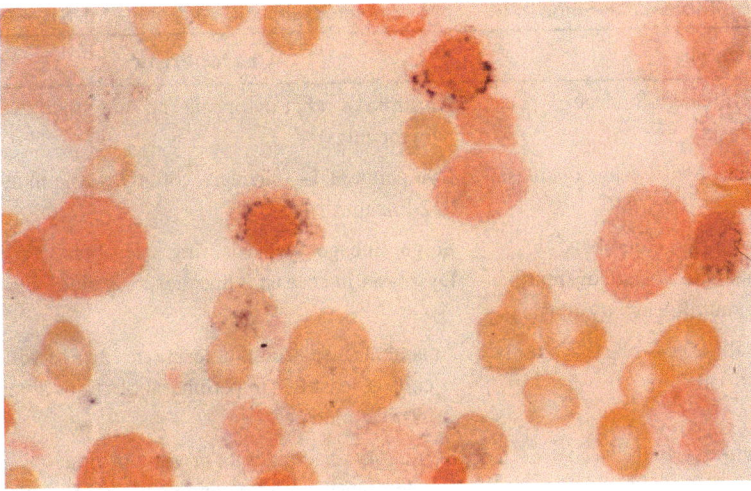

Fig. 6.10. BM aspirate film from a patient with myelodysplastic syndrome with single lineage dysplasia and ring sideroblasts, which have a ring of deep blue granules surrounding the nucleus. The film has been stained with a Prussian blue, or Perls' stain, which stains haemosiderin.

chemotherapy or irradiation and these patients may be younger. These conditions vary in their severity. Some cause chronic anaemia or other cytopenia but are compatible with survival for many years. Others are much closer to AML with cytopenia being combined with an increase of blast cells in the peripheral blood, bone marrow or both; however, the increase in blast cells is less than that in AML. Some of the types of MDS are summarised in Table 6.3 (WHO classification — 2016). You certainly do not need to know the categories of MDS, as the classification is continuously evolving (for instance, in the WHO 2022 classification, more molecular subtypes are defined, e.g. MDS with ringed sideroblasts is relabelled as myelodysplastic neoplasia with low blasts and an *SF3B1* mutation) — this table is just to show the range of abnormalities that can be present. The prognosis is worse for cases that result from previous chemotherapy and for those with increased blast cells or Auer rods. MDS progresses over time. Patients with MDS can die of complications of cytopenia, such as infection or haemorrhage, or death can occur when the disease evolves into AML. This type of AML responds poorly to treatment.

Table 6.3.   Some of the types of myelodysplastic syndrome (MDS)*.

Classification	Characteristics
MDS with single lineage dysplasia	Anaemia or other cytopenia (no more than two cytopenias)[†]
MDS with multilineage dysplasia	Cytopenia of 1–3 lineages with dysplasia in at last 2 lineages[†]

MDS with ring sideroblasts
  With single lineage dysplasia
  With multilineage dysplasia
	Single lineage dysplasia, ring sideroblasts[†,‡]
	Dysplasia in at least 2 lineages, ring sideroblasts[†,‡]

MDS with excess blasts (MDS-EB)	Anaemia, dysplasia in at least one lineage with blast cells at least 2% in peripheral blood or at last 5% in bone marrow[§]
MDS with isolated del(5q)	Refractory anaemia with or without ring sideroblasts with 5q– and possibly one other cytogenetic abnormality[†,¶]
Therapy-related MDS	MDS following cytotoxic chemotherapy or irradiation, often has multilineage dysplasia and may have an increase of blast cells or Auer rods
MDS, unclassified	Cases that do not meet the criteria for the above categories

*You do not need to know any details.

[†]With no increase in blast cells or Auer rods (an Auer rod is a cytoplasmic inclusion resulting from fusion of primary granules of cells of the neutrophil lineage).

[‡]Ring sideroblasts constitute at least 15% of erythroblasts or at least 5% if a specific mutation (in *SF3B1*) is present.

[§]Divided into MDS-EB-1 and MDS-EB-2, depending on the degree of increase in blast cells and the presence or absence of Auer rods.

[¶]But not –7 or del(7q).

Clinical features

Common clinical features result from anaemia including fatigue, breathlessness and ankle swelling. Patients with a low neutrophil count or with a normal count but defective neutrophil function may be susceptible to infection. Patients with thrombocytopenia or defective platelet function are subject to bruising and bleeding.

On physical examination there may be pallor, bruising, petechiae and sometimes splenomegaly.

Laboratory features and diagnosis

The blood film usually shows either a normocytic or macrocytic anaemia with a variable degree of anisocytosis and poikilocytosis. In sideroblastic anaemia there is usually a major population of macrocytes and a minor population of hypochromic microcytes giving a dimorphic blood film (Fig. 6.11); some cells contain Pappenheimer bodies, small navy blue inclusions that represent haemosiderin (Fig. 6.12). In addition to hyposegmented and hypogranular neutrophils, there may be some blast cells (Fig. 6.13). Platelets are often reduced in number and they may have reduced granules or be larger than normal.

The bone marrow is hypercellular with dysplastic changes in one or more lineages and sometimes an increase of blast cells. Iron stores are often increased and ring sideroblasts may be present.

Cytogenetic analysis may show an acquired clonal chromosomal abnormality, which helps to confirm the diagnosis. In the type of MDS designated MDS with isolated del(5q), also known as the 5q– syndrome, the clonal abnormality is an interstitial deletion of part of the long arm of

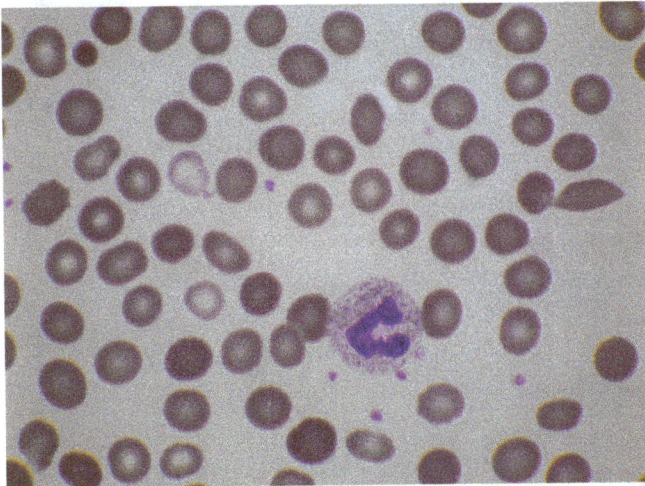

Fig. 6.11. PB film from a patient with myelodysplastic syndrome with single lineage dysplasia and ring sideroblasts showing a major red cell population of well-haemoglobinised macrocytes and a minor population (two cells) of hypochromic microcytes. This is referred to as a dimorphic blood film. MGG.

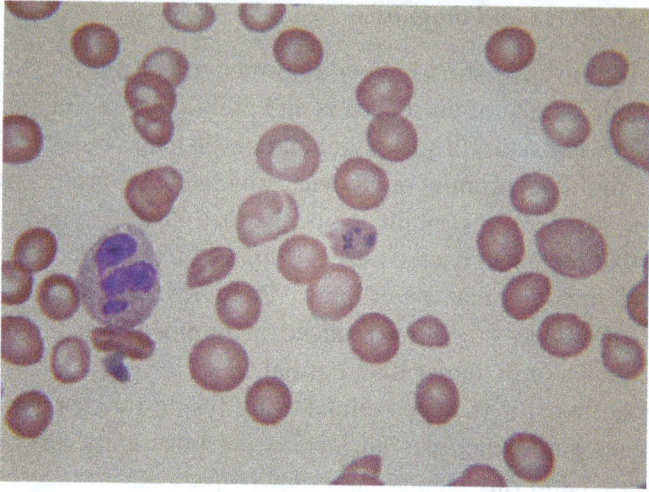

Fig. 6.12. PB film from a patient with myelodysplastic syndrome with excess blasts (who had sideroblastic erythropoiesis) showing a red cell (centre) containing Pappenheimer bodies. There are also macrocytes. MGG.

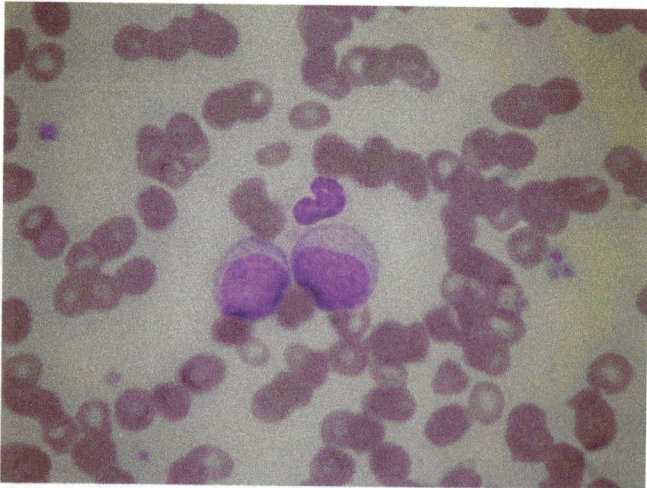

Fig. 6.13. PB film from a patient with myelodysplastic syndrome with excess blasts showing two blast cells and a hypogranular neutrophil band form. MGG.

chromosome 5. Other cytogenetic abnormalities can also be present including three copies of chromosome 8 (trisomy 8) or loss of one copy of chromosome 7 (monosomy 7) or loss of part of the long arm of chromosome 7, del(7q).

Management

Management may be symptomatic (palliative) or directed at prolonging life. Occasionally, in younger, fitter patients, treatment may be directed at cure. Prognostic scores, such as the Revised International Prognostic Scoring System (IPSS-R) and the Molecular International Prognostic Scoring System (IPSS-M), are used to stratify the risk of patients with MDS and thus help in selecting appropriate treatment.

Symptomatic management includes use of blood transfusion or erythropoietin injections for anaemia. Erythropoietin may be more efficacious in combination with granulocyte colony-stimulating factor. Platelet infusions are used, when needed, for bleeding. Infections require antibiotics. Active management, directed at life prolongation, involves cytotoxic chemotherapy in high-risk MDS. Azacitidine is licensed for MDS patients with a high-risk IPSS-R score. As this is a disease particularly of the elderly, active treatment is not always indicated. Patients with the 5q– syndrome are particularly responsive to lenalidomide. Luspatercept is an erythroid maturation agent that exerts its effect in the later stages of erythropoiesis and has shown promise in achieving transfusion independence in low-risk MDS, particularly with SF3B1 mutations. Immunosuppressive treatment can be of use, particularly in patients with a hypocellular bone marrow. In younger, fitter patients, haemopoietic stem cell transplantation should be considered since it offers the possibility of cure.

In patients with an otherwise good prognosis who are dependent on blood transfusions, tissue damage from iron overload can become a problem. This can be managed by chelation therapy.

Conclusions

The cause of anaemia or pancytopenia is often suggested by the clinical history and physical examination. In other circumstances, the blood film suggests a diagnosis. When the likely cause is not at all apparent, extensive investigation may be needed including haematological and biochemical tests, a bone marrow aspirate and trephine biopsy and imaging investigations.

Test Case 6.1

A 56-year-old woman presents with a lump in her breast and is found to have a carcinoma of the breast with metastasis to axillary lymph nodes. She is treated with surgery, radiotherapy and cytotoxic chemotherapy and makes a good recovery. However seven years later, during routine follow up, she complains of fatigue and ankle swelling. Other than pallor, no abnormality is found on physical examination, so some blood tests are done. A full blood count shows: WBC $3.5 \times 10^9/l$, neutrophil count $1.0 \times 10^9/l$, Hb 90 g/l (normal range (NR) 118–148), MCV 105 fl (NR 82–98) and platelet count $96 \times 10^9/l$. The blood film is reported as showing hypogranular 'Pelger' neutrophils, a dimorphic red cell population (normochromic macrocytic cells and hypochromic microcytic cells) with Pappenheimer bodies in some erythrocytes and occasional blast cells. Liver and renal function, calcium and phosphate are all normal.

Questions

1. What is your differential diagnosis and what is the most likely diagnosis?
2. Is her past medical history relevant?
3. What should be done next?

Write down your answers before checking the correct answer (page 405) and re-reading any relevant part of the chapter.

7

Leucocytosis, Leucopenia and Reactive Changes in White Cells

Donald Macdonald

What Do You Need To Know?

☞ The causes of a high white cell count and of increased numbers of neutrophils, lymphocytes and eosinophils
☞ The causes of a low white cell count, neutropenia and lymphopenia
☞ The reactive changes that occur in the blood in infection and inflammation

Leucocytosis

Leucocytosis means an increase in the white blood cell count (WBC). It is most often due to an increase in either neutrophils or lymphocytes but occasionally the number of eosinophils is sufficiently increased to cause an increase in the WBC. It is not useful to think about the causes of leucocytosis. Rather one must think about the causes of an increased number of cells of a specific cell type. It is the absolute number of cells that must be assessed rather than the percentage. For each cell type it is necessary to relate the patient's count to a normal range, and when necessary to a range for a specific age, gender or ethnic group.

Neutrophilia

Neutrophilia means an increase in the absolute number of circulating neutrophils. The normal range is higher in neonates than at other times of life; it is higher during pregnancy and even higher during labour and in the early post-partum period. The normal range is somewhat higher in women than in men. Neutrophil counts in people of African ancestry are often lower than in those of other ethnic origins.

Neutrophilia can be a physiological response to vigorous exercise, as neutrophils that are marginated against the endothelium of blood vessels are mobilised into the circulating neutrophil pool. The same thing can happen in an epileptic convulsion or following injection of adrenaline (epinephrine). Neutrophilia is also a common, non-specific response to infection (particularly bacterial infection), inflammation (including gout and acute inflammation in connective tissue disorders) and tissue damage or necrosis (infarction, trauma, surgery or burns). The neutrophil count is increased by corticosteroid administration, as a response to blood loss or haemolysis and as a rebound phenomenon following previously low levels.

When there is neutrophilia as a response to infection or tissue inflammation or damage there are often accompanying morphological changes such as toxic granulation, Döhle bodies and vacuolation (Fig. 7.1). 'Toxic granulation' is not specifically related to any toxin but refers to heavy granulation as a reactive change. Döhle bodies are small oval blue-grey cytoplasmic inclusions that contain aggregates of ribosomes; they indicate cytoplasmic immaturity. These reactive changes may be accompanied by a left shift. This term indicates that the proportion of non-lobulated neutrophils (neutrophil band forms) is increased; often there are also neutrophil precursors in the circulation. The presence of neutrophil vacuolation correlates strongly with bacterial infection but otherwise these reactive changes are not specific for infection. Occasionally, however, phagocytosed bacteria are seen within neutrophils, permitting rapid confirmation of the diagnosis of infection (Fig. 7.2).

Uncommonly, neutrophilia occurs as a feature of a haematological neoplasm, the neutrophils being part of the leukaemic clone of cells. This can occur in chronic myeloid leukaemia and in the myeloproliferative neoplasms (see Chapter 9). In these cases reactive changes are absent.

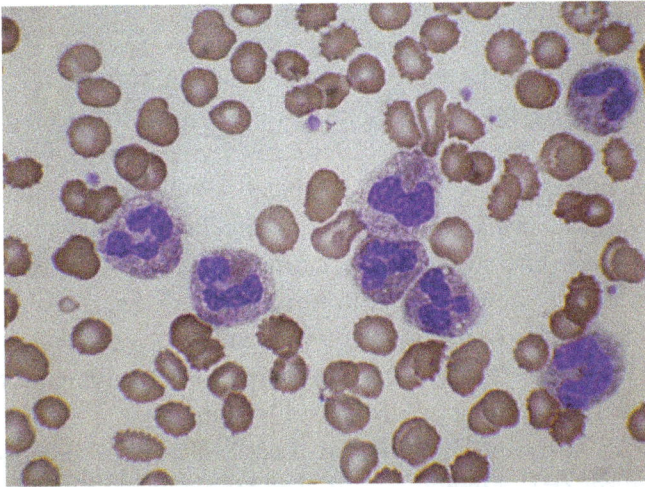

Fig. 7.1. Peripheral blood (PB) film from a patient with a bacterial infection showing neutrophilia, toxic granulation and mild neutrophil vacuolation. Two of the cells are band forms so there is therefore also a left shift. May–Grünwald–Giemsa stain (MGG).

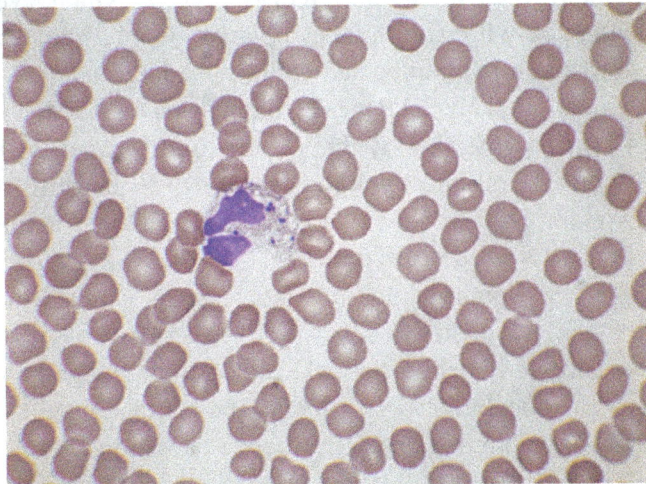

Fig. 7.2. PB film from a patient with meningococcal septicaemia showing a neutrophil that has phagocytosed meningococci. Note that there are no platelets in the film. There is severe thrombocytopenia as a result of platelet consumption through disseminated intravascular coagulation. MGG.

Lymphocytosis

Lymphocytosis means an increase in the absolute number of circulating lymphocytes. The lymphocyte count is higher in children than in adults but there are no gender or ethnic differences. Lymphocytosis is a common response to viral infection. It is also typical of whooping cough (Fig 7.3) and is sometimes seen in other bacterial infections including brucellosis and tuberculosis, and also in toxoplasmosis (infection by a protozoan parasite). Children often respond to infections, even bacterial infections, with lymphocytosis. Acute stress, for example, myocardial infarction, trauma or sickle cell crisis, can cause a sharp rise in the lymphocyte count; this is of brief duration and is followed by lymphopenia. There may be lymphocytosis early in the course of illness related to human immuno-deficiency virus (HIV) infection, followed by lymphopenia as the disease progresses. The lymphocyte count is also increased after removal of the spleen. Allergic reactions to drugs can cause lymphocytosis.

During a lymphocyte response to viral infection there are sometimes striking changes in the cytological features of the lymphocytes. These reactive lymphocytes are often referred to as 'atypical lymphocytes'. They are increased in size with basophilic cytoplasm, cytoplasmic margins that appear to flow around adjoining red cells and a large nucleus that may have a prominent nucleolus. Atypical lymphocytes are particularly characteristic of primary infection by the Epstein–Barr virus (EBV) but they also occur in other viral infections (cytomegalovirus, hepatitis A, adenovirus and primary HIV infection), rickettsial infections, toxoplasmosis and hypersensitivity reactions to drugs.

In children and young adults, lymphocytosis is almost always reactive. In older adults, lymphocytosis may be the result of a lymphoid neoplasm, either chronic lymphocytic leukaemia or non-Hodgkin lymphoma (see Chapter 8). The lymphocytes then have characteristic cytological features that differ from those seen in reactive conditions.

Infectious mononucleosis

Infectious mononucleosis or 'glandular fever' is an illness resulting from primary EBV infection. It usually occurs in adolescents and young adults.

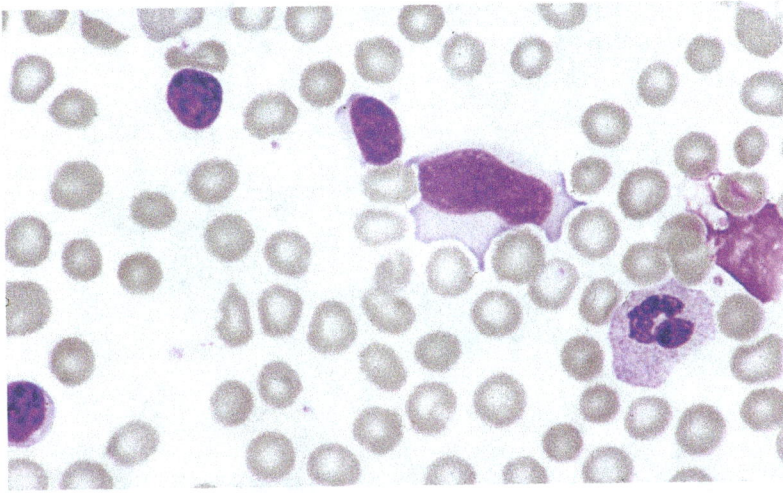

Fig. 7.3. PB film from a child with pertussis (whooping cough) showing lymphocytosis. Most of the lymphocytes are mature small lymphocytes but there is one large atypical lymphocyte with a deeply basophilic cytoplasmic margin; it appears to be flowing around adjacent red cells. The photograph also shows a neutrophil and a smear cell (a crushed lymphocyte). MGG.

Clinical features include fever, pharyngitis, tonsillar enlargement, lymphadenopathy and sometimes splenomegaly, jaundice or a rash. A diagnostically important laboratory feature is lymphocytosis, characterised by numerous atypical lymphocytes (Fig. 7.4). A minority of patients are anaemic as a result of the production of an autoantibody directed at the i red cell antigen. This is an agglutinating antibody acting at low temperatures so that red cell agglutinates are seen in blood films; it is referred to as a cold agglutinin. Some patients have thrombocytopenia.

Diagnosis is usually suspected from the blood film features in an appropriate clinical context. It can be confirmed by demonstration of a specific type of heterophile antibody: one directed at an antigen of another species. In this case, the antibody agglutinates sheep or horse red cells, is absorbed by ox red cells and is not absorbed by guinea pig kidney. Simple laboratory tests are available that show these rather curious serological specificities. The diagnosis can also be confirmed by demonstrating

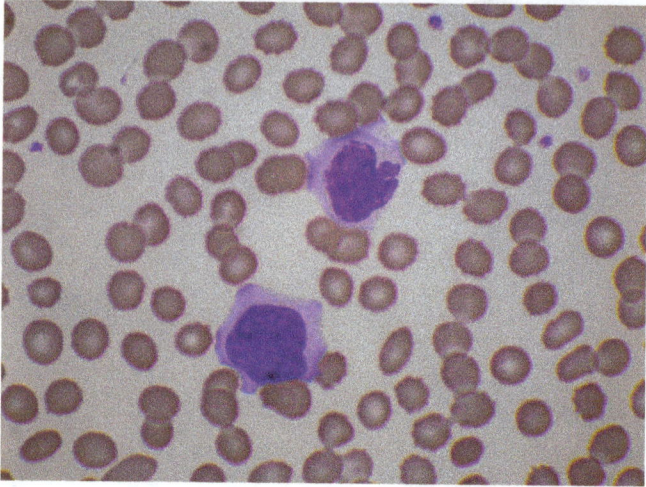

Fig. 7.4. PB film from a patient with infectious mononucleosis showing two atypical lymphocytes. These cells are enlarged in size, have large, irregularly shaped nuclei and have plentiful basophilic cytoplasm that appears to be flowing around adjacent red cells. The irregular shape of the red cells (crenation) is due to delay in making the blood film. MGG.

immunoglobulin (Ig) M antibodies to EBV viral capsid antigen, but this test is not necessary if the heterophile antibody is detected.

Eosinophilia

Eosinophilia means an increase in the absolute number of eosinophils in the circulation (Fig. 7.5). There is no gender or ethnic variation; higher counts previously observed in underdeveloped countries are likely the result of parasitic infections. A minor increase in the eosinophil count is common in individuals with allergic rhinitis (hayfever), asthma or eczema. Aside from these atopic conditions, a marked increase is also seen in other skin conditions, parasitic infections, allergic reactions to drugs, in some connective tissue disorders (e.g. eosinophilic granulomatosis with poly-angiitis, previously known as the Churg–Strauss syndrome) and as a reaction to lymphoma or other neoplasm. Much less often the eosinophils themselves belong to a clone of neoplastic cells; if they are the dominant cell type, the term 'eosinophilic leukaemia' is used.

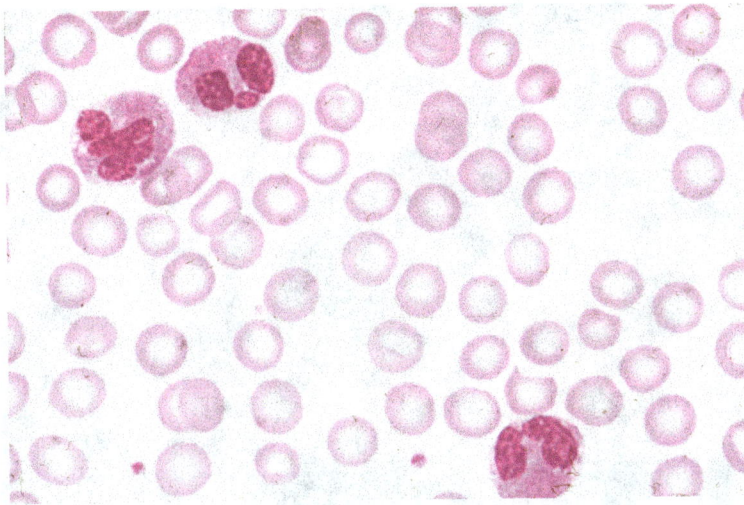

Fig. 7.5. PB film showing reactive eosinophilia. The nuclei are more lobulated than those of normal eosinophils and there are small cytoplasmic vacuoles. Minor morphological changes are common in reactive eosinophilia. MGG.

The cause of eosinophilia is often readily apparent from the clinical history and physical examination. If this is not so, the possibility of a drug reaction or parasitic infection should be considered. The parasites that cause eosinophilia are mainly nematodes (roundworms) and trematodes (flukes) that invade tissues (Figs. 7.6 and 7.7). Rarely the cause is detected in a blood film when microfilariae are seen (Fig. 7.7). Usually diagnosis requires examination of stools for ova, cysts and parasites. Examination of urine if schistosomiasis is also a possibility and serological tests may be required for antibodies to the more elusive parasites.

Monocytosis

Monocytosis is an increase in the number of monocytes in the circulation. It usually results from bacterial infection, including chronic infections such as tuberculosis and brucellosis. Following the more usual bacterial infections, it takes longer to appear than neutrophilia. Monocyte numbers can also be increased in inflammatory conditions, carcinoma and as a feature of leukaemia.

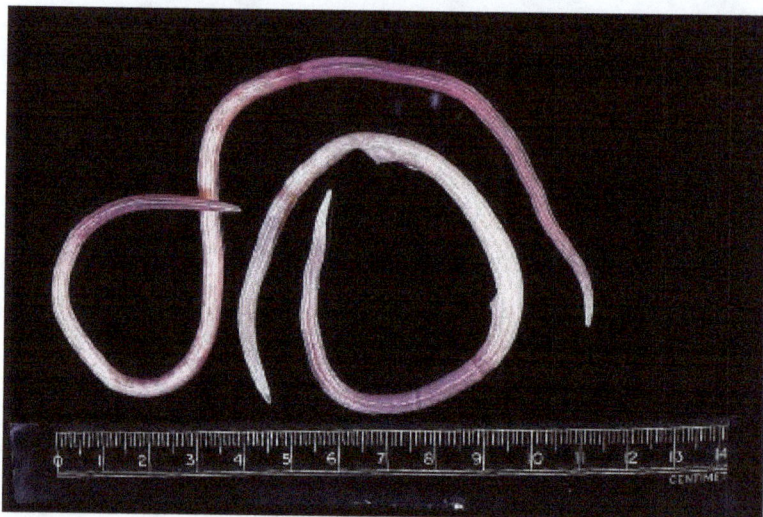

Fig. 7.6. Adult *Ascaris lumbricoides*. Eosinophilia in ascariasis is maximal during the stage of larval migration through the lungs. Reproduced with permission from W Peters and G Pasvol *Atlas of Tropical Medicine and Parasitology*, 6th Edn, Elsevier, 2007.

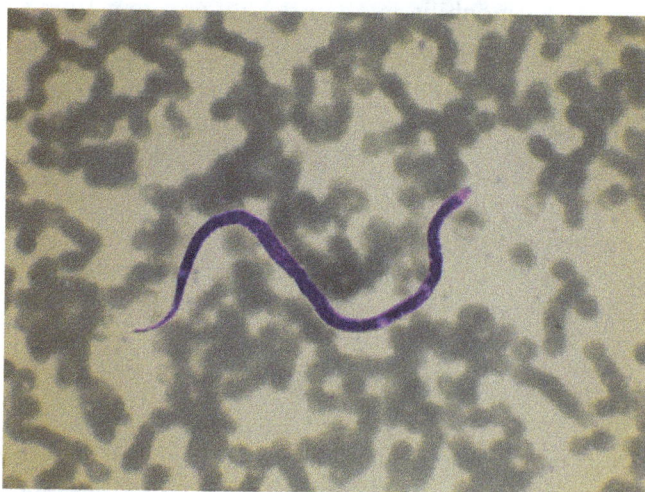

Fig. 7.7. Microfilaria of *Loa loa* in a blood film. MGG.

Basophilia

Basophilia is an increase in the number of circulating basophils (but note that the same word also means an increased uptake of basic dyes by cytoplasm). Reactive basophilia is uncommon, but basophilia is a useful diagnostic feature in myeloproliferative neoplasms and certain leukaemias in which the basophils are part of the leukaemic clone.

Leucoerythroblastic blood response

This term means that there are nucleated red cells and neutrophil precursors in the peripheral blood film. In the neonatal period this is a normal phenomenon but at other times of life it can be diagnostically useful. It is a useful clue to the presence of bone marrow metastases or bone marrow fibrosis, including primary myelofibrosis. However, it can also occur as a physiological response to acute blood loss, haemolysis or hypoxia.

Leucopenia

Leucopenia means a decrease in the WBC. It can be the result of a reduction in the neutrophil count, the lymphocyte count or both. As with leucocytosis, it is important to note which cell lineage is decreased.

Neutropenia

Neutropenia means a decrease in the absolute neutrophil count below the normal range, i.e. below what would be expected in a healthy individual of the same age, gender and ethnic origin. Neutropenia can be the result of a failure of bone marrow production, peripheral destruction or sequestration. Neutropenia may be multifactorial. For example, in severe bacterial infection there may be rapid migration of neutrophils to tissues, with the bone marrow being unable to produce cells at a sufficient rate to maintain circulating numbers.

When neutropenia is due to a failure of neutrophil production other lineages are also often affected. Failed production can be induced by drugs (for example, those used in the treatment of malignant conditions) or irradiation or be the result of an intrinsic disorder of the bone marrow or bone marrow infiltration. Replacement of the bone marrow by abnormal cells will cause neutropenia if it is sufficiently extensive but neutropenia is most likely when there is also an intrinsic defect in haemopoietic stem cells so that differentiation to neutrophils is impaired. Neutropenia is therefore characteristic of the myelodysplastic syndromes (see Chapter 6) and acute myeloid leukaemia (see Chapter 8).

Neutrophils may be destroyed in the circulation as a result of an idiosyncratic reaction to a drug (e.g. sulphonamides or antithyroid drugs) or due to the action of an autoantibody. Neither of these is common but it is important to suspect and detect drug-induced neutropenia since continuing the drug may lead to death from overwhelming infection. Patients with severe drug-induced neutropenia, known as agranulocytosis, may have virtually no neutrophils in the peripheral blood and usually present with fever due to infection, particularly respiratory tract infection.

Sequestration of aggregated neutrophils in the lungs can occur when the circulating blood is exposed to a foreign surface, as in haemodialysis. This phenomenon is transient and has no clinical consequences.

The cause of neutropenia is often apparent from the clinical history including the drug history. The blood film may provide clues, showing dysplastic features in the myelodysplastic syndromes and acute myeloid leukaemia and a leucoerythroblastic blood film when there is bone marrow infiltration. The film often also shows reactive changes in the remaining neutrophils since secondary infection is common.

Lymphopenia

Lymphopenia or lymphocytopenia means a reduction in the absolute number of circulating lymphocytes. It is a common non-specific occurrence, being part of the body's response to stress including trauma, surgery and infection. The lymphocyte count is lowered by corticosteroids, irradiation and the administration of cytotoxic or immunosuppressive drugs. Sometimes it is of serious significance, as it can be a feature of congenital and acquired immune deficiency syndromes, including the acquired immune deficiency syndrome (AIDS) resulting from HIV infection.

Conclusions

An increase or decrease of a specific type of leucocyte may have an obvious cause when clinical features are considered or the blood film may offer diagnostic clues. In other patients a bone marrow examination or additional tests are needed.

Test Case 7.1

A 36-year-old Somalian asylum seeker recently arrived in the UK, has a health assessment, which includes blood tests and a chest radiograph. His FBC shows: WBC 3.7×10^9/l, neutrophil count 1.2×10^9/l, lymphocyte count 1.2×10^9/l, eosinophil count 1.3×10^9/l, and platelet count 196×10^9/l. Hb and red cell indices (normal ranges in brackets) are:

RBC 3.71×10^{12}/l (4.32–5.66)
Hb 80 g/l (133–167)
Hct 0.26 l/l (0.39–0.50)
MCV 70 fl (82–98)
MCH 21.5 pg (27.3–32.6)
MCHC 310 g/l (316–349)

Questions

1. What is the likely cause of the anaemia?
2. Is there any other abnormality in the blood count that suggests an underlying cause?
3. How do you interpret the neutrophil count?

You may need to look up normal ranges for white cell counts. Write down your answers before checking the correct answer (page 405) and re-reading any relevant part of the chapter.

Test Case 7.2

A 25-year-old woman has recently been prescribed carbimazole for thyrotoxicosis. She is also taking an oral contraceptive. She presents to her GP with pharyngitis and a high fever. She looks very unwell so he does a blood count. This shows a WBC of $2.5 \times 10^9/l$ and a neutrophil count of $0.1 \times 10^9/l$. The Hb and platelet count are normal. The blood film shows marked toxic granulation. No immature cells are present.

Questions

1. What is the most likely diagnosis?
2. What action should be taken?

Write down your answers before checking the correct answer (page 406) and re-reading any relevant part of the chapter.

8

Blood Cancer Pathology: Lymphoma and Acute Leukaemia

Donald Macdonald

What Do You Need To Know?

☞ Diagnosis of haematolymphoid neoplasms (blood cancers) requires morphology, immunophenotype and genetic studies combined in an integrated assessment

☞ Classification is based on the malignant cell: lineage (myeloid or lymphoid), the stage of maturation (precursor or mature cell) and often the causative mutation

☞ Blood cancers are due to acquired somatic DNA aberrations (mutations and chromosomal translocations). The specific cancer type is determined by the nature of the DNA change(s) and the haematolymphoid cell type affected

☞ The main clinical and diagnostic features of Hodgkin and non-Hodgkin lymphomas, plus acute myeloid and lymphoid leukaemias

☞ Management of blood cancers requires both supportive care and cancer-directed treatment

☞ Emergency scenarios in blood cancers: sepsis, haemorrhage, thrombosis, biochemical disturbance. Their management and the importance of local neutropenic sepsis protocols

The Nature of Blood Cancers

The WHO classification of haematolymphoid tumours sets the internationally accepted criteria for the diagnosis of haematolymphoid neoplasms, the blood cancers. How the common blood cancers fit within the WHO classification is detailed as follows. The major groups are: acute leukaemia of myeloid or lymphoid lineage (AML or ALL), chronic leukaemia of myeloid or lymphoid lineage (CML or CLL), lymphoma, both Hodgkin and non-Hodgkin lymphomas (HL and NHL), plasma cell myeloma (multiple myeloma), myeloproliferative neoplasms (MPN) and myelodysplastic syndromes (MDS).

The first section of this chapter introduces the basic pathology of all blood cancer types and the importance of morphology, immunophenotyping and genetic studies in haematology diagnostics. The final section of the chapter deals with clinical aspects of lymphoma, CLL and acute leukaemias. Subsequent chapters deal with MPN (Chapter 9) and multiple myeloma (Chapter 10).

The distinction between lymphoma and leukaemia can cause confusion. In historical descriptions of blood cancers, it was recognised that, with some conditions, the malignant cell population involved mainly blood and bone marrow (BM), and this was designated as leukaemia (meaning 'white blood'). In conditions where the malignant cells involved lymph nodes and/or tissue, the term lymphoma was used. It is now appreciated that there is a degree of overlap in many conditions, and although the terms leukaemia and lymphoma both remain in use, it is better to understand the disorders based on the biology of the malignant cells rather than just their anatomical distribution.

Blood cancer diagnosis and classification is complex. Familiarity with the principles of the WHO classification system makes it easier to understand the link between molecular pathogenesis and clinical behaviour. The starting point is to appreciate that the goals of cancer diagnostic pathology are to identify the cell of origin (COO) of the malignancy, define the acquired somatic cell DNA mutation(s) responsible for transformation and set out diagnostic criteria for the condition. For example, a hepatocyte which has undergone malignant transformation and clonal expansion is the COO of hepatocellular cancer. The complexity of blood cancers simply reflects the complexity of normal lympho-haematopoiesis. A common

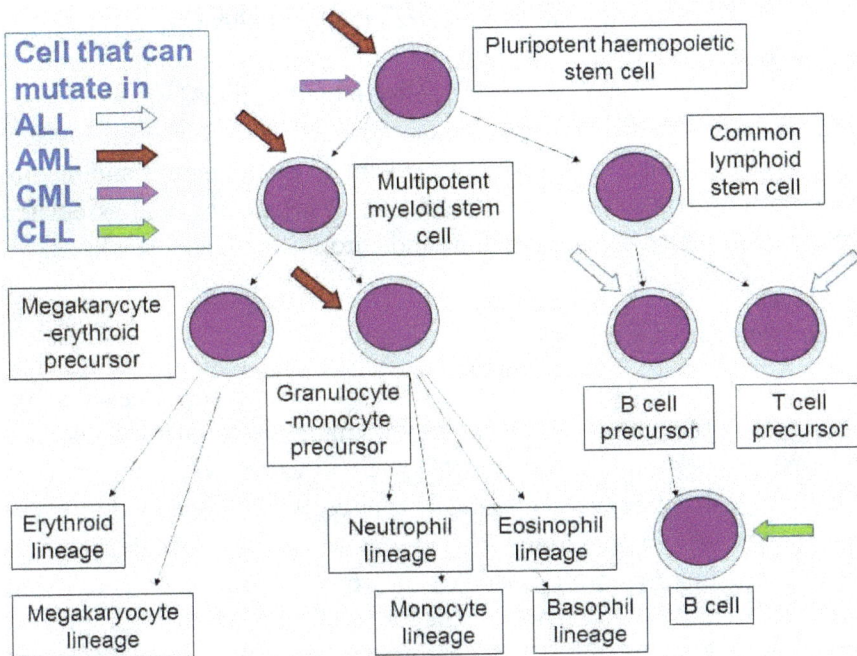

Fig. 8.1. The sites in the stem cell hierarchy where mutations can occur that give rise to acute myeloid leukaemia (AML), acute lymphoblastic leukaemia (ALL), chronic lymphocytic leukaemia (CLL) or chronic myeloid leukaemia (CML).

haematopoietic stem cell commits to becoming a myeloid or lymphoid stem cell and then undergoes lineage-specific differentiation to replenish the various mature blood cell types. Malignant transformation may occur at different stages in these processes; consequently, the COO of a blood cancer subtype is a lympho-haematopoietic precursor cell (Fig. 8.1).

Although malignant transformation causes clonal expansion of neoplastic cells either through increased proliferation and/or impaired apoptosis, blood-cancer-linked DNA aberrations can also affect the process of cellular differentiation. In conditions where the malignant transformation not only causes excess cell proliferation but also impairs cell differentiation, the malignant cells are arrested with an immature phenotype, i.e. blasts. In contrast, in other conditions where DNA aberrations arise in a precursor cell and cause excess cell proliferation but have no impact on cellular differentiation, the accumulating malignant cell population may differentiate to a mature blood cell phenotype. The WHO classification system aims to link the malignant cells to their normal equivalent cell type, such as plasma cells, in the disorder designated myeloma. In this classification, malignant cells are defined by: cell lineage, stage of maturation (precursor blast cells in acute leukaemias and mature blood cells in MPN and mature B- and T-cell neoplasms) and associated genetic aberrations (DNA mutations and chromosomal abnormalities).

Diagnosing Blood Cancers

Morphology alone cannot precisely define tumour types. Classification relies on a combination of morphology, immunophenotype and genetics (cytogenetics and molecular genetics). In practice, such expertise is brought together in regional diagnostic centres, where specialist laboratories analyse the biopsy sample and contribute their findings to an integrated pathology report. Based on this report, a diagnostic conclusion is reached. The WHO diagnostic categories of some of the major blood cancers are set out in Table 8.1. Many more subtypes are defined, but such detailed knowledge is beyond the requirements of a core curriculum.

Table 8.1. A list of the major WHO classified haematolymphoid neoplasms.

Lymphoid neoplasms	
Precursor B-cell neoplasms	**Precursor T-cell neoplasms**
(1) B-acute lymphoblastic leukaemia (ALL)	(1) T-acute lymphoblastic leukaemia (T-ALL)
Mature B-cell neoplasms	**Mature T- & NK/T-cell neoplasms**
(1) B-NHL	(1) T-NHL & NK/T-cell
• Burkitt lymphoma (BL)	• Peripheral T-cell lymphoma *NOS (PTCL)
• Diffuse large B-cell lymphoma (DLBCL)	• Anaplastic large cell lymphoma (ALCL)
• Primary DLBCL of CNS (PCNSL)	• Adult T-cell leukaemia/lymphoma (ATLL)
• Mantle cell lymphoma (MCL)	
• Follicular lymphoma (FL)	• Enteropathy-associated T-cell lymphoma (EATL)
• Chronic lymphocytic leukaemia/ small lymphocytic lymphoma (CLL/ SLL)	
• Marginal zone lymphoma (MZL)	• Mycosis fungoides/Sézary syndrome (MF/SS)

Table 8.1.   (*Continued*)

• Extranodal MZL of mucosal lymphoid tissue (MALT lymphoma) • Lymphoplasmacytic lymphoma/ Waldenström macroglobulinaemia (LPL/WM) • Hairy cell leukaemia (HCL)	• Nasal NK/T-cell lymphoma • Hepatosplenic T-cell lymphoma

(2) Plasma cell myeloma
(3) Hodgkin lymphoma
   • Classical Hodgkin lymphoma (cHL)
   • Nodular lymphocyte predominant
   • Hodgkin lymphoma (NLPHL)

Myeloid neoplasm

Precursor myeloid neoplasms

(1) Acute myeloid leukaemia (AML) including acute promyelocytic leukaemia (APML)

Myeloproliferative neoplasms

(1) Myeloproliferative neoplasms (MPN)
   • Chronic myeloid leukaemia *BCR::ABL1* positive (CML)
   • Polycythaemia vera (PV)
   • Primary myelofibrosis (PMF)
   • Essential thrombocythaemia (ET)
(2) Myelodysplastic syndromes (MDS)
   • MDS with defining genetic abnormality
   • MDS morphologically defined (low or increased blasts)
(3) MDS/MPN overlap
   • Chronic myelomonocytic leukaemia (CMML)

---

*NOS, not otherwise specified.
Note: Many more subtypes are recognised. In NHL the WHO defined subtype generally predicts clinical course. For example: Highly aggressive (ALL & BL), aggressive (DLBCL & MCL), indolent (FL, CLL, MZL). See page 166.

Morphology

The detailed morphology of specific conditions is described in the relevant section; however, an appreciation of the diagnostic approach taken and the importance of the correct type of biopsy is useful. Biopsies/

samples are taken from involved tissue, commonly the BM, peripheral blood or lymph nodes. Of note, 40% of lymphomas are extranodal, and such cases require a biopsy of the affected site, e.g. skin (often T-cell tumours); central nervous system (CNS), including brain, eye and cerebrospinal fluid (CSF) (primary CNS lymphomas); gastrointestinal (GI) tract, including gastric extranodal marginal zone lymphoma (MZL) (also known as mucosa-associated or MALT lymphoma) or small bowel lymphomas. Indeed, any tissue may be involved in lymphoma.

Morphologists describe a tumour based on both the cytological features of individual cells and on the overall architecture of the tumour and its distribution within the involved tissue. When investigating leukaemia, both a BM aspirate and a trephine biopsy may be required. An aspirate can provide cytological details, such as whether the cells are primitive blast-like cells, mature cells or a mixture and how they differ from their normal counterparts. The trephine core biopsy provides fewer cytological details but reveals details of architecture and features, such as the distribution of malignant cells within the marrow, e.g. the paratrabecular distribution of follicular lymphoma cells or clustering of malignant plasma cells. It may also reveal reactive fibrosis and/or invasion by metastatic non-haematopoietic cancers, such as breast or prostate tumours.

For lymphoma diagnosis, it is essential to consider the tumour architecture. The morphological descriptions will include cytological terms such as large, small or cleaved cells, but key information often relates to the distribution pattern of malignant cells within the node, e.g. diffuse, follicular or confined to the marginal zone. The correct biopsy type for a suspected lymphoma diagnosis must retain the tumour architecture (a wide-bore core or a surgical lymph node excision). Fine needle aspiration (FNA) of lymph nodes is inadequate and should be reserved for detecting non-lymphoid material, such as mycobacteria or metastatic carcinoma involving nodes.

Immunophenotyping in blood cancers

In many tumour types, immunophenotype is needed to reliably define lineage and stage of maturation, e.g. distinguishing between B- and T-lineage disorders. The immunophenotype of a malignant cell generally

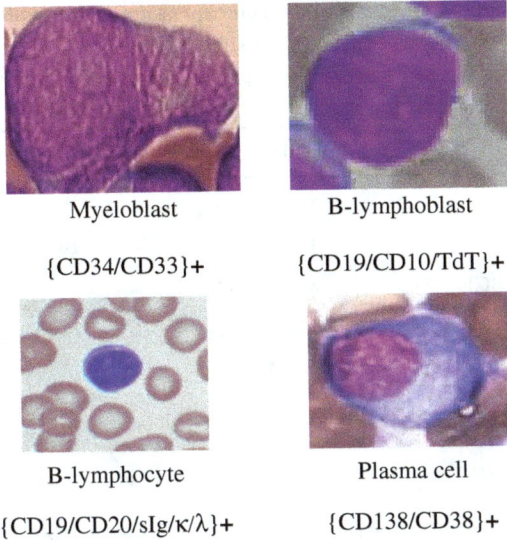

Myeloblast	B-lymphoblast
{CD34/CD33}+	{CD19/CD10/TdT}+
B-lymphocyte	Plasma cell
{CD19/CD20/sIg/κ/λ}+	{CD138/CD38}+

Fig. 8.2. Typical antigen expression profile of (normal or neoplastic) selected lympho-haematopoietic cell types. TdT terminal deoxynucleotidyl transferase, sIg cell surface immunoglobulin, κ/λ kappa or lambda Ig light chains.

remains fairly faithful to that of its normal counterpart. Immunophenotyping makes use of combinations of labelled monoclonal antibodies (a panel) to determine antigen expression on the malignant cells and thereby define the lineage, stage of maturation and any aberrant gain or loss of antigen expression (Fig. 8.2).

The expression of typical B-lymphoid markers, CD19 and CD20, helps to confirm the lineage of a B-cell neoplasm. Similarly, neoplastic cells that express CD34 are characteristic of leukaemic blasts, as CD34 is an antigen that is expressed in haematopoietic stem cells but subsequently downregulated at later stages of differentiation. In B-lymphoid development, the protein terminal deoxynucleotidyl transferase (TdT) is expressed only in precursor cells and cell surface immunoglobulin (sIg) only at later stages of maturation; this can help to distinguish between precursor and mature B-cell neoplasms. Precursor B-ALL cells are TdT+/sIg-, whereas in a mature B-cell lymphoproliferative disorder cells are usually TdT-/sIg+ (Fig. 8.2 and Table 8.2).

Table 8.2. Pattern of antigen expression seen in lymph-oproliferative neoplasms. For subtypes (e.g. CLL, FL, etc.) see Table 8.1. Ki67 % is the percentage of cells preparing to divide and is a marker of cell proliferation.

	TdT	CD20	CD10	CD5	Other
CLL	–	+		+	Weak sIg
FL	–	+	+	–	BCL2
DLBCL	–	+	+/–	–	
MCL	–	+	–	+	Cyclin D1
BL	–	+	+		Ki67>95%
B-ALL	+	+/–	+	–	

While the immune profile is generally close to that of normal equivalent cells, certain antigens may differ; this is called aberrant gain or loss of expression. The antigen CD7 is present on normal mature T lymphocytes but is often lost from expression in mature T-cell neoplasms. In CLL, the peripheral blood circulating leukaemic B lymphocytes aberrantly express CD5 (not expressed on circulating normal mature B lymphocytes).

Two techniques are used for immunophenotyping: flow cytometry and immunohistochemistry. In flow cytometry, monoclonal antibodies (MoAb) are tagged to different fluorophores, each emitting light of a specific wavelength. By careful selection of different MoAb/fluorophore combinations, it is possible to simultaneously determine the expression of three or more antigens on a single cell. Cells are suspended in a liquid medium, incubated with a panel of monoclonal antibodies and then washed to leave only the bound antibody. Labelled cells are passed as a single cell suspension through a chamber and exposed to a laser light beam. For each cell, five parameters can be determined: size (forward scatter of the light beam), granularity (side scatter) and antigen expression profiles (different light wavelengths emitted). Thousands of cells can be studied, and through computer analysis of the results, it is possible to gate or focus on a single cell type, e.g. the large cells typical of blasts (Fig. 8.3). The main limitation of flow cytometry in diagnostics is the requirement for a liquid cell suspension, thereby losing any insight into tumour architecture.

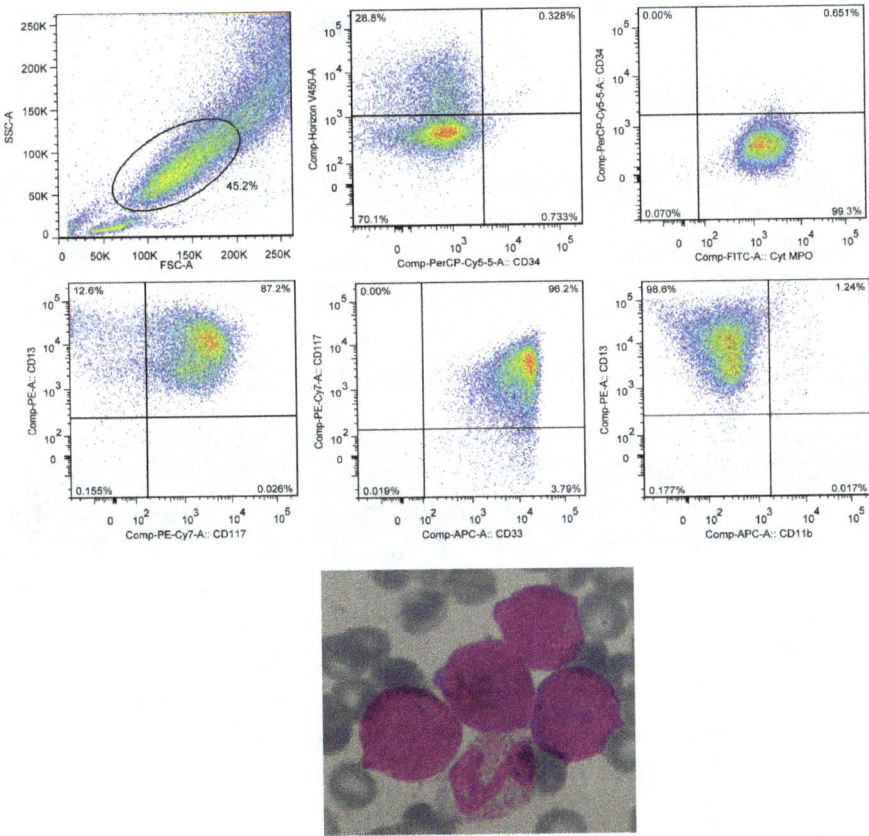

CD34- HLADR- MPO++ CD33+ CD13+CD11b-CD117+

Fig. 8.3. Flow cytometry in a case of acute promyelocytic leukaemia. Neoplastic promyelocytes 45.2% are identified by forward (fsc) and side scatter (ssc) (box upper left) Antigen expression is analysed on the gated promyelocytes using a panel of fluorescently labelled monoclonal antibodies. The threshold for antigen expression by cells is delineated, on the X-axis by the vertical line (to the right is positive) and on the y-axis by the horizontal line (above is positive) Image courtesy of Dr E Nadal and Dr Aris Chaidos. Imperial College London.

For solid tissue specimens obtained by whole node excision, immunohistochemistry can be performed. The biopsy specimen is fixed, embedded in paraffin wax and cut into slices using a microtome. The sections are then mounted on slides and incubated first with a MoAb against a specific antigen (primary antibody) and then with a secondary antibody attached to an enzymatic tag. Any bound primary antibody causes a reaction that allows visual detection. Although this technique can study only a single antigen per reaction, it retains tissue morphology. For example, if antigen-expressing malignant cells are confined to only one anatomical location, this may be informative, e.g. the marginal zone of a lymphoid follicle in MZLs. Abnormal expression of BCL2 protein in germinal centre B lymphocytes is a recognised finding in follicular lymphoma (Fig. 8.10).

Cytogenetics and Molecular Genetics in Blood Cancers

Blood cancers arise because of acquired somatic genetic changes in the lympho-haematopoietic precursors.

Before focusing on acquired mutations, one should note that, in a small proportion of cases, there is also a hereditary (germline) component. Some examples of inherited diseases with a predisposition to develop leukaemia or lymphoma include Down syndrome (ALL and acute megakaryoblastic leukaemia), Fanconi anaemia and dyskeratosis congenita (MDS and AML) and ataxia telangiectasia and Wiskott–Aldrich syndrome (NHL). In general, affected individuals carry a germline mutation in either a caretaker (DNA repair and maintenance of genetic integrity) or gatekeeper (regulation of cell cycle division) gene, which facilitates the early acquisition of transforming somatic mutation(s). Regarding familial links, recent whole genome studies in CLL families have identified candidate predisposition genes.

Somatic DNA mutations are well characterised. The acquisition of a new mutation (or chromosomal change) which provides a proliferative or survival advantage (driver mutation) results in clonal expansion; the progeny all carry the identical mutation. The new clone is then at risk of acquiring further mutations, repeating the process and emerging as subclones. When sufficient pathogenic mutations accumulate, a blood cancer arises, although the specific type is determined by the involved cell type (e.g. myeloid or lymphoid) and the function of the mutated gene(s) (e.g. tyrosine kinase, TK, or apoptosis regulation). This model of clonal evolution can be seen in the non-malignant clinical entities of monoclonal gammopathy of undetermined significance (MGUS) (see Chapter 10) and monoclonal B-cell lymphocytosis (MBL), both occurring in the elderly and carrying an annual risk of evolving to myeloma (in the case of MGUS) or CLL (in the case of MBL).

In the pathogenesis of blood cancers, a variety of mutations affecting different gene families are recognised. These include phenomena such as loss-of-function mutations affecting tumour suppressor and pro-apoptosis genes, gain-of-function mutations affecting TK genes causing constitutive activation and finally disruption of nuclear transcription factor genes. While most aberrations (DNA mutations and chromosomal disruptions) ultimately alter the amino acid sequence of the involved protein, the immunoglobulin gene translocations found in mature B-lymphoproliferative neoplasms result in overexpression of a normal (unmutated) proto-oncogene by changing the gene promoter.

Both cytogenetic and molecular genetic studies are helpful in diagnosing blood cancers. In comparison to non-haematological cancers, chromosomal aberrations are common, both structural (translocations, inversions or deletions) and numerical (aneuploidy). Cytogenetic studies, such as karyotyping, can detect any aneuploidy or overt translocation, but this is technically demanding and requires mitotically active metaphase cells. If in a particular case a specific chromosomal aberration is suspected, then a focused approach of fluorescence *in situ* hybridisation (FISH) may be simpler. DNA sequence-specific probes are fluorescently labelled and hybridised to cells. FISH can be used to confirm the presence of a predicted chromosomal aberration in both metaphase and interphase (mitotically inactive) cells. Interphase FISH is useful to study indolent, slowly dividing tumour types (Fig. 8.4).

The detection of DNA mutation(s) requires molecular biology techniques. Common investigations include reverse transcription polymerase chain reaction (RT-PCR) to detect and quantify novel fusion mRNAs, such as *BCR::ABL1* in CML, and Sanger DNA sequencing to confirm suspected DNA point mutations, such as *JAK2* V617F in polycythaemia vera (PV) or the *TP53* mutation. Increasingly, next-generation sequencing (NGS) — massive parallel DNA analysis of a panel of genes frequently mutated in acute leukaemia — is performed at diagnosis. In the future, this approach will offer the prospect of personalised therapy guided by the mutation profile of an individual.

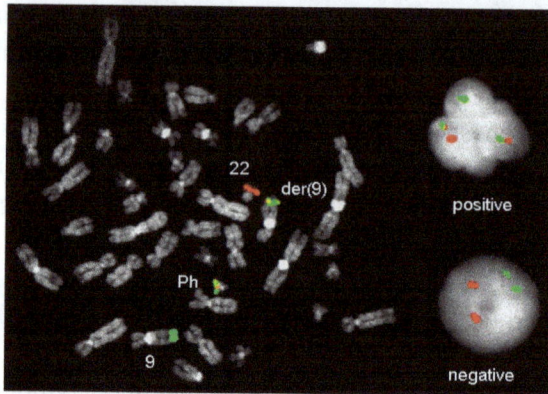

Fig. 8.4. Fluorescence *in situ* hybridisation (FISH) analysis of metaphase and interphase bone marrow cells from a patient with chronic myeloid leukaemia to demonstrate the t(9;22) *BCR::ABL1* fusion, the Philadelphia chromosome. Probes spanning the *BCR* locus (red) and the *ABL1* locus (green) are hybridised. The unrearranged chromosomes display a green (Ch 9), or red (Ch 22) signal. The translocated chromosomes; Philadelphia der(22) and der(9) display fusion signals (red-yellow-green).

Genetics of myeloid malignancies

Normal myeloid development requires both cellular proliferation and differentiation; these processes are under genetic control and can be disturbed by acquired genetic aberrations. Chromosomal aneuploidy (hyperdiploidy, hypodiploidy and monosomy) is common in acute leukaemia and impacts greatly on prognosis. The mode of action is complex and, in contrast to structural abnormalities, poorly understood.

Structural chromosomal changes are common. In myeloid neoplasms, chromosomal aberrations generally create a novel oncogenic fusion gene. The chromosomal breakpoints occur within an exon or intron of the two involved genes. The derivative chromosome created by the exchange of material has a new genomic structure with 5' exons from one gene lying upstream of 3' exons from the translocation partner. This new structure is transcribed and spliced into a fusion mRNA, which is then translated into a novel oncogenic fusion protein (Fig. 8.5). Note that a different chromosomal anatomy, further described in the following sections, is

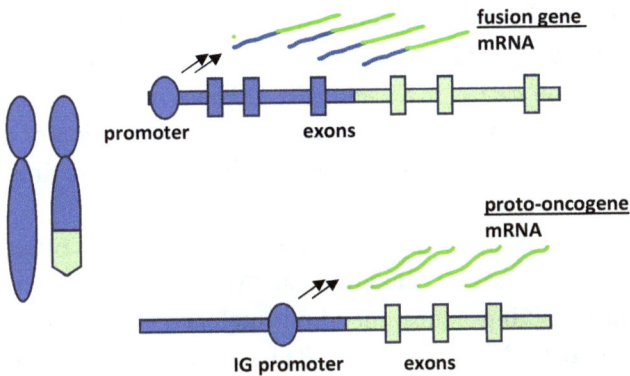

Fig. 8.5. Blood cancer associated translocations generate either, fusion genes or deregulated proto-oncogenes. Fusion genes occur in acute Leukaemia (AML, ALL) and CML, in which chromosome breakpoint occurs within two partner genes. On the derivative chromosome a novel fusion mRNA is transcribed. Deregulated proto-oncogenes occur in mature B-cell lymphoproliferative disorders (B-NHL). Breakpoints involve immunoglobulin loci (IGHeavy chain, IGkappa or IGlambda) the translocation partner is a normal proto-oncogene. The IG promoter drives increased expression of the normal (unmutated) proto-oncogene.

seen in translocations associated with mature B-cell lymphoproliferative disorders.

In addition to chromosomal aberrations, DNA point mutations and small deletions are also seen in myeloid disorders. Examples include *JAK*2 V617F in PV and *FLT3* internal tandem duplications in AML.

Precursor myeloid neoplasms and myeloproliferative neoplasms: Genetic differences

Acute myeloid leukaemia is characterised by a short natural history, with death from infection or haemorrhage, often within weeks of diagnosis if appropriate treatment is not given. The BM becomes entirely populated by immature precursor cells (myeloblasts) that proliferate but fail to differentiate. In contrast, MPN, including CML, are chronic disorders compatible with survival for many years. In these disorders, although proliferation is abnormal, differentiation is relatively unaffected, leading to an excess of mature cells that may retain normal function and protect against infection.

At the molecular level, chronic myeloproliferative disorders are often associated with activating mutations of cell surface receptor or cytoplasmic TK genes, e.g. *FLT3*, *JAK2* and *ABL1*. These mutations constitutively drive cellular proliferation but are not key in the regulation of differentiation. This gives rise to excessive clonal proliferation but no impairment of differentiation, which is an MPN disease phenotype.

In acute myeloid leukaemia, TK gene mutations are often accompanied by a second class of mutation, an AML-associated chromosomal translocation involving genes encoding nuclear DNA-binding transcription factors, e.g. *RUNX1* and *RARA*. This combination of activation of a TK gene (a class 1 mutation) driving proliferation and a DNA transcription factor mutation blocking maturation (a class 2 mutation) gives rise to excessive clonal proliferation with the cells blocked and unable to differentiate, which is an AML disease phenotype.

Genetics of lymphoid malignancies

A glance at the WHO classification (see Table 8.1) reveals that lymphoid neoplasms have many more subtypes than myeloid, this reflects the greater complexity of normal lymphoid development, an essential feature of our adaptive immune system. Normal B cells arise in the BM as precursor cells (B lymphoblasts) and then circulate into lymph nodes, where they enter germinal centres (GCs). In the GC, normal B cells undergo rapid cell proliferation, selection by antigen response and elimination by apoptosis of unresponsive or self-reacting B cells. Mature B cells may be classified as pre- or post-GC cells. The post-GC B lymphocytes emerge and may circulate as memory cells or mature into antibody-secreting plasma cells in the BM or on mucosal surfaces (Fig. 8.6). This complex development pathway explains the variety of lymphoid neoplasms. Similar processes occur during T-cell maturation in the thymus.

Immune cells (T and B lymphocytes) exhibit partial genomic instability. In normal development, this is seen as DNA cutting, excision and recombination of the immunoglobulin (*IG*) and T-cell receptor complex genes. In B lymphocytes, DNA recombination occurs at two developmental stages. In the genetic loci of the immunoglobulin heavy chain (*IGH*, chromosome 14q32) gene and in the kappa (*IGK*, chromosome 2p12) and

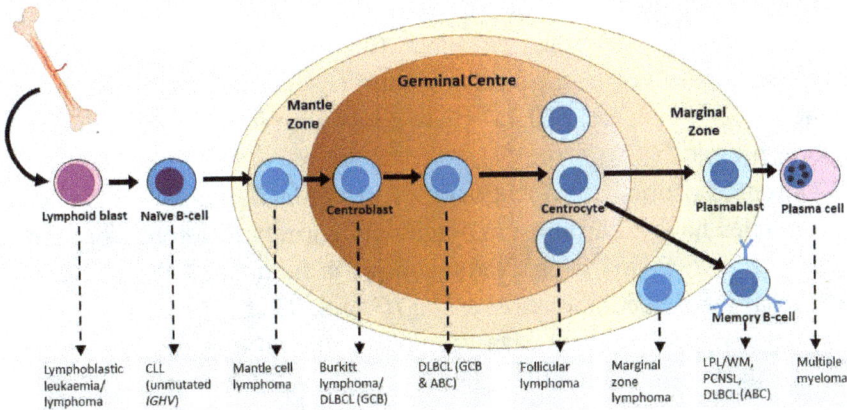

Fig. 8.6. The course of normal B-cell development. Mature B-cells leave the bone marrow and enter the circulation, eventually entering lymph nodes via high endothelial venules. Here, they become activated by exposure to antigens, and proliferate inside the GCs of lymphoid follicles. Activated B cells then undergo further affinity maturation through somatic hypermutation of the immunoglobulin heavy chain variable region (*IGHV*), Some of these activated B cells differentiate into memory B cells, or into antibody-producing plasma cells. The developmental stage at which different lymphoproliferative neoplasms arise is indicated by the dotted arrows. Using gene expression profiling, cases of B-NHL subtype DLBCL can be divided into those showing a profile similar to normal germinal centre B-cells (GCB) or to activated B-cells (ABC). Image courtesy of Dr Edward Bataillard, Imperial College London.

lambda (*IGL*, chromosome 22q11) light chain genes, variable, diversity and joining gene segments are recombined, and if successful, then the heavy and light chains produced by the cell are assembled into a complete immunoglobulin molecule. A second DNA recombination event occurs during class switching when the primary immune response of IgM antibody production switches to IgG, IgA, IgD or IgE production. T lymphocytes undergo a similar process at the T-cell receptor genes (*TRA, TRB, TRG, TRD*) to produce α/β and less commonly γ/δ T lymphocytes, but they do not undergo a second recombination event equivalent to class switching. Further partial genomic instability during germinal centre lymphoid development occurs with somatic DNA hypermutation of the *IG* gene sequences encoding the antibody variable region, which refines antibody specificity. In lymphoproliferative neoplasms, sequencing of the variable gene can determine whether the cell is pre-germinal centre (*IGHV* unmutated) or post-germinal centre (*IGHV* mutated), which is of prognostic significance in CLL, where cases with *IGHV* unmutated have a poorer prognosis.

The chromosomal translocations seen in mature B-lymphoproliferative malignancies have a chromosomal anatomy entirely different from those that give rise to fusion genes. Pathogenesis is fundamentally an error in the normal DNA recombination at the *IG* loci. There is reciprocal chromosomal material exchanged between one of the *IG* loci, most frequently *IGH* at 14q32, less frequently either *IGK* at 2p12 or *IGL* at 22q11, and a range of partner loci, which leads to the translocation of a proto-oncogene into the position normally occupied by a successfully rearranged *IG* gene. The translocated proto-oncogene now lies in proximity to the *IG* promoter sequence, which drives high levels of gene expression in mature B cells — an oncogenic event (Fig. 8.5).

The *IG* gene translocation partner determines which cellular process is disrupted, e.g. Cyclin D1 *(CCND1)* cell cycle control, *BCL2* apoptosis (Fig. 8.10) and *MYC* multiple pathways, including proliferation and apoptosis. Finally, the stage of maturation of the affected B cell also determines the disease phenotype, e.g. plasma cells/myeloma or GC lymphocytes/ NHL.

In addition to chromosomal translocations, NGS sequencing has identified a variety of DNA mutations in mature B-lymphoproliferative disorders. Some are disease specific, such as *BRAF* V600E in hairy cell leukaemia and *MYD88* L265P in Waldenström macroglobulinaemia. Other mutations are seen at increased frequency and impact prognosis in certain conditions, e.g. *TP53* in CLL and *NOTCH1* and *SF3B1* mutations in other conditions (Table 8.3).

Clinicopathological Features and Management of Blood Cancers

Having reviewed blood cancer pathology and molecular genetics, the following sections deal with the clinical aspects of lymphoma and acute leukaemia. It should be emphasised that, as a junior doctor, one is not expected to know the details of blood cancer treatment protocols.

Table 8.3. Examples of chromosomal translocations and DNA mutations that are present in various mature B-cell lymphoproliferative disorders. For lymphoma subtypes DLBCL, LPL/WM, CLL see Table 8.1.

Translocation/Genes	Lymphoma
t(8;14) *IGH::MYC*	Burkitt lymphoma
t(14;18) *IGH::BCL2*	Follicular lymphoma (80%) DLBCL (34%)
t(3;14) *IGH::BCL6*	DLBCL (62%)
t(11;14) *IGH::CCND1*	Mantle cell lymphoma
Mutations	
MYD88 L265P	LPL/WM
TP53	CLL (early stage 5%, late stage 30%)

However, it is highly possible that, in a general medical setting, one may encounter either a patient with a suspected blood cancer diagnosis or a haematology patient admitted as a medical emergency. Therefore, it is important to be aware of the potentially serious clinical scenarios and the need to take advice and act quickly in these situations. Emergency and supportive care protocols are vital when dealing with blood cancers.

Haematology patients are at risk of morbidity and mortality from the complications of infection, haemorrhage, thrombosis, biochemical disturbance and renal and neurological sequelae. These may present suddenly and progress rapidly; it is only through good supportive care that patients can have any prospect of surviving the disease and the challenges of cancer-directed treatments. Supportive care includes blood product support and any specialist requirements, such as irradiated products. Infection is a major cause of morbidity and mortality in haemato-oncology patients; management involves both prevention and treatment. In indolent lymphoid disorders, prevention is based on vaccination schedules and drug prophylaxis against herpes zoster reactivation or *Pneumocystis jirovecii* infection. Relevant viral serology, hepatitis B, hepatitis C, HIV, human T-cell lymphotropic virus 1 (HTLV-1), Epstein–Barr virus (EBV) and cytomegalovirus (CMV) must be determined, and where results are of concern, they should be acted upon. In the treatment of infection, most haemato-oncology patients are, to a varying degree, immunocompromised, with the most profoundly so being neutropenic and post-transplant patients. Clinical vigilance, with early antibiotic treatment and compliance with all local infection protocols, especially for neutropenic fever, is essential.

In some scenarios, biochemical risks are a major threat — renal failure in myeloma or tumour lysis syndrome in aggressive disorders, such as acute leukaemia and Burkitt lymphoma or in CLL commencing venetoclax. Awareness of the risks, close monitoring of biochemistry results and rapid intervention are all important to avoid irreversible renal damage or death from electrolyte disturbance (Box 8.1).

Box 8.1
Tumour lysis syndrome (an oncology emergency)

Occurrence

Aggressive (high LDH) lymphoma and acute leukaemia with high-burden disease.
CLL (indolent disorder) if treated with venetoclax.

Pathogenesis

Tumour cell death releases potassium, phosphate and uric acid. Causes nephropathy, nephrocalcinosis, acute renal failure, electrolyte disturbance and death.

Diagnosis

Elevated: K, PO_4, urate. Low Ca.
Rising creatinine and urea.

Prevention and management

Aware of high-risk scenarios and typical biochemistry findings.
Hydration plus allopurinol or rasburicase (the latter contraindicated in G6PD deficiency).
Follow guidelines for management of acute hyperkalaemia and hyperphosphataemia.

Major Subtypes of Lymphoma and Chronic Lymphocytic Leukaemia

The relative frequency of the more common lymphoma subtypes, including CLL, is shown in Fig. 8.7.

Non-Hodgkin lymphoma: Incidence and aetiology

NHL constitutes 4% of all cancers. The European incidence is 19 per 100,000 per year. The neoplastic cells generally involve lymph nodes, but as normal lymphocytes circulate widely throughout tissues, lymphomas can develop in any tissue or organ, e.g. kidney, gut, adrenals, breast or skin; they also arise in immune-privileged sites, such as the eye and brain (primary CNS lymphoma) or testis. Lymphoma is seen worldwide but with geographical variations in the frequency of certain subtypes: nasal NK/T lymphomas are common in the Far East, endemic Burkitt lymphoma involving the jaw is seen in children in sub-Saharan African and adult T-cell leukaemia/lymphoma (ATLL) occurs in populations with a high frequency of HTLV-1 infection.

In most lymphoma cases, there is no obvious cause or explanation why it developed. Some inherited diseases have a predisposition to lymphoma, and there are also a set of well-recognised acquired risk factors linked to specific NHL subtypes, such as MZL involving mucosa-associated lymphoid tissue (MALT) in anatomical sites, e.g. gastric, parotid or thyroid. Alternatively, some factors are associated with an

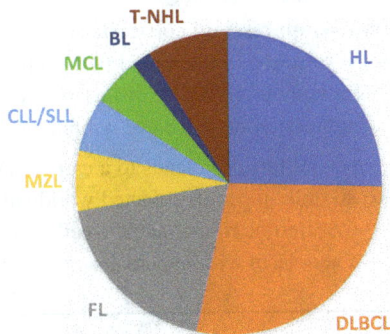

Fig. 8.7. Relative frequency of the more common lymphoma subtypes and CLL. For the definitions of abbreviations, see Table 8.1.

increased risk of various lymphoma subtypes, including both HL and NHL. Common to all risk factors is perturbation of the normal immune system: chronic antigenic stimulation, HTLV-1 retroviral infection and a loss of normal T-lymphocyte function, with the possible contribution of EBV-driven B-cell lymphocytosis (Table 8.4).

Table 8.4. Aetiological factors associated with lymphoma development. EBV, Epstein–Barr virus. HTLV-1, human T-cell lymphotropic virus 1.

Aetiology	Lymphoma notes
Inherited disorders	**Inherited diseases,** such as Wiskott–Aldrich syndrome, ataxia telangiectasia and severe combined immunodeficiency, all have an increased risk of NHL. CLL has a recognised familial association. Whole genome sequencing in affected families has identified linked genes.
Chronic antigenic stimulation	Lymphocyte proliferation is initially antigen dependent, but autonomous clones may emerge, progressing to NHL; examples include: **B-NHL:** extra-nodal marginal zone lymphoma (MZL) subtype gastric MZL (MALT) with *H. pylori* infection or parotid NHL with Sjögren syndrome. *H. pylori* eradication can result in lymphoma remission. **T-NHL:** enteropathy-associated T-cell lymphoma (EATL) in coeliac disease.
Loss of T-cell function	**EBV carrier state** may change phase, causing B-lymphocyte proliferation. Loss of T-cell function fails to eliminate proliferating B lymphocytes expressing EBV antigens. **HIV infection** is associated with an increased risk of lymphoma related to low T lymphocyte counts. **T-cell immunosuppression:** corticosteroids or ciclosporin to prevent solid organ rejection is associated with an increased risk of post-transplant lymphoproliferative disorders (PTLDs). Reducing immunosuppression may achieve lymphoma remission.
HTLV-1 retroviral infection	**HTLV-1** retroviral infection leads to a carrier state. It is estimated that there are 20 million people infected worldwide. Decades-long latency with a 1–6% lifetime risk of adult T-cell leukaemia lymphoma. An aggressive neoplasm with hypercalcaemia is a common clinical feature.

Clinical presentation and initial investigation

The most common presentation is with painless progressive lymphadenopathy, which may be localised to one nodal region or generalised, with or without splenomegaly. Lymphadenopathy may be superficial, deep-seated or both. In cases where the lymphomatous mass is deep-seated, the presentation may be delayed until there is impact on nearby tissue, either by direct infiltration, e.g. lung, liver or brain, or commonly by extrinsic compression of a viscus or vessel, e.g. bile duct, ureters, GI tract or vena cava (Fig. 8.8). Once lymphoma is suspected, a full blood count (FBC) is first checked to exclude CLL (associated with lymphadenopathy but can be diagnosed on a peripheral blood sample). At this stage, a node biopsy is required; this should be a wide-bore core biopsy or lymph node excision. A biopsy of deep-seated nodal masses, such as intra-abdominal or thoracic, may be challenging and require imaging guidance or surgical expertise.

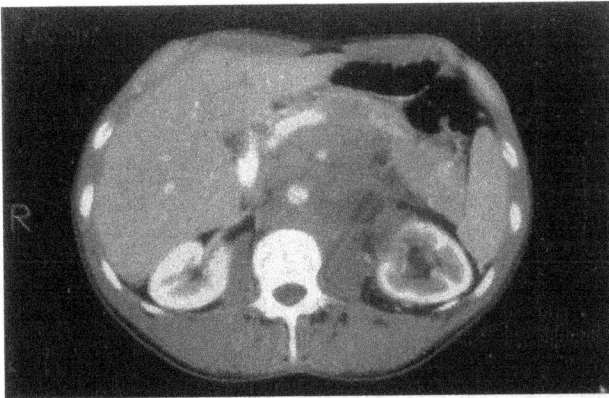

Fig. 8.8. CT scan of the abdomen after administration of oral and intravenous contrast medium. There is a mass of lymphomatous lymph nodes surrounding the aorta. Note that there is also hydronephrosis of the left kidney as a result of ureteric obstruction by the lymphoma.

Systemic symptoms of weight loss, drenching night sweats and fever may be seen with aggressive lymphoma subtypes. Pruritus may occur. Dysfunction of the normal immune system can cause infective problems, such as recurrent sino-pulmonary infection or herpes zoster reactivation. Other immune-mediated associations include autoimmune haemolytic anaemia (AIHA), cryoglobulinaemia and, in Waldenström macroglobulinaemia, an immunoglobulin (Ig)M paraprotein causing plasma hyperviscosity.

NHL diagnosis staging and baseline information

Once a tissue diagnosis is established, prior to treatment planning, it is essential to collect key baseline information. This includes: disease extent (anatomical staging), laboratory results that impact prognosis and therapy options, patient demographics, performance status and co-morbidities.

In both NHL and HL, staging is based on ^{18}F-fluorodeoxyglucose positron-emission tomography (PET) scanning or computed tomography (CT) scanning. The current approach is termed Ann Arbor staging, with stages I–IV depending on the extent of the disease, and as A or B depending on the absence or presence of specific B symptoms (fever >38°C, weight loss of more than 10% in six months or night sweats). Thus, a lymphoma would be IA if it were confined to a single lymph node region and there were no symptoms, whereas it would be stage IVB if there were involvement of lymph nodes, spleen, liver and BM with B symptoms (Fig. 8.9).

A BM biopsy is performed when required. Examination of CSF for the presence of malignant cells is indicated in some scenarios, such as neurological symptoms or signs at presentation, or in cases of NHL with aggressive histology, extra-nodal involvement and/or elevated lactate dehydrogenase (LDH) levels. The results not only impact staging, but if detected, additional CNS-directed treatment using intra-thecal or high-dose intravenous (IV) methotrexate will be required.

Baseline laboratory results for immunoglobulins, paraprotein, erythrocyte sedimentation rate (ESR) and LDH should be determined. The LDH level is raised in more aggressive lymphomas and is a useful prognostic marker. Viral screening for HIV and hepatitis B and C is required

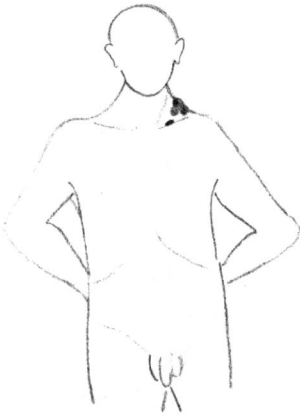

Stage I. Disease confined to a single lymph node region or lymphoid structure (e.g. spleen, thymus or and Waldeyer's ring)

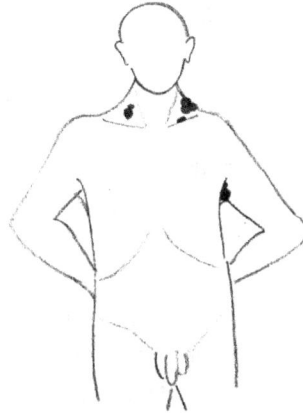

Stage II. Involvement of two or more lymphoid regions or structures, but with disease confined to one side of the diaphragm

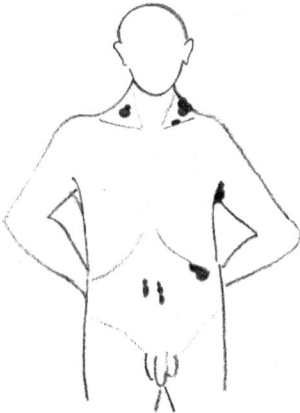

Stage III. Disease on both sides of the diaphragm but with no more than limited contiguous involvement of non-lymphoid organs

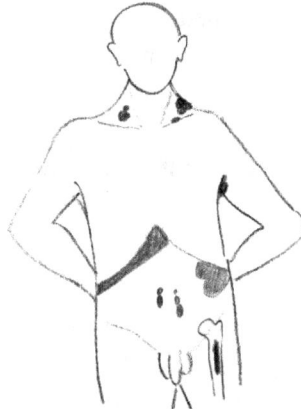

Stage IV. Involvement of nonlymphoid organs such as liver, lung or bone marrow

Stage A   No symptoms meeting the criteria for stage B disease
Stage B   Having fever, drenching night sweats or significant weight loss (e.g. loss of more than 10% of body weight in the preceding six months)
The subscript E indicates that there is limited extra-nodal disease contiguous with known nodal disease.

Fig. 8.9.   Staging of lymphoma using the Ann Arbor staging system.

in all cases and for HTLV-1 in T-cell malignancies, as results may alter treatment. Hepatitis B carriers who receive lymphoma chemotherapy need prophylaxis to prevent viral reactivation that can lead to hepatic failure. If the plan involves the use of certain drugs with toxicity profiles, then baseline cardiac assessment electrocardiogram (ECG), cardiac ECHO (anthracyclines) and pulmonary function tests (bleomycin) are required.

Age, performance status and co-morbidities will impact the lymphoma-directed treatment options; drug toxicity encountered with the most intensive regimens may not be tolerated by frailer patients. In appropriate cases, fertility preservation should be discussed; males may opt for sperm cryopreservation. The options for female patients are complex, much less secure and beyond the scope of this text.

The concept of indolent and aggressive lymphomas

The WHO-defined lymphoma entities follow very different clinical courses, with more rapid tumour growth being observed in aggressive disorders. Clinicians often use the WHO pathological diagnosis as a starting point to predict the course and to plan a treatment strategy. Lymphoma subtypes can be grouped into those predicted to behave in a highly aggressive, aggressive or indolent manner. An alternative terminology consists of high grade (aggressive and highly aggressive) or low grade (indolent). Table 8.1 provides some examples.

The predicted clinical course of an indolent lymphoma is of a slowly growing neoplasm with survival of up to 10–20 years or more. They are generally incurable by chemotherapy, and the usual strategy at diagnosis is monitoring, with treatment only started when lymphoma-related clinical problems are imminent or have arisen, e.g. obstruction or organ impairment. Indolent lymphomas typically respond to treatment and enter a period of remission but recur, requiring further lines of treatment, until they ultimately become refractory.

The predicted behaviour of an aggressive lymphoma is more rapid progression with grave clinical consequences. Unlike most indolent lymphomas, they are potentially curable, so treatment is initiated at diagnosis. The prospect of a cure is determined by subtypes and defined prognostic variables.

The final group — highly aggressive lymphomas — includes Burkitt lymphoma (BL) and the precursor lymphoid neoplasms. BL is the most rapidly proliferating of all human cancers; it requires urgent treatment with multidrug immunochemotherapy, following which high cure rates can be achieved.

Common NHL subtypes

The prognosis and treatment of different NHL subtypes vary. Several helpful prognostic scoring systems are available. Although the details of these are not required for a core curriculum, they are useful to illustrate the outlook for different disorders and highlight the main adverse factors (Table 8.5).

Diffuse large B-cell lymphoma

Diffuse large B-cell lymphoma (DLBCL) is the most common subtype of NHL, representing about 35% of cases. It occurs at all ages. Histologically, the lymph node is effaced by sheets of large B cells.

Table 8.5. Prognostic scoring systems for NHL subtypes, DLBCL, FL and CLL (Table 8.1) IPI International prognostic index, B_2M Beta 2 microglobulin, *TP53mt* mutated, ECOG PS Eastern cooperative oncology group performance status, *IGHV*unmt unmutated, OS overall survival, PFS progression free survival.

DLBCL IPI	FL IPI	CLL IPI
Adverse factors	Adverse factors	Adverse factors
• Age >60	• Age >60	• Age >65
• LDH raised	• LDH raised	• B_2M raised
• Stage III/IV	• Stage III/IV	• *TP53mt*/17p del
• ECOG PS ≥ 2	• Hb <120 g/l	• *IGHV* unmt
• >1 extra nodal	• Nodal areas >4	• Rai/Binet advanced stage
10yr OS (%)	Median PFS (mo)	5yr OS (%)
Good (0–1) 91	Low (0–1) 84	Low (0–1) 93
Low int (2) 81	Int (2) 70	Int (2–3) 79
High int (3) 65	High (≥3) 42	High (4–6) 63
Poor (4–5) 59		V high (7–10) 23

A variety of translocations and mutations underlie this heterogenous disorder. As an aggressive lymphoma, treatment with combination immunochemotherapy is started at diagnosis using regimens such as rituximab cyclophosphamide, doxorubicin (hydroxydaunorubicin), vincristine (Oncovin) and prednisolone (R-CHOP), given in six cycles. Overall, 60% of patients are cured. The International Prognostic Index (IPI) (Table 8.5) provides the prognostic details. Relapse is an ominous event, but salvage therapies with curative potential are available. Current options include high-dose chemotherapy supported by autologous stem cell rescue or CAR-T cell therapy (see Chapter 14). Novel approaches using bispecific T-cell-engaging antibodies show efficacy, but clinical trials will determine the optimal approach to relapsed disease.

DLBCL is quite a varied disease, and in some cases, malignant cells are confined to a specific anatomical site, e.g. the mediastinum in primary mediastinal B-cell lymphoma (PMBL) or the brain and/or eye in PCNSL. PCNSL lymphoma requires different forms of immunochemotherapy using agents such as methotrexate and cytarabine that cross the blood–brain barrier.

Follicular lymphoma

Follicular lymphoma is the second-most common B-cell lymphoma, representing about 25% of cases of NHL. This is an indolent (low-grade) lymphoma, which is usually in widespread stage III or IV at diagnosis. Chromosomal translocation t(14:18) results in dysregulated expression of the *BCL2* gene, which has an anti-apoptosis function (Fig. 8.10). A lymph node biopsy demonstrates small cells with clefted nuclei and a follicular growth pattern (Fig. 8.10). Immunohistochemistry is essential to making a reliable distinction from reactive follicular hyperplasia as a response to antigenic stimulation. In follicular lymphoma, BCL2 is expressed by the cells that form follicles, while in reactive hyperplasia it is not.

Occasionally, follicular lymphoma is localised (stage I) and can be cured by radiotherapy; however, for higher-stage disease, the strategy involves monitoring until treatment is required. The current standard of care is immunochemotherapy, including an anti-CD20 monoclonal

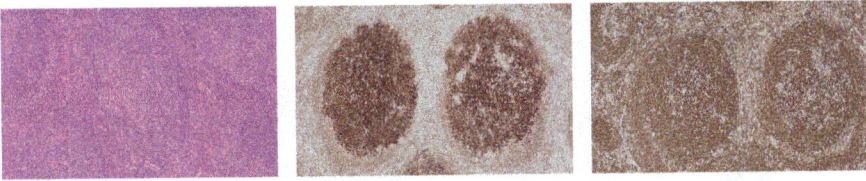

Fig. 8.10.   A lymph node involved by follicular lymphoma showing neoplastic follicles (x4 magnification). Left: Haematoxylin and Eosin (H and E). Centre: neoplastic follicles showing strong expression for CD10, which is a germinal centre marker. Right: neoplastic follicles show strong expression for BCL2 confirming a diagnosis of follicular lymphoma. Images courtesy of Dr Rashpal Flora, Imperial College NHS Trust.

antibody (rituximab or obinutuzumab) and cytotoxic agents, such as bendamustine, or combination regimens, such as CHOP or COP (with the omission of hydroxydaunorubicin). The predicted clinical course is that of an indolent lymphoma — incurable — but survival may be measured in decades. Prognostic details are provided by the FL-IPI (Table 8.5).

Burkitt lymphoma

Burkitt lymphoma is a highly aggressive lymphoma due to the chromosomal translocation dysregulating expression of the *MYC* gene. This lymphoma occurs in an endemic form in children in Africa, sporadically in developed countries and with an increased incidence in HIV carriers. Endemic BL results from an interaction between malaria and EBV, and it usually presents with a tumour of the mandible or maxilla. The EBV virus is also implicated in a proportion of cases of sporadic and HIV-related BL. The sporadic form can involve the abdominal cavity, breasts, ovaries and other sites.

On biopsy, the lymph node is obliterated by infiltrating lymphoma cells with prominent mitoses and apoptotic cells; within this infiltrate, scattered macrophages stand out, giving a 'starry sky' appearance. This distinctive histological appearance reflects the high rates of proliferation and cell death. The Ki-67 proliferation index (an immunohistochemistry marker of dividing cells) is greater than 95%. When there are circulating lymphoma cells in the peripheral blood, they have strongly basophilic, vacuolated cytoplasm, which suggests the diagnosis (see Fig. 8.11). Treatment is

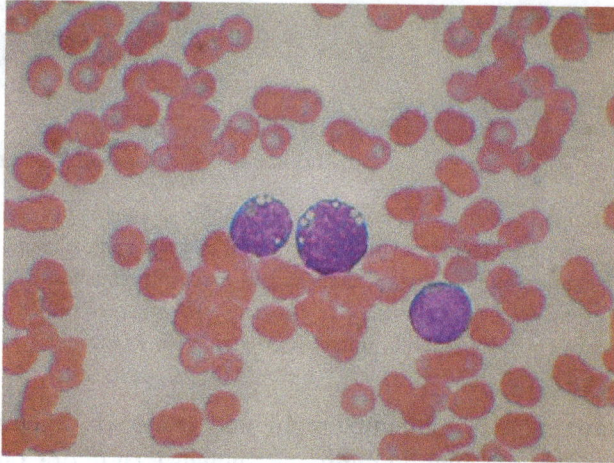

Fig. 8.11. PB film from a patient with Burkitt lymphoma (May–Grünwald–Giemsa (MGG) stain).

urgent, involving multiagent chemotherapy and CNS-directed therapy. Tumour lysis syndrome is a common complication when therapy starts. Cure rates of 90% can be achieved.

Extranodal marginal zone lymphoma and post-transplant lymphoproliferative disorders

Details regarding the morphology, prognosis and therapy of all the WHO-recognised subtypes are beyond the requirements of a core curriculum. Exceptions include the extra-nodal MZLs (previously known as MALT lymphomas). These develop in a scenario of chronic antigenic stimulation; common sites and associated immune activation are gastric (*H. pylori* infection), thyroid (Hashimoto disease) and parotid (Sjögren syndrome). They are indolent lymphomas. Eradication of *H. pylori* infection by antibiotic therapy may lead to lymphoma regression.

PTLDs are seen in patients receiving T-cell immune suppression to prevent graft rejection of heart, lung, kidney, haematopoietic stem cells, etc. The histological subtype varies but is commonly DLBCL. Management of this disorder is complex and fraught. Reduction of immune suppression may lead to lymphoma remission; however, in clinical practice, the challenge is to balance the need to preserve the transplanted organ against the risks of reducing immunosuppression or administering lymphoma-directed immunochemotherapy to already immunosuppressed patients.

T-cell lymphomas

T-cell lymphomas (10% of all lymphomas) are less common than B-cell lymphomas. They are a heterogeneous group of diseases varying in clinical course, from indolent to highly aggressive disorders. They are generally incurable but often characterised by responsive disease, which recurrently relapses until ultimately becoming refractory.

Some show a predilection for the skin, mycosis fungoides (MF) and Sézary syndrome (SS). MF often presents as limited skin plaques, which respond to topical therapy such as psoralen-sensitised light therapy (PUVA). Long-term control may be achieved through a topical approach; however, progression to systemic disease has a poor prognosis. SS is characterised by erythroderma and peripheral blood circulating malignant cells. These have a typical morphology of cerebriform nuclei with a T-lymphocyte immunophenotype.

The small bowel is involved by enteropathy-associated T-cell lymphoma, which is related to coeliac disease. This is a highly aggressive lymphoma subtype with a poor prognosis.

One distinctive NHL subtype is ATLL, associated with HTLV-1 infection. Serology for HTLV-1 should be performed when ATLL is a possibility, e.g. in patients with typical haematological features and in all patients with a T-cell lymphoma. The virus is endemic in Japan, the Caribbean, South America, Sub-Saharan Africa, Romania, Iran and other areas. ATLL is an aggressive neoplasm, so there may be systemic symptoms, and most patients with ATLL have circulating lymphoma cells, which are distinctive for their lobulated, sometimes flower-shaped, nuclei. ATLL is strongly associated with malignant hypercalcaemia. The condition is poorly responsive to combination chemotherapy treatment regimens.

Chronic lymphocytic leukaemia

Chronic lymphocytic leukaemia occurs from early middle age onwards but is predominantly a disease of the elderly. The median age at presentation is in the early 70s. It is the most common leukaemia in Western Europe and North America, with an incidence of about 4.7 per 100,000 per year and a male predominance (1.3:1). CLL is often preceded by MBL, where there is a low level of circulating B lymphocytes with a CLL immunophenotype; progression to CLL occurs in 1% of cases per annum. Small lymphocytic lymphoma (SLL) and CLL are biologically the same disease. In SLL, the clonal B lymphocytes are confined to lymph nodes with little or no blood and marrow involvement. Management is the same as that adopted for CLL.

Clinical features

In many patients with CLL, the diagnosis is an incidental FBC finding in an asymptomatic patient. With more advanced disease, there is lymphadenopathy (Fig. 8.12), splenomegaly, hepatomegaly and increased susceptibility to infection. Infections are the result of hypogammaglobulinaemia and impaired cell-mediated immunity. Herpes zoster ('shingles') is common, as are sino-pulmonary infections with *S. pneumonia* and *H. influenzae*. Other immune complications may develop, such as AIHA, immune thrombocytopenia (ITP) and pure red cell aplasia.

Haematological features

Initially, there is lymphocytosis with an otherwise normal blood count. With more advanced disease and more extensive BM infiltration, there is normocytic normochromic anaemia and thrombocytopenia.

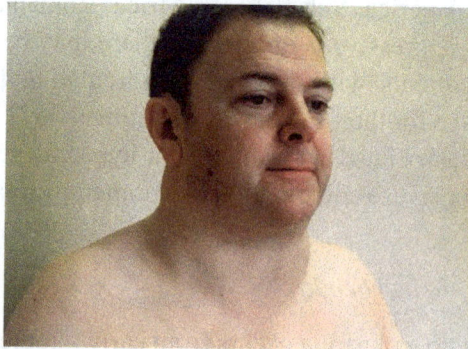

Fig. 8.12. Cervical lymphadenopathy in a patient with CLL.

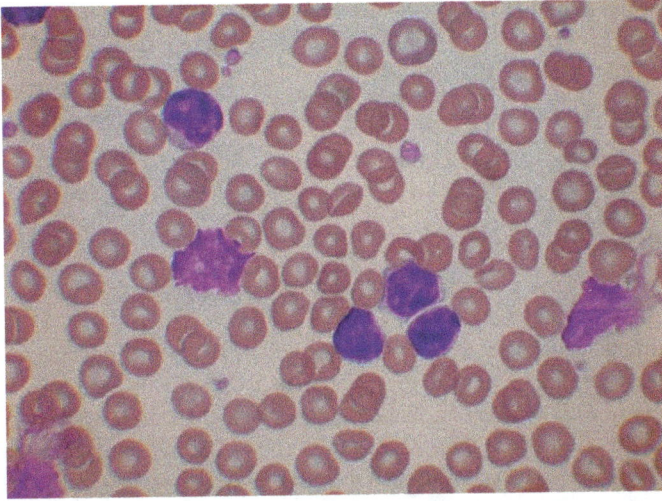

Fig. 8.13. PB film from a patient with CLL showing four small mature small lymphocytes and three smear cells (MGG stain).

The blood film shows a monotonous population of mature small lymphocytes with clumped chromatin and scanty cytoplasm (Fig. 8.13). These cells are more fragile than normal, leading to the formation of characteristic 'smear cells' when a blood film is spread. A BM aspirate is not necessary for diagnosis if the immunophenotype is typical (Fig. 8.14).

CLL behaves as an indolent lymphoma, with a median survival between 10 and 12 years; the clinical staging systems of Binet or Rai may be helpful. The most informative prognostic scoring system is CLL IPI (Table 8.4). In CLL, the poorest prognosis is associated with aberrations affecting the tumour suppressor gene *TP53*, either chromosome deletion, del(17p) or DNA mutation.

In a small number of CLL patients, transformation to a condition that resembles a large B-cell lymphoma is possible, which is known as Richter syndrome. This has a grave prognosis.

Optimal management of CLL is based on supportive care and the timing and choice of treatment. Central to supportive care is vaccination against pneumococcus, seasonal flu and severe acute respiratory syndrome-coronavirus-2 (SARS-CoV-2). Live vaccines are avoided. Bacterial

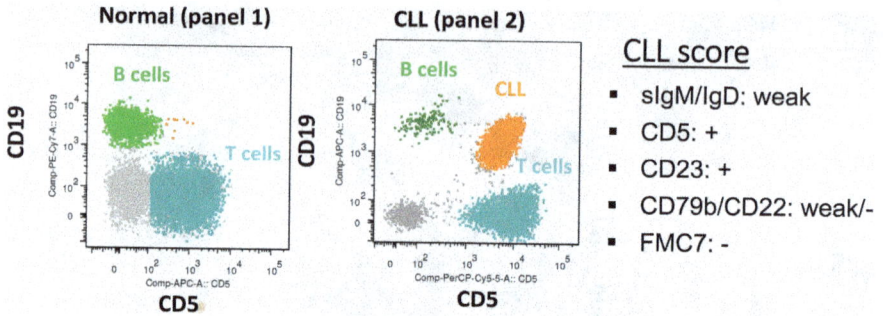

Fig. 8.14. Immunophenotyping in CLL. Two colour flow cytometry gating on peripheral blood lymphocytes. Panel 1: normal presentation of T cells (CD5+) and B cells (CD19+). Panel 2: a case of CLL showing an abnormal population of CD5+ B cells (CD19/5+) typical of CLL. The CLL score used in diagnosis shows the full antigen profile of CLL. Courtesy of Dr Aristeidis Chaidos, Imperial College.

infection needs early antibiotic therapy, and recurrent respiratory infections associated with hypogammaglobulinaemia may respond to immunoglobulin replacement therapy. Herpes zoster reactivation requires full-dose aciclovir treatment, and to prevent its reactivation, prophylaxis may be needed.

Regarding CLL directed treatment, the strategy is monitoring only unless or until therapy is required. Indications include a rapidly doubling (<6 months) lymphocyte count, progressive cytopenia due to CLL burden in the BM (anaemia, thrombocytopenia and neutropenia), critical lymphadenopathy and/or B symptoms. Autoimmune cytopenias should first be treated using immune-directed treatment, e.g. corticosteroids.

CLL-targeted therapies using either a Bruton tyrosine kinase (BTK) inhibitor (acalbrutinib or ibrutinib) or a BCL2 inhibitor (venetoclax) are now commonly used as first-line treatments, replacing traditional immunochemotherapy regimens. Venetoclax treatment must be initiated cautiously due to the risk of causing tumour lysis syndrome. These targeted agents generally achieve an excellent response but with variable duration. Recurrence requiring further lines of therapy often has a poorer or less durable response and is associated with a higher burden of *TP53*-disrupted cells.

Hodgkin lymphoma

In HL, the malignant cells are of B-cell origin. HL is divided into classical Hodgkin lymphoma (95% cHL) and nodular lymphocyte-predominant Hodgkin lymphoma (5% NLPHL). NLPHL is closer in nature to an indolent B-NHL and is managed using the same treatment strategy and regimens.

The incidence of cHL is 3 per 100,000 per year. It occurs at all ages in Western countries from adolescence onwards but earlier in developing countries. There are strong aetiological links to EBV, and there is a clear increase in EBV-related cases in patients with HIV infection. There is a bimodal age distribution, with EBV-related cases accounting for the increased incidence in older patients. cHL spreads contiguously through the normal lymphatic pathways. Presentation is usually with lymphadenopathy, although extensive mediastinal disease may present with a cough or as an oncological emergency, such as superior vena cava obstruction. Systemic symptoms are common, and in addition to the recognised B symptoms, there can be pain induced by alcohol consumption or pruritus.

cHL is unusual in that the neoplastic cells are only a minority of cells in the involved tissue, the majority being polyclonal lymphocytes, eosinophils, fibroblasts and other reactive cells. The neoplastic cells are distinctive, large mononuclear cells with large nucleoli (Hodgkin cells) or large binucleated or polylobated cells, also with large nucleoli (Reed–Sternberg cells) (Fig. 8.15). Immunohistochemistry is important in the diagnosis. Although the neoplastic cells are of B-cell origin, they often fail to express common B-cell antigens and instead express CD30 and usually CD15. cHL is subdivided into four types based on the reactive features surrounding the neoplastic cells: nodular sclerosis (NS, 40%), lymphocyte rich (LR, 15%), mixed cellularity (MC, 30%) and lymphocyte depleted (LD, 15%). The NS subtype is characterised by sclerotic reticulin bands traversing the lymph node to create a nodular appearance. This subtype accounts for most cases of cHL in young adults and explains the bimodal age distribution. The other subtypes, LR, MC and LD, differ in the number of reactive lymphocytes present in the involved node. Increased numbers are associated with a better prognosis: five-year overall survival (OS) for LR is 70%, and for LD, it is 20%.

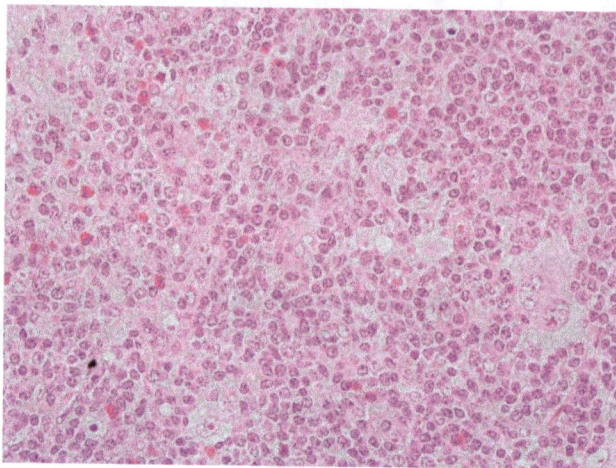

Fig. 8.15. Section of a lymph node biopsy specimen from a patient with Hodgkin lymphoma (H&E stain), showing a giant binucleated Reed–Sternberg cell (right) and several mononuclear Hodgkin cells. Note the characteristic large eosinophilic nucleoli in both the Reed–Sternberg cells and the mononuclear Hodgkin cells. The background cells are mainly lymphocytes and eosinophils.

Management of cHL

The overall cure rate of cHL is 80%, though the individual prognosis varies according to the anatomical stage of disease and the presence or absence of recognised risk factors. PET-CT scanning of the chest, abdomen and pelvis is critical to determining the stage using the Ann Arbor staging system (Fig. 8.9). A BM biopsy is not generally needed. Based on staging, patients are categorised as early (stages I–IIA) or advanced (stages IIB–IV). Other prognostic factors include: age >50 years, mediastinal involvement >0.35 of thoracic diameter, markedly raised ESR and B symptoms and >4 nodal areas in stage II. These factors can be incorporated into scoring systems to identify early favourable and early unfavourable disease. All patients receive chemotherapy between two and six cycles, depending on stage and risk factors. A regimen of doxorubicin, bleomycin, vinblastine and dacarbazine (ABVD) is commonly used. The finding of a complete metabolic response (CMR) on interim PET-CT scan after two cycles of ABVD is predictive of a good long-term outcome.

The ABVD regimen provides high cure rates and preserves fertility (which is important in the female NS subtype demographic). Of concern with ABVD is the risk of bleomycin-induced pulmonary fibrosis.

Consolidating chemotherapy with the addition of radiotherapy can be considered which is termed combined modality treatment (CMT). CMT reduces the chance of Hodgkin recurrence within the radiation field but may damage 'bystander' normal tissues; in patients receiving mediastinal radiotherapy, this can cause long-term myocardial, coronary artery intimal and lung fibrosis. As a single modality, both chemotherapy and radiotherapy are mutagenic, but cumulatively, they carry a much greater risk of causing secondary leukaemias and skin cancer, and for very young women who receive mediastinal radiotherapy, there is a major risk of secondary breast cancer. Current practice strives to achieve high cure rates using only chemotherapy, reserving radiotherapy for certain scenarios such as bulky or chemotherapy-refractory sites of disease. These dilemmas are illustrated by the observation that of the 20% of patients who fail to achieve a cure for cHL, death in the first 10 years after diagnosis is mainly due to relapsed refractory cHL, whereas beyond 10 years, death is largely the result of therapy-related complications, as described above.

Relapsed disease requires salvage therapy; such treatment has curative potential, but the results are inferior to good first-line treatment. Effective approaches include high-dose chemotherapy with autologous stem cell rescue. Other approaches include immunomodulatory therapy using programmed death-1 (PD1) immune checkpoint inhibitors or the CD30-targeting antibody–drug conjugate brentuximab vedotin.

Acute Leukaemias

Acute leukaemias are examples of precursor cell neoplasms. They are characterised by the accumulation of blasts in the BM and often in peripheral blood. The natural history (in the absence of treatment) of acute leukaemias involves the effacement of normal BM by blasts, leading to marrow failure and death within weeks. The investigation of a suspected case of acute leukaemia is always a matter of urgency, as patients require supportive care with blood products and antibiotics to prevent death from bleeding, overwhelming infection or leukaemia complications, such as leucostasis, while time is taken to establish a precise diagnosis. AML and ALL occur at all ages, though AML is mainly a disorder of adults, while ALL is the most common leukaemia of childhood.

Acute myeloid leukaemia

The incidence of AML is 3.5 per 100,000 per year. The median age at diagnosis is 65 years. The incidence rises 10-fold from 1 to 10/100,000 per year between the ages of 20 and 70. AML may occur in childhood but represents only 10% of childhood leukaemia.

In most cases, there is no obvious explanation as to why AML has developed. Inherited risk factors include Down syndrome with an increased risk of AML, acute megakaryoblastic leukaemia and ALL, Fanconi anaemia and other inherited BM failure syndromes. Non-syndromic germline mutations in *RUNX1* are associated with leukaemia development. Environmental risk factors include benzene and radiation. Previous treatment with chemotherapy and/or radiotherapy increases the risk of AML, which is designated as therapy-related or cytotoxic-related AML.

Clinical presentation

At presentation, clinical features result from the proliferation of leukaemic cells; although arising in the BM, myeloblasts may involve blood and other tissues, including the skin and gums, particularly when there is monocytic differentiation. Patients with very high white blood cell (WBC) counts may experience obstruction of small blood vessels by leukaemic cells, known as leucostasis. This can lead to a stroke or respiratory impairment. Other clinical features result from bone-marrow failure. These include fatigue, dyspnoea, bruising, bleeding, petechiae and fever. Bacterial infections of the mouth and pharynx are common and can cause cervical lymphadenopathy. Acute promyelocytic leukaemia is often complicated by disseminated intravascular coagulation (DIC) and the activation of fibrinolysis so that there is prominent bleeding and bruising, for example bruising appearing spontaneously or at venepuncture sites.

There is anaemia and thrombocytopenia. Usually, the WBC count is increased as a result of considerable numbers of blast cells in the peripheral blood, although some patients may have a few or no circulating blast cells, leading to a low WBC count. Blast cells may be myeloblasts, monoblasts or both. Less often, they may also be megakaryoblasts or primitive erythroid cells. The neutrophil count is usually reduced, and neutrophils can show dysplastic features.

Diagnosis and differential diagnosis

The main differential diagnoses of AML are ALL and BM failure for any other reason. In many patients, the diagnosis is obvious from the clinical features plus the blood count and blood film, where blast cells with granules or rod-shaped cytoplasmic structures known as Auer rods (Fig. 8.16) identify the cells as being of myeloid lineage.

All patients require a BM aspirate (Fig. 8.17), which is examined for morphology to determine the percentage of blast cells and is assessed by immunophenotyping. The typical myeloid blast immunophenotype is CD34/CD33/CD13/CD117 positive. Expression of other antigens, such as

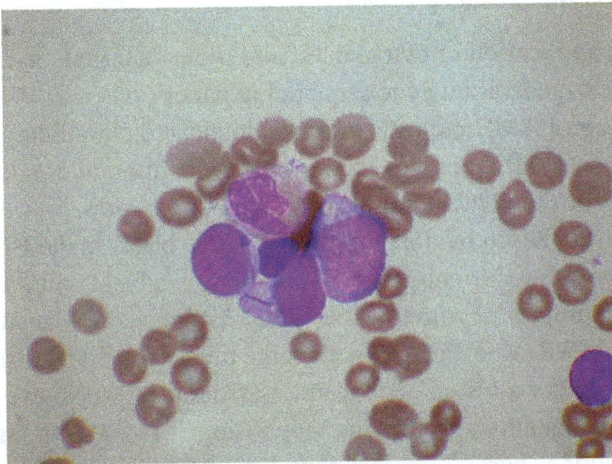

Fig. 8.16. A neutrophil and three blast cells; one of the blast cells has an Auer rod, indicating that these cells are myeloblasts and the diagnosis is AML (MGG stain).

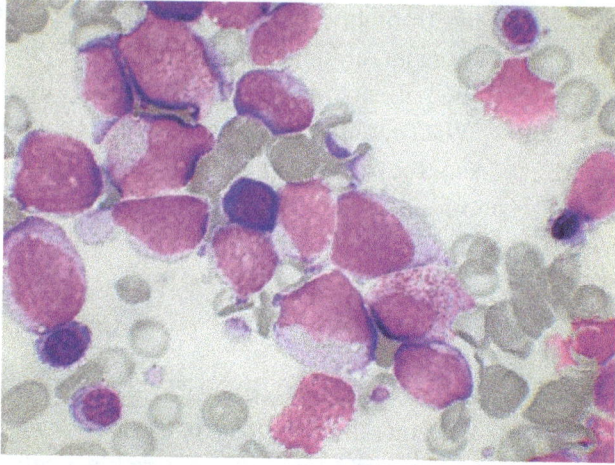

Fig. 8.17. Bone marrow aspirate in acute monoblastic leukaemia. Monoblasts are large cells with few, if any, granules. Their lineage can be confirmed by immunophenotyping.

glycophorin (erythroid) or CD11 (monocytoid), indicates a degree of lineage differentiation.

Classification and genetics

The routine application of cytogenetic and molecular genetic analyses, in particular next-generation gene sequencing panels, has resulted in a better understanding of AML biology, more sophisticated classification systems of the different AML subtypes, better prognostication and more complex treatment algorithms, including novel targeted therapies.

AML is diagnosed by the presence of >20% blasts in the BM. In cases with a recognised recurrent genetic abnormality, a blast count of >10% is sufficient. Examples of some of the WHO-recognised AML subtypes are noted in Table 8.6. Many are defined by the presence of a recurrent genetic abnormality, either a fusion gene resulting from a chromosomal translocation or a gene mutation, such as nucleophosmin 1 (*NPM1* mutated in 30% of AML) and/or a short internal tandem duplication (ITD), which alters the sequence of the FMS-like TK receptor gene (*FLT3*) (*FLT3*-ITD in 10% of cases of AML).

Table 8.6. Examples of WHO-categorised subtypes of acute myeloid leukaemia.

WHO classification of AML (some examples)
AML with recurrent genetic abnormalities
AML t(8;21) *RUNX1::RUNX1T1*
AML inv(16) *CBFB::MYH11*
APML t(15;17) *PML::RARA*
AML mutated *NPM1*
AML NOS (not otherwise specified)
Acute myelomonocytic leukaemia
Acute erythroid leukaemia
Cytotoxic–related AML
AML prognosis by genetic aberration
Favourable
t(8;21) *RUNX1::RUNX1T1*
inv(16) *CBFB::MYH11*
mt*NPM1*, No *FLT3*-ITD
Intermediate
FLT3 ITD
Cytogenetic abnormality not classed as favourable or adverse
Adverse
Chromosomal monosomy
Complex karyotype
TP53 mutation

An attempted cure for AML requires intensive leukaemia-directed treatment. The decision for an individual patient is complex. Two factors primarily impact the AML prognosis: patient age and the leukaemia-associated genetic abnormality. In patients aged over 70, there is a 3% prospect of a cure due to a higher proportion of poor-risk genetic abnormalities and a higher risk of treatment-related mortality with intensive regimens. In many scenarios involving elderly patients or younger patients with cytotoxic-related AML, which has a poor outlook, providing only, best supportive care may be most appropriate.

In patients under the age of 60, a long-term cure can be achieved in 40% of cases. The goal of treatment is to achieve remission, defined as fewer than 5% blasts in the BM, through induction chemotherapy. Traditional induction regimens consist of two blocks of intensive chemotherapy using an anthracycline and cytarabine. Remission can be achieved in up to 80% of cases, but relapse is common without further consolidation treatment. For some favourable-risk AML subtypes, such as *NPM1*-mutated AML without *FLT3*-ITD or the core binding factor leukaemias (*RUNX1::RUNX1T1* and *CBFB::MYH11*), treatment with chemotherapy alone may be sufficient for a cure. Patients are assessed after completion of chemotherapy for any evidence of measurable residual disease (MRD) in the BM using sensitive methods, such as quantitative PCR, and those patients who achieve undetectable MRD are monitored for molecular relapse.

However, for the majority of patients with intermediate- or unfavourable-risk AML (or favourable-risk AML with detectable MRD after induction chemotherapy), allogeneic stem cell transplantation offers the only possibility of a cure and long-term survival. The decision for stem cell transplantation is a complex one and must balance the reduced risk of leukaemia relapse against the high 10–30% transplant-related mortality (see Chapter 14).

The advent of hypomethylating agents (such as azacitidine and decitabine) and the BCL2 inhibitor venetoclax has dramatically changed the treatment landscape for AML and now presents a viable and better-tolerated treatment option for older patients, compared to standard intensive chemotherapy. Outcomes have improved further thanks to novel targeted inhibitors, such as FLT3 inhibitors (for patients with *FLT3*-ITD), selective IDH inhibitors, and the antibody-drug conjugate gemtuzumab ozogamicin.

Acute promyelocytic leukaemia

Acute promyelocytic leukaemia (APML) is associated with a t(15;17) translocation, which creates a fusion gene, *PML::RARA*. This subtype features a distinctive biology, clinical course and treatment. The retinoic acid receptor α (RARA) is a nuclear transcription-regulating protein, active in normal haemopoietic cellular differentiation. The *PML::RARA*

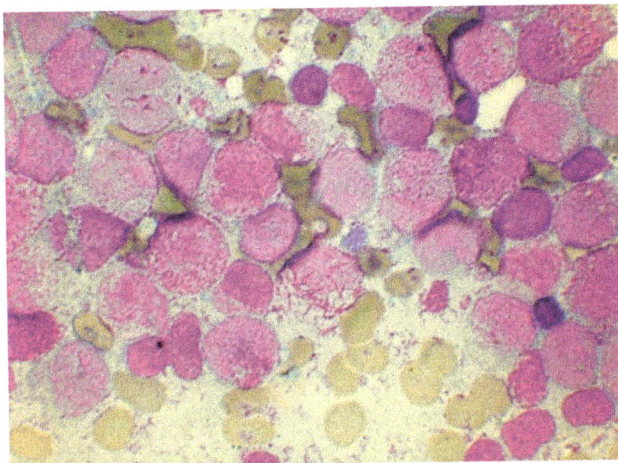

Fig. 8.18.   Bone marrow aspirate in acute promyelocytic leukaemia (MGG stain). Most of the cells are abnormal promyelocytes with brightly staining granules. One cell at the centre contains multiple Auer rods, a characteristic feature of this subtype of AML.

fusion protein blocks cellular differentiation. In APML, the leukaemic cells are arrested at the promyelocyte stage of differentiation (Fig. 8.18). These cells release the contents of the large cytoplasmic granules into the circulation, leading to coagulopathy with DIC and hyperfibrinolysis (see Chapter 11). The clinical features include bleeding from multiple sites with a risk of fatal pulmonary or cerebral haemorrhage. In APML, at presentation, DIC occurs in 40% of cases and is associated with early haemorrhagic death in 10–20% of cases. This is a medical emergency and requires vigorous supportive care with fresh frozen plasma and platelet transfusions. Leukaemia treatment consists of a combination of all-*trans*-retinoic acid (ATRA) and arsenic trioxide (As_2O_3), completely avoiding chemotherapy, to overcome the differentiation block and allow the maturation of the promyelocytes. This can be complicated by the ATRA syndrome of fever, hypoxia with pulmonary infiltrates and fluid overload; however, the syndrome generally responds to corticosteroid therapy. Following differentiation therapy, further cycles of As_2O_3 reduce the risk of recurrence. Untreated APML has a median survival of 1 month; however, with urgent and good haematology care, cure rates may reach 90%.

Acute lymphoblastic leukaemia

Acute lymphoblastic leukaemia (ALL) is predominantly a childhood disease, with a peak incidence around the age of 2–5. The prognosis in children is relatively good, with about 85% of children being cured by modern treatment. Cases also occur in adult life, with the prognosis in adults being significantly worse than in children. In children, the five-year survival rate is about 90%. In young adults, it is 60–70%, falling to about 40% in older adults and as low as 15% in those over the age of 65 years.

ALL is not a single disease but rather a heterogeneous group of disorders. The majority of cases, about 75–80%, are of B lineage, with the remainder being of T lineage. The current WHO classification is based on associated recurrent genetic abnormalities. Many subtypes are recognised, and some examples are shown in Table 8.7. The associated genetic abnormalities determine the prognosis and optimal treatment.

Clinical features

Clinical features can result either from the direct effects of the proliferation of leukaemic cells or from BM impairment because of the crowding out of normal haemopoietic cells. Presenting features that are the direct result of tissue infiltration by leukaemic cells include bone pain, lymphadenopathy, hepatomegaly and splenomegaly. Less often, there is testicular infiltration, leading to enlargement of one or both testes, or CNS infiltration, usually

Table 8.7. Examples of WHO-categorised subtypes of acute lymphoblastic leukaemia. The karyotype has a major impact on prognosis.

WHO classification of ALL (some examples)
ALL with recurrent genetic abnormalities:
ALL t(9;22) *BCR::ABL1*
ALL t(12;21) *ETV6::RUNX1*
ALL with hyperdiploidy
ALL with hypodiploidy
ALL NOS (not otherwise specified)

leading to cranial nerve palsies. Renal infiltration can result in abdominal enlargement and impaired renal function. Patients with a very high WBC count may suffer renal failure and a tumour lysis syndrome; this may be present pre-treatment but is more often precipitated by chemotherapy. In patients with T-ALL, chest radiography may show an enlargement of the thymus as a result of thymic infiltration by lymphoblasts. Presenting features resulting from impaired BM function include pallor, petechiae and bruising.

Haematological features

There is usually anaemia and thrombocytopenia. In the majority of patients, leukaemic lymphoblasts circulate in the blood (Fig. 8.19). In a minority of patients, there are no circulating lymphoblasts, and the diagnosis is made when a BM aspirate is performed to look for a cause of cytopenia.

Diagnosis and differential diagnosis

In children with cytopenia without circulating lymphoblasts, the differential diagnosis includes other causes of BM failure. However, if there is only isolated thrombocytopenia, a diagnosis of autoimmune or post-infection thrombocytopenia is much more likely, and ALL is unlikely. Once blast cells are detected in the blood or BM (Fig. 8.20), the differential diagnosis is between ALL and AML. Immunophenotyping is essential to confirm a provisional diagnosis of ALL. The typical immunophenotype of B-ALL is TdT, CD19 and CD22 positive and CD10 positive (Table 8.2). Karyotyping is essential, and because of the prognostic and therapeutic importance of the t(9;22) translocation, it is also necessary to perform molecular analysis for the *BCR::ABL1* fusion gene, particularly in adults.

Prognosis and treatment

As in all haematological malignancies, treatment involves supportive care to compensate for the impaired BM function and leukaemia-directed combination chemotherapy. In all cases, and particularly in young children,

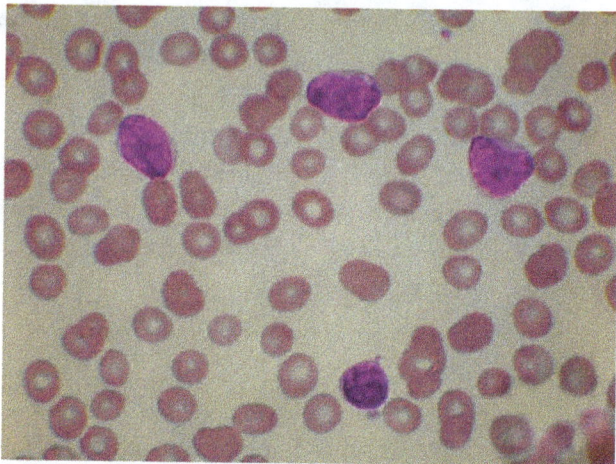

Fig. 8.19. Peripheral blood (PB) film in ALL showing three blast cells and a lymphocyte (MGG stain).

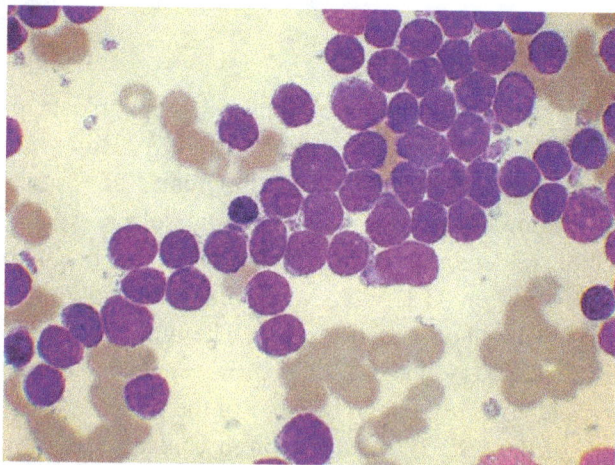

Fig. 8.20. Bone marrow aspirate film in ALL showing complete replacement of normal haemopoietic cells by leukaemic lymphoblasts (MGG stain).

supportive care includes an indwelling central venous catheter, plus attention to blood product support, antibiotics, anti-fungals, fluids and electrolytes to prevent disease- or therapy-related death.

In childhood B-ALL, long-term cure rates of 90% can be achieved. In adult ALL, the prospect of a cure is significantly lower, at 5% in patients aged greater than 70. Adult ALL has a higher proportion of poor-risk genetic abnormalities, in particular t(9;22) *BCR::ABL1*. Philadelphia-positive ALL constitutes 20–30% of adult ALL (*cf.* paediatric ALL, 3–5%).

The management of childhood ALL is complex. A key principle is to stratify cases into standard and high risk based on age (standard risk: 1–10 years), presenting WBC (standard-risk WBC $<50 \times 10^9/l$) and genetics. Details of genetic stratification are beyond a core curriculum, but key points are as follows: a hyperdiploid karyotype is favourable, while a hypodiploid karyotype is prognostically unfavourable. The presence of the Philadelphia chromosome/*BCR::ABL1* confers an extremely poor prognosis. ALL treatment has four components: remission induction combination chemotherapy, consolidation chemotherapy, maintenance oral chemotherapy for 2–3 years and CNS-directed treatment. Because of the risk of CNS disease, therapy with intrathecal methotrexate or high-dose intravenous methotrexate, combined with cytarabine to cross the blood–brain barrier, is given to all patients. Despite seemingly successful first-line treatment, some patients will suffer an ALL relapse. Salvage treatment using either allogeneic stem cell transplantation or CAR-T therapy may achieve a cure in a proportion of relapsed childhood ALL cases.

In childhood ALL, effort is focused on better defining prognosis and response monitoring. The goals are to decrease treatment intensity and avoid, where possible, long-term toxicity, such as myocardial damage from anthracyclines, infertility and therapy-related AML, in children with good-risk disease, while improving the outcome for children with poor-risk disease.

The management of adult ALL is based on the same four components as in childhood ALL. Key differences are the addition of imatinib, an ABL1 kinase inhibitor, to chemotherapy regimens for all Philadelphia-positive ALL. In view of the poorer prognosis of adult ALL and those with Philadelphia-positive ALL, adults who are considered to have an adequate performance status may undergo stem cell transplantation in first remission.

Test Case 8.1

A 65-year-old man undergoes a blood count and a biochemical screening following admission to hospital with a myocardial infarction. Unexpectedly, his blood count shows a lymphocytosis. He is re-examined, and no lymphadenopathy, hepatomegaly or splenomegaly is found, so the blood count is repeated the next day. It shows: WBC $49 \times 10^9/l$, neutrophil count $6.1 \times 10^9/l$, lymphocyte count $42 \times 10^9/l$ and monocyte count $0.9 \times 10^9/l$. The Hb and platelet counts are normal. Immunophenotyping is done with the following results:

Kappa 85% (weak expression), lambda 5% (moderate expression), CD19 88%, CD2 (a T-cell marker) 10%, CD5 94%, CD23 82%, FMC7 negative and CD79b negative.

Questions

1. What is the most likely diagnosis and why?
2. Does the patient need any treatment for this condition at present?
Write down your answers before checking the correct answer (page 406) or re-reading any other relevant part of the chapter.

Test Case 8.2

A 4-year-old child is noted to be pale and listless by his mother. He is an only child and has previously been well. His GP finds him to have abdominal enlargement, lymphadenopathy and bruising, and refers him urgently to a hospital. An FBC shows: WBC of $146 \times 10^9/l$, neutrophil count $1.3 \times 10^9/l$, blast cells $144.7 \times 10^9/l$, Hb 87 g/l and platelet count $86 \times 10^9/l$. Immunophenotyping is done with the following results:

TdT 92%, CD10 89%, CD19 87%, CD22 89% and CD3 1%.

Questions

1. What is the most likely diagnosis and why?
2. What other tests are needed?

Write down your answers before checking the correct answer (page 406) or re-reading any relevant part of the chapter.

9

Myeloproliferative Neoplasms

Donald Macdonald

What Do You Need To Know?

☞ Myeloproliferative neoplasms are characterised by an abnormal FBC result with an elevated myeloid blood cell count (Hb, platelets or granulocytes), although in later stages of primary myelofibrosis, pancytopenia ensues

☞ The differential diagnoses of myeloproliferative neoplasms include reactive (secondary) causes of an elevated myeloid cell count

☞ A diagnostic approach to distinguish polycythaemia vera from secondary polycythaemia

☞ Myeloproliferative neoplasms (*BCR::ABL1* negative): polycythaemia vera, essential thromobocythaemia and primary myelofibrosis; clinicopathological features and principles of management

☞ Myeloproliferative neoplasm (*BCR::ABL1* positive): Chronic myeloid leukaemia; clinicopathological features and principles of management

☞ Chronic myelomonocytic leukaemia: clinicopathological features and principles of management

Myeloproliferative Neoplasms and Secondary Causes of Elevated Blood Cell Counts

Through a process of differentiation, the myeloid stem cell gives rise to mature myeloid lineage cells, which include erythrocytes, megakaryocytes/platelets, granulocytes (eosinophils, neutrophils and basophils) and monocytes. The precursor cells of each lineage are found in the bone marrow and can be recognised morphologically, e.g. myeloblasts, promyelocytes and myelocytes or erythroblasts in their early, intermediate and late forms. This chapter is focused on myeloproliferative neoplasms (MPN), which are clonal neoplastic myeloid disorders where the main cellular perturbation consists of excessive, autonomous proliferation of one or more myeloid lineages. In MPN, there is generally effective maturation, resulting in an excess of mature cells in the peripheral blood. In all the MPN, there is a variable risk of evolution to a terminal acute leukaemia phase. The MPN are grouped as *BCR::ABL1*-negative MPN: polycythaemia vera (PV), essential thrombocythemia (ET) and primary myelofibrosis (PMF). The final entity is *BCR::ABL1*-positive, chronic myeloid leukaemia (CML).

MDS and MDS/MPN Overlap Syndromes

Other disorders recognised by the World Health Organization (WHO) classification system are the myelodysplastic syndromes (MDS) and MDS/MPN overlap syndromes. Although both clonal myeloid disorders, MDS and MDS/MPN differ from the MPNs in that haemopoiesis is ineffective in at least one lineage. The bone marrow is often hypercellular in MDS, but there is increased death of haemopoietic cells in the bone marrow so that, despite the hypercellular marrow, there is inadequate production of mature cells of one or more lineages, which leads to peripheral blood cytopenia. MDS have been discussed in Chapter 6. There is also an MDS/MPN overlap category in which there is effective production of cells of one lineage, whereas another lineage shows ineffective haemopoiesis, and is often morphologically dysplastic. For example, there could be a marked elevation of the platelet count associated with sideroblastic anaemia or marked monocytosis associated with neutropenia. Chronic myelomonocytic leukaemia (CMML) is an example.

Raised cell count: Distinguishing MPN from a reactive/secondary cause

A common clinical scenario is an FBC result showing raised haemoglobin concentration (Hb), haematocrit (Hct), platelet count or granulocyte count. Such a finding requires investigation to determine if this is an MPN or a reactive elevation.

Polycythaemia

Polycythaemia refers to an increase in the red blood cell count (RBC), Hb and Hct. An unexplained raised Hct (i.e. >0.52 for males and >0.48 for females) should prompt an investigation to determine the cause. It is important to understand the distinction between pseudopolycythaemia (relative polycythaemia) and true polycythaemia and, if true polycythaemia, the distinction between primary (PV) and secondary polycythaemia.

In pseudopolycythaemia, the red cell mass (RCM) is normal and plasma volume is reduced. This may be seen in patients with any or all of the following risk factors: overweight, excessive alcohol consumption or diuretic therapy. The risk of thrombotic complications arising from an abnormal Hct reading is low, and the clinical approach involves addressing, where possible, the contributing factors. In practice, pseudopolycythaemia is diagnosed after the careful exclusion of true polycythaemia. Technically, pseudopolycythaemia can be confirmed by radio-isotope studies of RCM and plasma volume; however, such investigations are now rarely performed.

True polycythaemia: Secondary causes

True polycythaemia (in which RCM is raised but plasma volume is normal) may be primary (neoplastic, PV) or secondary (reactive). The secondary causes fall into two main groups: those with an **appropriate** elevation of erythropoietin (EPO) and those with an **inappropriate** elevation of EPO. EPO is appropriately elevated in any scenario causing hypoxia in the juxtatubular cells of the kidney, including: living at high altitude, cardiac or pulmonary diseases severe enough to produce hypoxia, renal artery stenosis and, rarely, high-affinity haemoglobinopathies. Causes of secondary polycythaemia with inappropriate EPO elevation include: misuse of EPO or androgenic steroids, secretion of EPO by renal and hepatic cell carcinomas, cerebellar hemangioblastoma and polycystic kidney disease.

An elevation of the Hct is associated with an increase in whole blood viscosity, and if the Hct rises above 0.60, a steep rise in viscosity occurs, which can impair blood flow and therefore tissue oxygenation. The raised Hct in secondary polycythaemia will also cause a thrombotic risk, though less severe than the risks in PV. Secondary polycythaemia that results from inappropriate EPO synthesis is never beneficial, and management involves correcting the Hct, ideally by venesection and identifying the cause, e.g. relevant clinical history to determine hormone use and imaging of the kidneys and liver to identify tumours. The management of cases with an appropriate elevation of EPO level must be tailored to the patient. The aim is to identify a balance between the beneficial effects of increased oxygen-carrying capacity in a severely hypoxic patient and the harmful effects of increased whole-blood viscosity. Figure 9.1 provides a simple guide to the classification of polycythaemia.

Myeloproliferative neoplasms (BCR::ABL1 negative)

These MPN are characterised by the **effective** production of mature cells, at least in the early stages of the disease. The three most important disorders are polycythaemia vera, essential thrombocythaemia and primary myelofibrosis. They are closely related, often showing the same acquired molecular genetic abnormalities (Table 9.1).

All these conditions show a greater or lesser tendency to transform into acute myeloid leukaemia (AML). In addition, PV and ET can evolve into myelofibrosis, with possible further disease evolution to AML (Fig. 9.2).

Polycythaemia vera

Polycythaemia vera is an MPN that is characterised by elevated levels of RBC, Hb and Hct, with or without an increase in the white blood cell

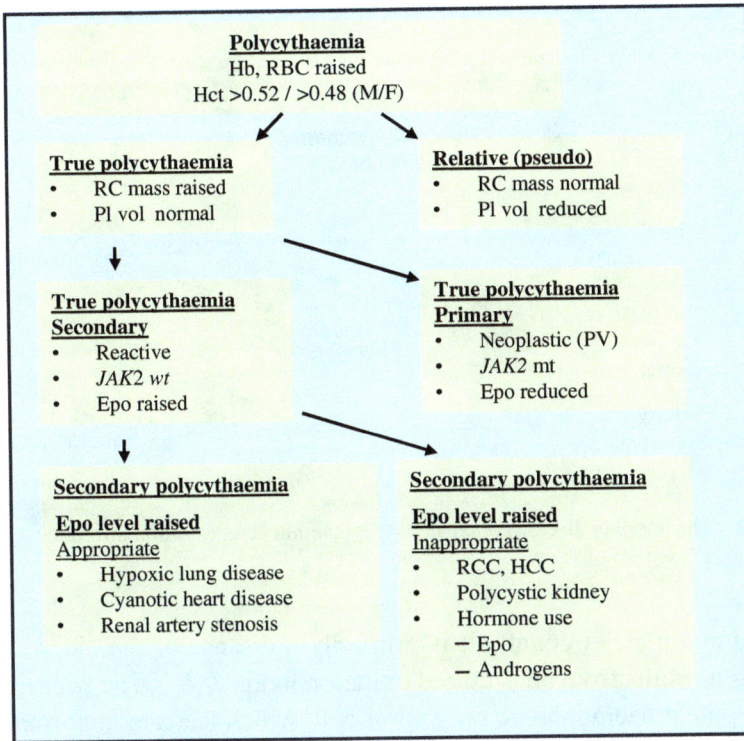

Fig. 9.1. Guide to polycythaemia. RCM (red cell mass); RC (red cell); Pl (plasma); PV (polycythaemia vera), *JAK2* Janus Kinase 2, *JAK2* mt (mutant) wt (wild type/no mutation) RCC and HCC (renal cell and hepatic cell cancer).

Table 9.1. Shows the frequency of mutations involving the genes *JAK2, CALR* and *MPL* in the MPN: PV (polycythaemia vera), ET (essential thrombocythaemia) and PMF (primary myelofibrosis).

	JAK2 (%)	*CALR* (%)	*MPL* (%)
PV	100		
ET	65	25	3
PMF	65	25	7

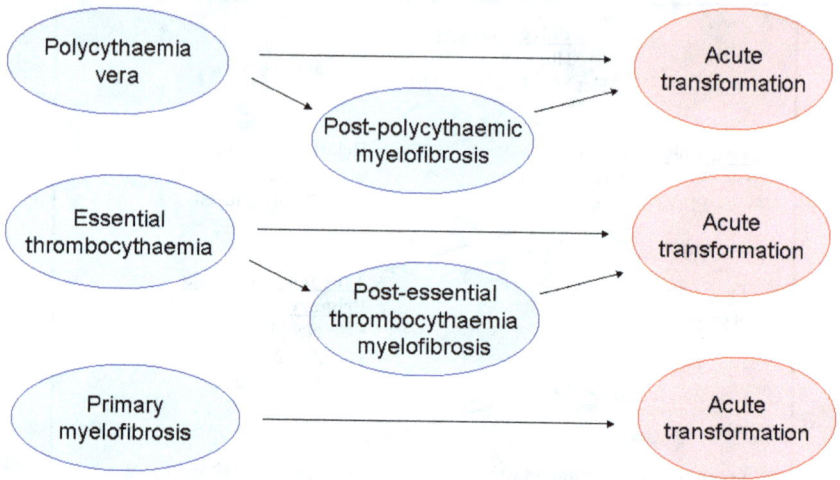

Fig. 9.2. The possible disease course in polycythaemia vera, essential thrombocythaemia and primary myelofibrosis.

(WBC) and platelet counts. It is primarily a disease of the elderly. This condition results from an acquired mutation in the *JAK2* gene occurring in a multipotent haemopoietic progenitor cell, which leads to abnormal proliferation signals without the need for erythropoietin to bind to erythropoietin receptors. In about 95% of patients, this is a point mutation, *JAK2* V617F, in exon 14 of the gene. In another 5% of patients, there is a mutation in exon 12.

Clinical features

Patients with polycythaemia usually have a plethoric complexion with conjunctival injection. The most prominent clinical features result from impaired circulation and thrombosis; they include headache, dizziness, transient ischaemic attacks, stroke, peripheral gangrene (Fig. 9.3), myocardial infarction and venous thromboembolism. The spleen may be enlarged by several centimetres below the left costal margin. Thrombosis of the hepatic vein can lead to hepatomegaly, jaundice and ascites (known as Budd–Chiari syndrome). The portal vein and the mesenteric veins are also prone to thrombosis. There is an increased incidence of peptic

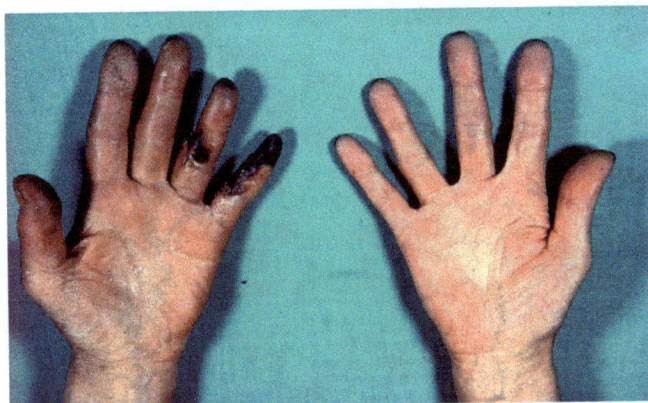

Fig. 9.3. Clinical photograph of the hands of a patient with polycythaemia vera showing poor circulation in the thumb and fingers of one hand with gangrene of two digits and impending gangrene of the others.

ulceration, and some patients suffer from itchiness, particularly after a hot bath; both of these clinical features result from increased histamine secretion by basophils. There is an increased incidence of gastrointestinal haemorrhage. Some patients may suffer from gout since uric acid production is increased as a result of increased breakdown of nucleic acids.

Haematological features

Polycythaemia vera is characterised by increased RBC, Hb and Hct levels and, often, increased WBC, neutrophil, basophil and platelet counts as well. The blood film has a 'packed' appearance (Fig. 9.4). The bone marrow is hypercellular as a result of increased erythropoiesis. Granulopoiesis and megakaryocytes are also usually increased. Iron stores are typically absent, as all of the stored iron has been incorporated into the expanding red cell mass. Serum erythropoietin is low.

Diagnosis and differential diagnosis

The diagnosis of polycythaemia vera is based on the findings of a raised Hct level (>0.52 for males and >0.48 for females) and the presence of a

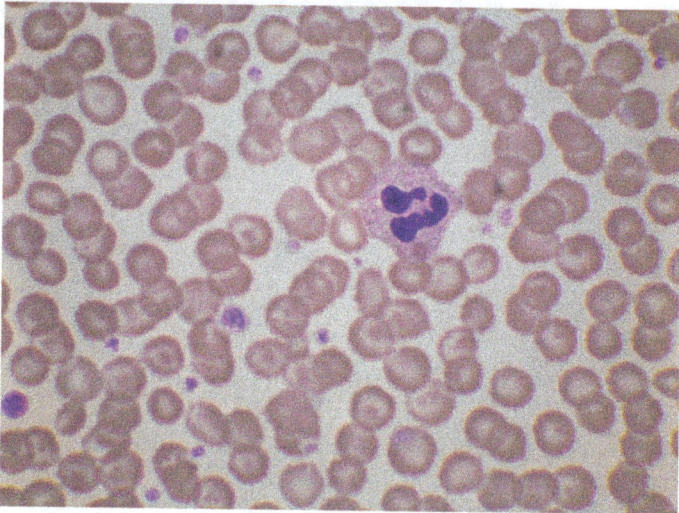

Fig. 9.4. Peripheral blood (PB) film in polycythaemia vera showing a 'packed film' (May–Grünwald–Giemsa (MGG) stain). The haemoglobin concentration (Hb) in this male patient was 202 g/l and the haematocrit was 0.61 l/l. There is also thrombocytosis (platelet count: 916×10^9/l) and some of the platelets are larger than normal. *JAK2* V617F was detected.

JAK2 mutation. EPO levels will be suppressed. The serum ferritin levels should be determined as iron deficiency can suppress the elevation of Hct and Hb, though the RBC count remains high, as do the WBC and platelet counts.

Management

It is necessary to correct polycythemia and any associated thrombocytosis, primarily to prevent cardiovascular accidents (CVAs) or other thrombotic events. If there is isolated polycythaemia, the Hb and Hct levels can be lowered through regular venesection (of about 450 ml of blood on each occasion) until they return to normal ranges. Repeated venesections lead to the depletion of iron stores, making infrequent venesections sufficient to maintain the Hct level at a target value of less than 0.45. Aspirin at a dose of 75–100 mg daily is prescribed. If the platelet or WBC count is also elevated, or if the patient cannot tolerate regular venesections, an oral antimetabolite, such as hydroxycarbamide, is used. More recently, targeted JAK2 inhibitors have been used to treat patients who are refractory to hydroxycarbamide. Although some patients develop myelofibrosis or AML, the median survival with treatment is 10–20 years.

A strategy to investigate an unexplained polycythaemia

Unexplained raised Hb and Hct (>0.52 for males and >0.48 for females) levels require investigation. The starting point should be a clinical assessment for any condition causing hypoxia, such as cyanotic heart disease or hypoxic lung disease; it may be helpful to check blood oxygen saturation or arterial oxygen levels. A family history of polycythaemia or consistently raised Hb on FBC results going back many years may suggest an inherited cause, such as high-affinity haemoglobin. In the absence of an obvious clinical explanation, initial laboratory studies should include a FBC, including red cell indices and differential count, blood film, iron studies, *JAK2* mutation analysis and serum EPO levels. The finding of a *JAK2* mutation and reduced EPO levels are indicative of PV. A polycythaemia with raised EPO levels and an absence of a *JAK2* mutation (note that both exons 14 and 12 must be screened) should prompt investigation for a secondary polycythaemia, including any history of EPO or androgen usage, along with imaging studies of the kidneys and liver to exclude an underlying neoplasm.

Thrombocytosis

Thrombocytosis (also referred to as thrombocythaemia) is an increase in the platelet count. Thrombocytosis is a common, non-specific reaction to infection and inflammation. Less often, it is the result of an MPN, which, in the case of isolated thrombocytosis, is designated as essential thrombocythaemia. Thrombocytosis may be primary or secondary (Box 9.1).

Some of the causes of thrombocytosis are shown in Table 9.2.

Essential thrombocythaemia

Essential thrombocythaemia is a haematological neoplasm, specifically an MPN, resulting from mutation in a multipotent haemopoietic progenitor cell. In about 65% of the cases, a *JAK2* mutation occurs. In around 25% of

---

Box 9.1
Classification of thrombocytosis

Primary	Intrinsic bone marrow disease (essential thrombocythaemia)
Redistributional	Platelets redistributed from splenic pool into general circulation when the spleen has been removed or is atrophic
Secondary	Normal bone marrow response to extrinsic stimulus, e.g. infection, inflammation or malignancy

Table 9.2. Some causes of thrombocytosis.

Mechanism	Cause
Reactive thrombocytosis	Infection
	Inflammation (e.g. inflammatory bowel disease, acute episodes in rheumatoid arthritis)
	Surgery or trauma
	Haemorrhage
	Haemolysis
	Malignant disease (e.g. carcinoma of lung)
	Iron deficiency
	Rebound following recovery from bone marrow suppression
Altered distribution of platelets	Post-splenectomy or hyposplenism
Intrinsic bone marrow disease	Essential thrombocythaemia
	Polycythaemia vera (many cases)
	Primary myelofibrosis (early stages of disease)
	Chronic myeloid leukaemia (many cases)
	Myelodysplastic/myeloproliferative neoplasms (some cases)

patients, there is a mutation in the *CALR* gene, and in another 3% in the *MPL* gene, which encodes the membrane receptor for thrombopoietin (Table 9.1).

Clinical features

Diagnosis is often incidental when a blood count is done for an unrelated condition or as part of a routine health check. Other patients present with either vascular insufficiency or thrombosis, e.g. stroke or peripheral gangrene (Fig. 9.5). Microvascular involvement can lead to transient ischaemic attacks, disturbances of hearing and vision, recurrent headaches and erythromelalgia. Paradoxically, patients with very high platelet counts can present with haemorrhage; this is caused by the uptake of large multimers of von Willebrand factor by platelets, leading to acquired von Willebrand disease.

Haematological features

The blood film and count show thrombocytosis without polycythaemia (Fig. 9.6). Platelet size is increased. The WBC, neutrophil and basophil counts may be elevated, whereas the RBC, Hb and Hct levels are normal. The bone marrow shows an increase in megakaryocytes, which appear larger than normal and form clusters.

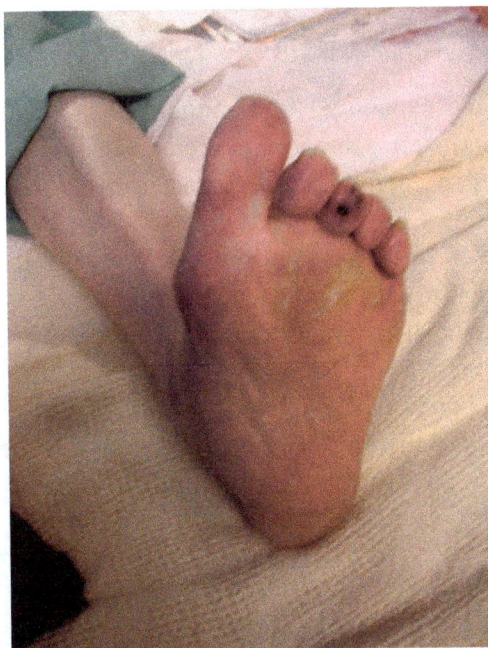

Fig. 9.5. Gangrene of the toes in a patient with essential thrombocythaemia.

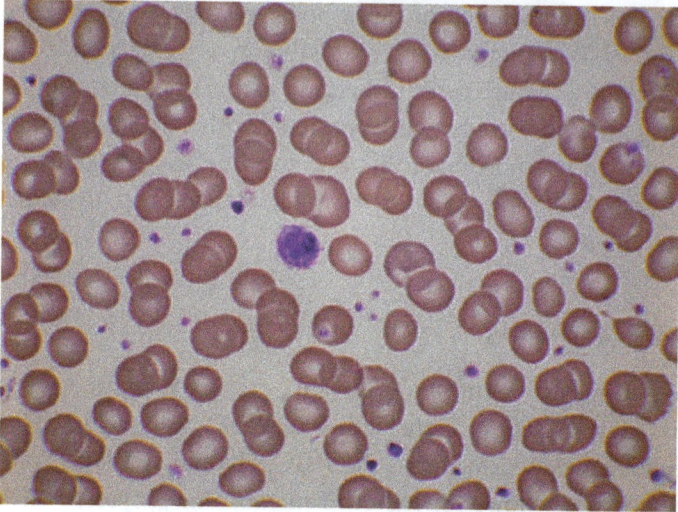

Fig. 9.6. PB film in a patient with essential thrombocythaemia showing thrombocytosis and one giant platelet (MGG stain). The platelet count was $1297 \times 10^9/l$ with the white cell count, haemoglobin concentration (Hb) and mean cell volume being normal.

Diagnosis and differential diagnosis

The diagnosis is most soundly based on the demonstration of thrombocytosis with specific features supporting a diagnosis of an MPN, such as a relevant mutation. If there is a coexisting iron deficiency and a *JAK2* mutation, a diagnosis of PV cannot be excluded without the cautious administration of iron. If no mutation is demonstrated, the diagnosis is made by excluding the causes of reactive thrombocytosis and demonstrating typical ET-associated bone marrow histology. The early stages of primary myelofibrosis may be confused with ET, but they are distinguished based on bone marrow histology. CML can present with isolated thrombocytosis; it is therefore important to exclude the presence of a *BCR::ABL1* fusion gene.

Management

The prognosis of ET is favourable; survival is approximately 20 years. Transformation to myelofibrosis or AML is quite infrequent, and life expectancy is comparable to that of an age-matched population. Treatment involves administering 75 mg of aspirin daily, unless there is clinically significant acquired von Willebrand disease. In patients with very marked thrombocytosis (e.g. a platelet count of 2,000–3,000 × 10^9/l), particularly with any history of bruising or haemorrhage, the count should be lowered by administering hydroxycarbamide before aspirin to avoid increasing the risk of haemorrhage. Cytoreduction using hydroxycarbamide is reserved for disease with higher-risk factors: age >60 years, previous history of thrombosis and platelet count >1,500 × 10^9/l. It is also important to correct, where possible, any other cardiovascular risk factors, such as smoking or hypertension. During pregnancy or if pregnancy is planned, α interferon is the most appropriate therapy; however, hydroxycarbamide should not be used.

Bone Marrow Fibrosis

Bone marrow fibrosis refers to the increased deposition of collagen and reticulin (a fibrillar protein composed of collagen III) in the bone marrow. Some of the causes of collagen fibrosis are shown in Table 9.3.

Table 9.3. Some causes of collagen fibrosis of the bone marrow.

Cause	Example
Myeloproliferative neoplasms	Primary myelofibrosis Post-polycythaemic myelofibrosis Post-essential thrombocythaemia myelofibrosis Chronic myeloid leukaemia (rarely)
Acute myeloid leukaemia	Specific subtypes (e.g. acute megakaryoblastic leukaemia)
Lymphoma	Non-Hodgkin lymphoma Hodgkin lymphoma
Non-haemopoietic neoplasms	Metastatic carcinoma, particularly carcinoma of the breast or prostate
Bone diseases	Paget disease, hyperparathyroidism, rickets, osteopetrosis (marble bone disease)

Primary myelofibrosis

Primary myelofibrosis, previously called 'idiopathic myelofibrosis', is an MPN in which the proliferation of a clone of cells derived from a mutated multipotent haemopoietic progenitor cells leads to reactive bone marrow fibrosis. It should be noted that myelofibrosis is a response to cytokines secreted by neoplastic myeloid cells (particularly megakaryocytes). There is also mobilisation of haemopoietic progenitor cells from the bone marrow, leading to extramedullary haemopoiesis, particularly in the liver and spleen. MPN-associated mutations are present (Table 9.1). Primary myelofibrosis predominantly affects the middle-aged and elderly.

Clinical features

Patients usually present with hepatosplenomegaly, bruising and symptoms of anaemia (Figs. 9.7 and 9.8). The enlargement of the spleen may be significantly pronounced. There may be fatigue, weight loss, fever and increased sweating.

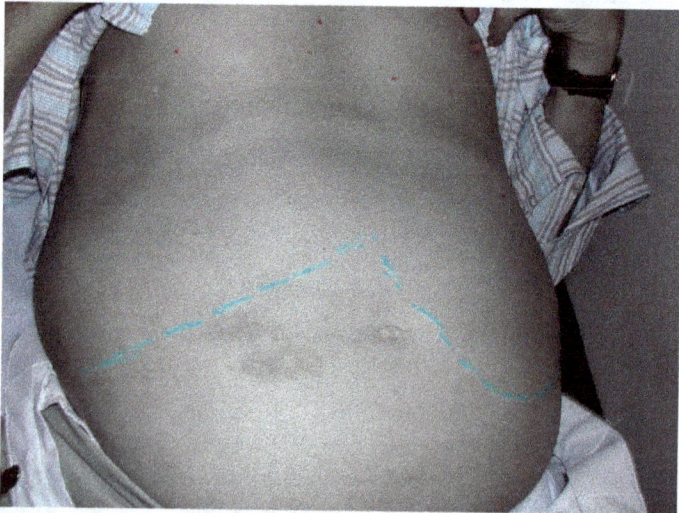

Fig. 9.7. The abdomen of a patient with primary myelofibrosis, with the size of the liver and spleen indicated. Note that there is also bruising.

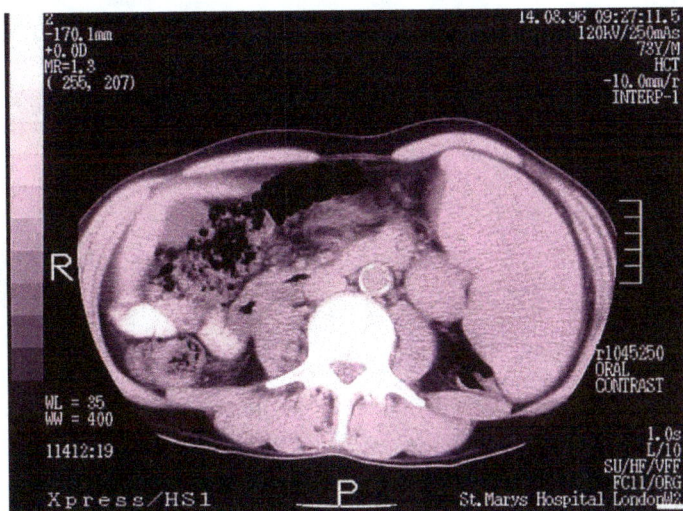

Fig. 9.8. Computed tomography (CT) scan of the abdomen in a patient with primary myelofibrosis showing highly pronounced splenomegaly. (There is also calcification in the wall of the aorta.)

Both haemorrhage and thrombosis can occur. In advanced disease, massive splenomegaly can cause hypersplenism, portal hypertension and ascites. Some patients may also suffer from gout.

Haematological features

The clinical course is variable. There may be an early proliferative phase with thrombocytosis and an increased WBC count. This will progress to a fibrotic phase with worsening anaemia, leucopenia and thrombocytopenia. Cytopenias result from inadequate bone marrow production; however, as progressive splenomegaly develops, hypersplenism plays a major role. The blood film is leucoerythroblastic (i.e. nucleated red blood cells and granulocyte precursors are present), and there are teardrop poikilocytes (Fig. 9.9). Because of bone marrow fibrosis, it may be impossible to aspirate bone marrow — a so-called dry tap. The diagnosis depends on the trephine biopsy histology, which demonstrates the fibrosis (Fig. 9.10). Late in the course of the disease, haemopoiesis becomes ineffective, and

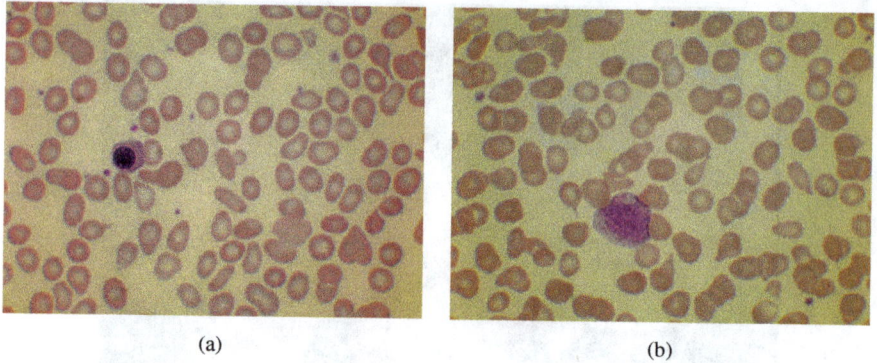

Fig. 9.9. PB film from a patient with primary myelofibrosis (MGG stain): (a) teardrop poikilocytes, elliptocytes and a nucleated red blood cell; (b) a myelocyte. Note that there are very few platelets.

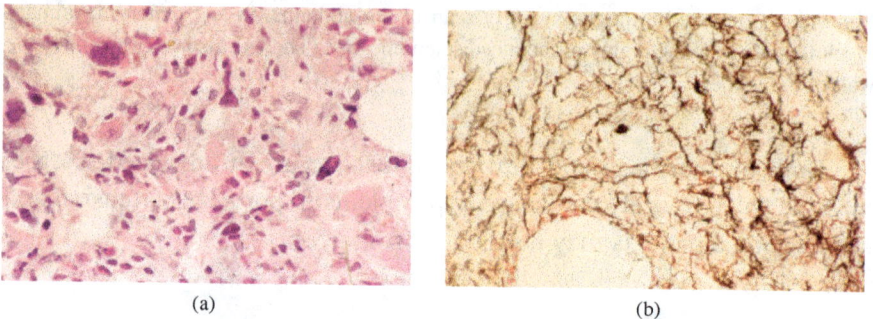

Fig. 9.10. Trephine biopsy sections from a patient with primary myelofibrosis: (a) megakaryocytes and other haemopoietic cells embedded in pale pink collagen on a haematoxylin and eosin stain; (b) increased reticulin deposition on a reticulin stain.

the lactate dehydrogenase is markedly elevated. Haemopoietic cells may be dysplastic.

Diagnosis and differential diagnosis

When the disease is advanced, the diagnosis is straightforward, based on clinical features, a leucoerythroblastic anaemia, a fibrotic bone marrow and detection of a relevant mutation.

Management

Of the *BCR::ABL1*-negative MPNs, PMF has the least favourable prognosis, with a median survival of 4–6 years. Clinical factors associated with poor prognosis include: older age, constitutional symptoms, anaemia, transfusion dependence, thrombocytopenia, leukocytosis, circulating blasts and a degree of bone marrow fibrosis. Newer prognostic scoring symptoms incorporate clinical features with genetic mutation analysis to stratify patients (genetically inspired prognostic scoring system (GIPSS)).

Allogeneic haemopoietic stem cell transplantation is the only potentially curative treatment and can be offered to a small number of younger patients with an adequate performance status and poor-risk disease. For the remainder, options include hydroxycarbamide (for thrombocytosis or painful splenomegaly) during the earlier proliferative phase, danazol (an anabolic steroid) or erythropoietin (for anaemia) and immune-modulatory drugs, thalidomide or lenalidomide. The management of more advanced disease is complex; options include ruxolitinib (a JAK2 inhibitor) or momelotinib (a combined JAK and activin A receptor type 1, ACVR1, inhibitor). Morbidity and mortality are most commonly due to haemorrhage, portal hypertension and varices, extra-medullary haematopoiesis or transformation to acute leukaemia.

Chronic Myeloid Leukaemia

CML is a rare leukaemia, with incidence in the UK being 1–2 per 100,000 per year. It is largely a disease of adults; the median age of presentation is 50 years, and there is a slight male preponderance. The condition usually arises *de novo*, though radiation exposure is a known risk factor. CML is characterised by the finding of the Philadelphia (Ph) chromosome and the resulting *BCR::ABL1* fusion gene (Figs. 9.12 and 8.4). Genetic studies of this condition have seen some of the most remarkable advances in scientific medicine. In sequence, the Ph chromosome was identified, molecular pathogenesis was elucidated, genetic-based diagnostics and monitoring were established and, ultimately, a targeted therapy that has transformed the outcome of this disorder was developed.

In CML, the natural history is that of a biphasic disease. An initial chronic phase is characterised by an expanded population of maturing granulocytic cells; the counts are well controlled with treatment, and systemic symptoms are absent. At presentation, 90% of patients are in the chronic phase. This evolves into a more advanced phase where the proportion of precursor blast cells progressively increases (accelerated phase: 10–19% blasts; blast crisis: >20%) and systemic symptoms are present. At advanced stages, the malignant cells are poorly responsive to treatment, and survival is short.

Clinical features

Nowadays, up to half of all patients are diagnosed with an incidental FBC before any symptoms appear. Where present, symptoms include fatigue, lethargy, bleeding, weight loss, splenic discomfort and increased sweating. The most common physical finding is splenomegaly; with more advanced disease, the liver is also enlarged. The high WBC count may impair blood flow, causing priapism or tinnitus.

Haematological features

There is an increase in the WBC count due to an increase in both granulocyte precursors (particularly myelocytes) and mature granulocytes — neutrophils, eosinophils and basophils (Fig. 9.11). The platelet count is usually normal or high. There may be anaemia, which is not usually severe. The bone marrow is intensely hypercellular due to an increase in granulocytic cells and megakaryocytes.

In the accelerated phase, there may be thrombocytopenia or refractory thrombocytosis; basophils are often increased. A blast crisis can either emerge suddenly from the chronic phase (particularly a lymphoblastic crisis) or follow an accelerated phase. Blast cells increase in number in the marrow and appear in the peripheral blood. Blast crisis can be myeloid, lymphoid or mixed lineage.

Diagnosis and differential diagnosis

A marked increase in neutrophils and myelocytes, a consistent increase in basophils and, usually, an increase in eosinophils make the differential

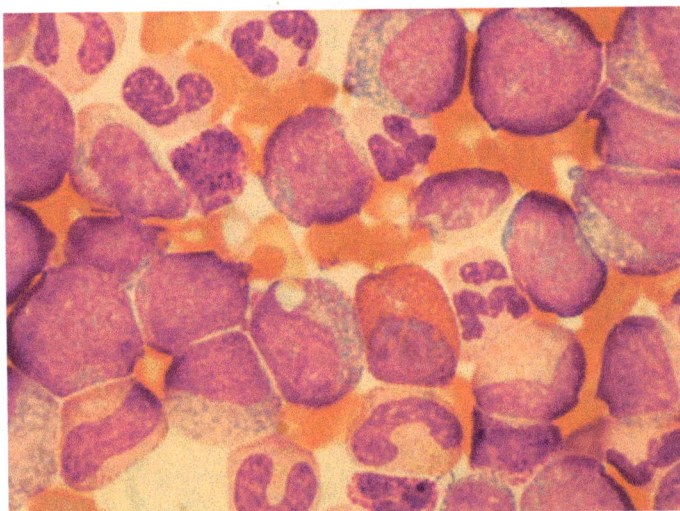

Fig. 9.11. PB film from a patient with chronic myeloid leukaemia with a very high WBC (MGG stain). There are mature cells and precursors of all three granulocytic lineages.

count extremely typical so that confusion with reactive neutrophilia is only likely in early cases that are detected incidentally. Confirmation of the diagnosis requires cytogenetic analysis (Fig. 9.12), fluorescence *in situ* hybridisation (FISH) analysis (Fig. 8.4) or molecular analysis to demonstrate the *BCR::ABL1* fusion gene.

The Ph chromosome results from a balanced reciprocal translocation between chromosomes 9 and 22, designated as t(9;22)(q34.1;q11.2). It leads to the formation of an oncogenic fusion gene, *BCR::ABL1*. At the molecular level, the breakpoint on chromosome 9 disrupts *ABL1*, a gene encoding a tyrosine kinase. On chromosome 22, the breakpoint disrupts the *BCR* gene. The translated fusion protein *BCR::ABL1* is a constitutively activated tyrosine kinase that promotes autonomous cell proliferation. Among the cases, there may be different genomic breakpoints. Such variations determine the number of *BCR* exons included in the fusion gene, resulting in several distinct BCR::ABL1 fusion proteins, defined by their molecular weight in kilodaltons. Examples include p210$^{BCR::ABL1}$ (the majority of CML cases and one-third of Ph-positive ALL cases) and p190$^{BCR::ABL1}$ (a minority of CML cases and two-thirds of Ph-positive ALL). Further details of Ph-positive ALL are described in Chapter 8.

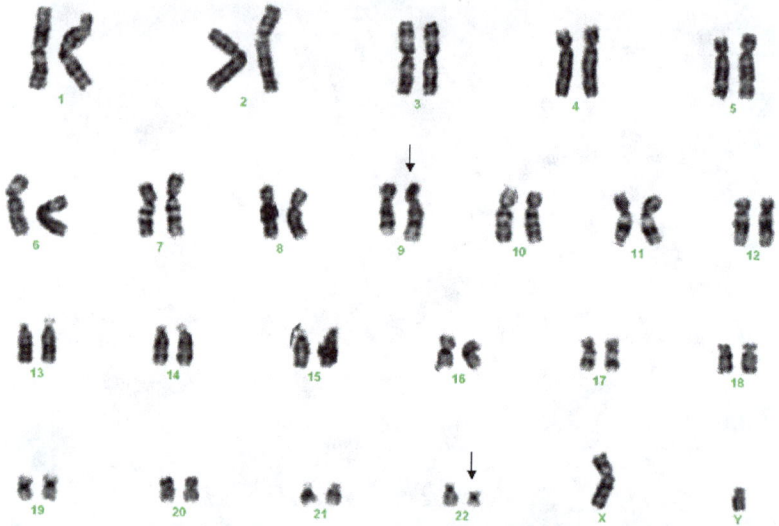

Fig. 9.12. Bone marrow karyogram of a patient with chronic myeloid leukaemia. The two abnormal chromosomes that have been formed as a result of the t(9;22)(q34.1;q11.2) translocation are marked with arrows. The derivative chromosome 22 with an abbreviated long arm is the Philadelphia (Ph) chromosome.

At diagnosis and during monitoring, RT-PCR techniques show greater sensitivity than cytogenetics, and they can also detect a fusion gene in rare cases with a cryptic chromosomal translocation. This has been used to develop quantitative RT-qPCR testing to monitor the proportion of residual leukaemic cells in patients on therapy. RT-qPCR can detect the presence of one leukaemic cell in 10^6 normal cells. If serial measurements of the *BCR::ABL1/ABL1* (leukaemic/normal cells) transcript ratio while on treatment reduce from 100% to 0.1% (a three-log reduction), this is defined as a major molecular response (MMR) to therapy.

Management

Prior to the mid-1990s, CML was mainly treated with hydroxycarbamide and, apart from a small proportion of patients eligible for allogeneic stem cell transplantation, CML was incurable, with a median survival of 5–6 years. The introduction of the oral ABL1 tyrosine kinase inhibitor (TKI) imatinib, followed by next-generation inhibitors, such as nilotinib and dasatanib, has dramatically improved outcomes to the extent that survival rates of patients with CML in the chronic phase are approaching those of age-matched normal controls. TKIs are generally ineffective in advanced-phase disease.

At diagnosis in the chronic phase, patients may be given a short course of treatment with hydroxycarbamide to bring down the elevated WBC count. Risk stratification using prognostic scores may be useful. TKI therapy is started, and the response is monitored at various milestones during treatment (at 3, 6, 12 months and thereafter regularly). The expectation regarding treatment is a gradual reduction in the size of the leukaemic clone. Response to treatment can be measured in terms of the haematological, cytogenetic and/or molecular response. A complete cytogenetic response (CCR) is defined as no Ph-positive metaphases detected in 20 cells. RT-qPCR monitoring measures the ratio of leukaemic (*BCR::ABL1*) to normal (*ABL1*) cDNA transcripts. A major molecular response (MR3) is a three-log *BCR::ABL1/ABL1* ratio reduction (0.1% residual leukaemia). Patients who achieve MR4 (four-log reduction) at 12 months might expect 100% leukaemia-free survival.

TKI treatment is usually continued indefinitely. In patients whose leukaemic clone develops resistance (rising *BCR::ABL1/ABL1* ratio) to multiple lines of TKI therapy and who progress to the advanced-phase disease, the prognosis is poor; however, allogeneic stem cell transplant may offer a small chance of cure.

For those patients who sustain a deep molecular response for more than three years and who meet other stringent criteria, clinical programmes using highly sensitive molecular monitoring may permit a trial of TKI discontinuation to determine whether a treatment-free remission can be sustained.

Chronic Myelomonocytic Leukaemia

The MDS/MPN category includes CMML, a chronic myeloid neoplasm resulting from mutation in a multipotent myeloid progenitor cell; it is characterised by monocytosis (i.e. a monocyte count of at least $1 \times 10^9/l$) and anaemia. It is predominantly a disease of the elderly. Transformation to AML can occur.

Clinical features

Patients may present with symptoms of anaemia or with other systemic symptoms, such as weight loss, fatigue and increased sweating. Some patients may exhibit infection or bleeding. Physical examination may show splenomegaly and, less often, hepatomegaly.

Haematological features

The blood count usually shows leucocytosis, anaemia and, sometimes, thrombocytopenia. Additionally, monocytosis is present (Fig. 9.13). The neutrophil count may be high, normal or low. There may be anisocytosis, poikilocytosis and dysplastic changes in neutrophils (such as hypolobulation and hypogranularity). The bone marrow aspirate shows increased cellularity. Dysplastic features can include sideroblastic erythropoiesis (the presence of erythroblasts with a ring of iron-containing granules around the nucleus). Blast cells may be increased in the blood and the bone marrow but are not as numerous as in AML (less than 20%). Cytogenetic analysis may reveal an acquired clonal abnormality, such as trisomy 8.

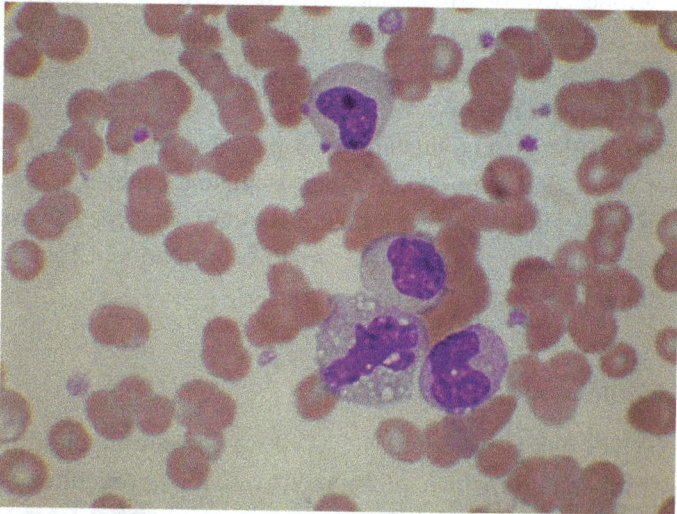

Fig. 9.13.   PB film from a patient with chronic myelomonocytic leukaemia (MGG stain), showing two monocytes (bottom) and two dysplastic neutrophils (top). The neutrophils are hypogranular with defective lobulation.

Diagnosis and differential diagnosis

The differential diagnosis includes a leukaemoid reaction due, for example to infection.

Management

Patients do not necessarily require treatment at diagnosis. If there are symptoms, a blood transfusion and chemotherapy may be beneficial.

Test Case 9.1

A 61-year-old man suffers from chronic obstructive pulmonary disease (COPD) and is on home oxygen therapy. He has recently developed frequent headaches and experiences pruritus after showering. A FBC reveals; Hb 190 g/l (130–175), haematocrit 52 (35–48), WBC 8×10^9/l (3.0–10.0), neutrophils 6×10^9/l (2.0–7.5), lymphocytes 1.5×10^9/l (1.5–4.0), platelets 350×10^9/l (150–400).

Questions

1. What is the most likely diagnosis?
2. Outline appropriate further investigation?
3. How should this be managed?

Write down your answers before checking the correct answer (page 407) and re-reading any relevant part of the chapter.

10

Multiple Myeloma

Aristeidis Chaidos

What Do You Need To Know?

☞ The clinicopathological features of multiple myeloma and other plasma cell disorders associated with paraproteins

☞ Emergencies in multiple myeloma

☞ Principles of treatment and supportive management in multiple myeloma

Introduction

Multiple myeloma is the second-most common blood cancer after lymphomas. It is a malignancy of the terminally differentiated, class-switched and immunoglobulin-secreting plasma cells homing to the bone marrow. The secreted IgG or IgA immunoglobulin is detected in the blood and is known as a paraprotein or M-spike. IgM paraproteins are produced in Waldenstrom's macroglobulinaemia and other low-grade B cell lymphomas. IgM-secreting multiple myeloma is very rare (<1%). Myeloma plasma cells produce an excess of monoclonal free kappa or lambda light chains that are present in serum, and through the kidney filtrate, they are excreted in urine. Bence Jones protein consists of monoclonal free light chains in urine.

The annual incidence of multiple myeloma in Caucasians is six per 100,000 population; however, it is twice as high among black individuals of African or Afro-Caribbean ancestry. The higher incidence in black populations and the sporadic cases of familial multiple myeloma indicate a potential genetic predisposition in myelomagenesis. Old age is another risk factor, and the median age at presentation is 67 years. Only 1% of multiple myeloma patients are younger than 40 years. Obesity is the only modifiable risk factor, with a risk ratio of 1.11 to 1.5, depending on body mass index.

The median overall survival of patients with multiple myeloma has increased from around 3.5 years in the 1990s to >7 years with modern therapies. At least one-third of multiple myeloma patients currently live with their disease beyond 10 years. Thus, the prevalence of multiple myeloma in the community is increasing, driven by advances in therapy and the ageing population. Although the aetiology remains unknown, multiple myeloma is always preceded by monoclonal gammopathy of undetermined significance (MGUS), its asymptomatic premalignant precursor.

Monoclonal gammopathy of undetermined significance

MGUS is the presence of serum paraprotein in concentrations up to 30 g/l and/or monoclonal serum free light chain in the absence of symptoms or end-organ damage. In MGUS, malignant plasma cells account for <10% of all bone marrow cells. MGUS is the most commonly known premalignant condition, occurring in 3–4% of individuals aged 50 years or older. The vast majority of MGUS remains asymptomatic long term, and the average annual risk for progression to multiple myeloma is <1%. MGUS does not require treatment, only clinical monitoring. The Mayo Clinic risk stratification uses the paraprotein concentration (>15 g/l), the subtype (non-IgG) and an abnormal serum free light chain ratio (kappa : lambda <0.26 or >1.65). The probability of progression is just 2% at 20 years for patients without risk factors but increases to 27% for those meeting all three criteria (Table 10.1).

Table 10.1. Plasma cell disorders with paraproteins.

	Laboratory features	Clinical presentation
MGUS	Paraprotein <30 g/l, bone marrow plasma cells <10%	No symptoms
Smouldering multiple myeloma	Paraprotein >30 g/l and/or bone marrow plasma cells 10–60%	No symptoms
Multiple myeloma	Bone marrow plasma cells >10% and myeloma-defining events (CRAB-SLiM)	Myeloma defining events: C: hypercalcaemia R: renal insufficiency A: anaemia B: one or more bone lytic lesions in imaging S: bone marrow plasma cells >60% Li: serum free light chain ratio >100 M: two or more focal lesions in MRI
Solitary Plasmacytoma	Biopsy-proven bone or soft tissue with clonal plasma cells Normal bone marrow Normal imaging beyond solitary lesion	No CRAB-SLiM
Plasma cell leukaemia	Presence of ≥5% circulating myeloma cells	Feature of aggressive myeloma
AL amyloidosis	MGUS and smouldering multiple myeloma or symptomatic multiple myeloma	Proteinuria, including nephrotic syndrome Heart failure Neuropathy Macroglossia Abnormal liver function
MGRS	MGUS or smouldering multiple myeloma	Renal insufficiency Proteinuria
POEMS	Clonal plasma cells in the bone marrow and/or paraprotein High serum VEGF Sclerotic bone lesions	Polyneuropathy Organomegaly Endocrinopathy Oedema or effusions Skin changes Papilloedema Thrombocytosis

Notes: MGUS: monoclonal gammopathy of undetermined significance, MGRS: monoclonal gammopathy of renal significance, POEMS: polyneuropathy, organomegaly, endocrinopathy, sclerotic bone lesions, VEGF: vascular endothelial growth factor.

Smouldering multiple myeloma

Smouldering myeloma is an asymptomatic precursor to multiple myeloma, which evolves from MGUS. It is characterised by 10–60% malignant plasma cells in the bone marrow and/or a serum paraprotein concentration of >30 g/l. The International Myeloma Working Group (IMWG) risk stratification system utilises three criteria: concentration of paraprotein (>20 g/l), marrow infiltration by myeloma plasma cells (>20%) and serum free light chain ratio (>20). Patients with 0–2 criteria are monitored for progression, similar to MGUS. High-risk patients meeting all three criteria have a 47% probability of progression to myeloma at two years. Management of this group remains a matter of controversy, and some studies advocate early treatment to avert progression.

The Pathogenesis of Multiple Myeloma: Genetics and Bone Marrow Microenvironment

Multiple myeloma is characterised by heterogeneous genetics and discrete molecular disease subtypes. Initiating genetic events occur early in myelomagenesis and are present in MGUS and smouldering multiple myeloma. In approximately 40% of patients, the initiating event is a translocation between the locus of heavy chain immunoglobulin genes in chromosome 14q32 and a partner oncogenic driver, commonly *CCND1* in t(11;14), *NSD2/FGFR3* in t(4;14), *MAF* in t(14;16), *MAFB* in t(14;20) and *CCND3* in t(6;14). In the remaining 60%, hyperdiploidy with additional copies of odd-numbered chromosomes (3, 5, 7, 9, 11, 15, 19 and 21) is the primary initiating genetic event. Common secondary genetic events include gain or amplification of chromosome 1q, deletions of chromosome 17p (*TP53* locus), deletions of 1p, *MYC* translocations (especially in hyperdiploid cases) and mutations of the *KRAS*, *NRAS*, *BRAF*, *DIS3* and *FAM46C* genes. In clinical practice, the initiating and main secondary genetic lesions of the malignant plasma cells are analysed using fluorescent in situ hybridisation (FISH) and incorporated into clinical staging and risk stratification systems.

Interactions between myeloma cells and the bone marrow microenvironment support tumour growth, resulting in morbidity and clinical symptoms. Homing of myeloma cells to the endosteal niche suppresses osteoblasts and, via RANKL, activates osteoclastic activity, causing bone resorption, osteolytic lesions, hypercalcaemia, bone pain and fractures (Figs. 10.3 and 10.4). Mesenchymal stromal cells and fibroblasts secrete pro-myeloma cytokines, such as IL-6; in turn, myeloma cells promote marrow angiogenesis and disrupt the normal haematopoietic niche. Multiple myeloma moulds an immunosuppressive microenvironment with Tregs, myeloid-derived suppressor cells, tumour-associated macrophages and impaired natural killer cell maturation, chemotaxis and killing. The multiple myeloma immune microenvironment underlies both the tumour immune evasion during the progression from MGUS and smouldering multiple myeloma to symptomatic disease and the immunodeficiency related infections.

Clinical Presentation and Diagnosis

The diagnostic hallmarks of multiple myeloma are hypercalcaemia, renal disease, anaemia and bone disease (described by the acronym CRAB). The IMWG updated the diagnostic criteria in 2014 to include various biomarkers, called SLiM: >60% plasma cells in bone marrow biopsy (S), serum free light chain ratio >100 (Li) and ≥2 lesions in CT or MRI scan (M). SLiM identifies asymptomatic patients with a high risk for progression (70–95% in two years), who may be managed as those who have symptomatic disease.

Bone lytic lesions are present in 80% of patients at diagnosis, predominantly affecting the proximal skeleton; spine, femurs, rib cage, sternum, humeri and skull. Back pain is common and acute may indicate spinal fracture (Figs. 10.3 and 10.4). Symptomatic anaemia with fatigue, lethargy and dyspnoea is present in 50% of cases, while drowsiness, polyuria and weakness suggest hypercalcaemia. Patients with a very high paraprotein concentration, particularly in IgA multiple myeloma, may develop headache and blurred vision from blood hyperviscosity.

Renal disease is another cardinal manifestation of multiple myeloma, affecting 25% of patients at diagnosis and up to 50% at relapse. It is defined by a serum creatinine level of >177 μmol/l (>2 mg/dl) or an estimated glomerular filtration rate of <40 ml/min. Myeloma kidney disease occurs when excessive amounts of free light chains (>500 mg/l) enter the glomerular filtrate and trigger proximal tubular inflammation and cast formation in the distal tubules. Hypercalcaemia, dehydration, infection and nephrotoxic drugs may contribute; however, only kidney injury from cast nephropathy is recognised as a CRAB diagnostic criterion. Kidney injury that is characterised by lower levels of serum free light chains and non-selective proteinuria (mainly albuminuria with low amounts of Bence Jones protein) indicates either kidney AL amyloidosis or another form of monoclonal gammopathy of renal significance (MGRS). These patients should undergo a kidney biopsy.

Recurrent bacterial and viral infections are often present at diagnosis and may worsen with treatment. Multiple myeloma patients may experience several episodes of varicella zoster virus reactivation, particularly during treatment with proteasome inhibitors. The antibody response to vaccination is suboptimal, and additional booster doses are often required. Severe bacterial and atypical infections are a major source of morbidity, seen with T-cell engagers (TCEs) and chimaeric antigen receptor (CAR)-T cell therapy and also as a result of lymphodepleting chemotherapy, prolonged cytopenias, corticosteroids, anti-IL6 and anti-IL1 drugs used in the management of cytokine release syndrome (CRS) and immune effector cell-associated neurological syndrome (ICANS). Common infections associated with immunotherapy include CMV and EBV reactivation, fungal infections and *Pneumocystis jirovecii* pneumonia; all of these were previously uncommon in myeloma patients.

Emergencies in multiple myeloma

Spinal cord compression or cauda equina from spinal fractures and/or vertebral plasmacytomas are common and require urgent treatment to prevent permanent neurological damage. Impending compression or neurological signs must be investigated urgently through a whole-spine MRI, laboratory tests and a neurosurgical assessment. A spinal mass biopsy may be indicated when the diagnosis of multiple myeloma is not known or uncertain. Unlike cord compression in metastatic solid cancer, spinal plasmacytomas respond very well to radiotherapy, high-dose steroids and systemic chemotherapy, while surgical decompression is usually reserved for bone fragments that compromise the spinal canal.

Hypercalcaemia should be treated with intravenous fluids, zoledronic acid infusion and high-dose steroids in anticipation of systemic chemotherapy. The anti-RANKL antibody denosumab may be used in refractory cases.

Renal failure from myeloma cast nephropathy is a devastating medical emergency; however, with early and appropriate systemic chemotherapy, fluids and electrolyte management, it is potentially reversible. Bortezomib-based triplet or quadruplet combinations aim for a rapid and substantial reduction of serum free light chain levels to permit renal recovery. Efficient treatment of cast nephropathy is of utmost importance, as patients already on renal replacement therapy have a substantially lower chance of overall survival.

Plasma cell disorders beyond multiple myeloma

Systemic AL amyloidosis results from monoclonal, misfolded light chains which form amyloid deposits in various organ targets. The neoplastic plasma cell clone may be small in volume, as in MGUS, or amyloidosis may coexist with symptomatic multiple myeloma. AL amyloidosis may affect several organs, most commonly the kidneys, myocardium, liver, spleen, peripheral nerves, GI tract, tongue and skin. Kidney AL amyloidosis presents with proteinuria, often in the nephrotic range, although renal function is less affected. Symptoms of unexplained heart failure and abnormal free light chains should be investigated for cardiac AL amyloidosis, which is the most severe manifestation and determinant of prognosis. Peripheral neuropathy, abnormal liver function and macroglossia are other clinical features of systemic AL amyloidosis.

MGRS is a group of rare kidney diseases caused by nephrotoxic paraproteins or free light chains. The neoplastic plasma cell burden does not meet haematological criteria for treatment (MGUS and smouldering multiple myeloma). An MGRS diagnosis requires a kidney biopsy. The most common types of MGRS are light chain deposition disease and proliferative glomerulonephritis with monoclonal immunoglobulin deposits.

POEMS is a rare disease characterised by serum paraprotein (almost always lambda subtype), clonal plasma cells in the bone marrow, polyneuropathy, organomegaly, sclerotic bone lesions, endocrinopathy and high blood VEGF levels (Table 10.1).

Laboratory features

Apart from normocytic anaemia, blood counts are preserved in multiple myeloma, while thrombocytopenia only develops in the advanced stages of the disease. When the paraprotein concentration is very high, the blood film background stains abnormally blue and erythrocytes form rouleaux. The erythrocyte sedimentation rate (ESR) is high, often >100 mm/hr, in the presence of high paraprotein and anaemia. Occasional circulating neoplastic plasma cells may be observed in the film but are more easily detected using flow cytometry, and their number holds prognostic significance. When circulating myeloma cells constitute ≥5% of the total white blood cells this condition is referred to as plasma cell leukaemia and it is a feature of aggressive disease.

Biochemical tests usually show elevated serum globulins and diminished albumin levels. Serum protein electrophoresis detects paraprotein as an abnormal band in the gamma or beta region and has a quantification sensitivity of around 2 g/l. Serum immunofixation identifies the subtypes of heavy chains and light chains with a higher sensitivity of around 0.25 g/l (Fig. 10.1). The serum levels of normal immunoglobulins are reduced, a condition known as immune paresis. The serum free light chain assay is an integral part of the myeloma workup and has replaced Bence Jones spot urine tests in screening. Light chain myelomas (20% of all cases) do not secrete a complete paraprotein, only monoclonal kappa or lambda free light chains. Non-secretory myeloma, which is characterised by an absence of serum paraprotein or monoclonal free light chains, is rare (1%). Serum urea, creatinine, uric acid and calcium form the essential biochemistry. The alkaline phosphatase is usually normal, and abnormality high values indicate either a bone fracture or liver AL amyloidosis. Finally, high serum LDH levels indicate proliferative disease, and LDH is a prognostic marker.

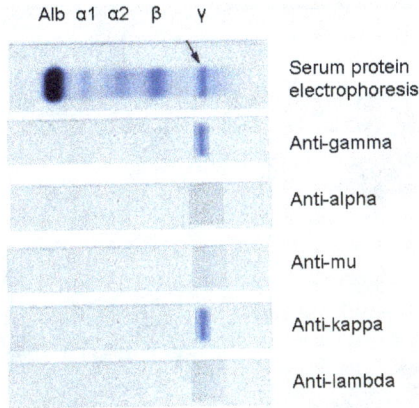

Fig. 10.1. Serum protein electrophoresis incorporated into a diagram to represent immunofixation. With anti-γ and anti-κ antisera, there is a discrete band corresponding to the band on electrophoresis showing the presence of an IgGκ paraprotein. With anti-α, anti-μ and anti-λ antisera, there is diffuse staining representing the background polyclonal immunoglobulins.

The examination of bone marrow films shows an excess of abnormal pleomorphic plasma cells, some of which are binucleated. Plasmablasts are often seen in aggressive or proliferative multiple myeloma. They have less condensed chromatin, obvious nucleoli and a higher nucleocytoplasmic ratio (Fig. 10.2). The extent of marrow infiltration is better assessed using a trephine bone marrow biopsy with immunohistochemistry for CD138, a specific marker of mature plasma cells. Amyloid deposits stain as red amorphous material with Congo Red and produce green birefringence under cross-polarised light. Next-generation flow cytometry in marrow aspirate samples may be used for measurable residual disease (MRD) assessment after treatment and produces results similar to those obtained with next-generation sequencing.

Imaging

Conventional X-ray skeletal surveys have low sensitivity, missing up to 25% of patients with lytic bone disease, and are nowadays considered obsolete in determining this condition. Instead, low-dose whole-body non-contrast CT scans effectively detect small lytic lesions and, with

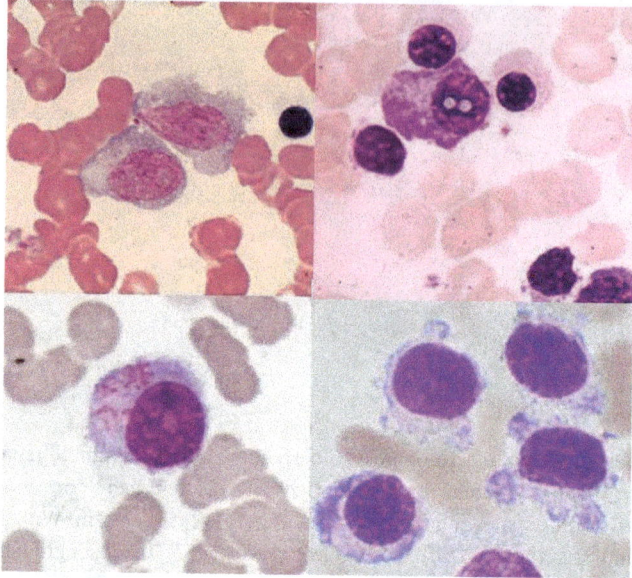

Fig. 10.2. BM aspirate films from four patients with multiple myeloma showing different cytological abnormalities: plasmablasts, a lack of chromatin condensation and nucleoli (top left); globules of immunoglobulin overlying nucleus (top right); cytoplasmic granules and crystals in a nucleolated myeloma cell (bottom left); and plasma cells with a high nucleocytoplasmic ratio and cytoplasmic blebs (bottom right).

some limitations, extra-skeletal deposits. Irradiation exposure from low-dose CT scans is comparable to that of conventional X-ray skeletal surveys. Therefore, CT is now the recommended modality for screening in MGUS or suspected multiple myeloma (Fig. 10.3). More sensitive techniques include the ^{18}F-FDG-PET-CT scan, which detects tumour cells with abnormally high glucose metabolism, and whole-body diffuse-weighted MRI, which analyses tissue water and fat composition and the movement of water molecules to provide information on cellularity. Whole-body MRI and ^{18}F-FDG-PET-CT scans accurately assess patterns of diffuse marrow infiltration and focal osseous lesions, which are dense myelomatous infiltrates and differ from osteolytic disease (Fig. 10.4). Both imaging techniques differentiate treated from untreated lesions, describe extramedullary plasmacytomas or bone expansile soft tissue and are integrated into both the diagnostic CRAB-SLiM criteria and MRD assessment.

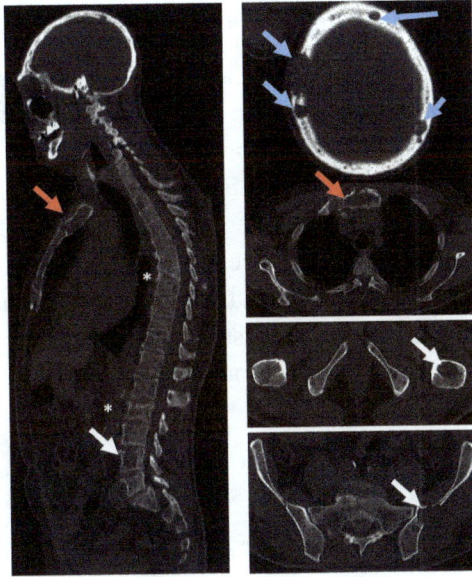

Fig. 10.3. Low-dose non contrast CT skeletal survey Sagittal and axial bone windows in a case of myeloma. Multiple lytic bone lesions, manubrium (red arrows), skull vault (blue arrows), femora, pelvis, spine (white arrows). Note several compression fractures in the spine (*). *Images courtesy of Prof Tara Barwick, Imperial College Healthcare NHS Trust.*

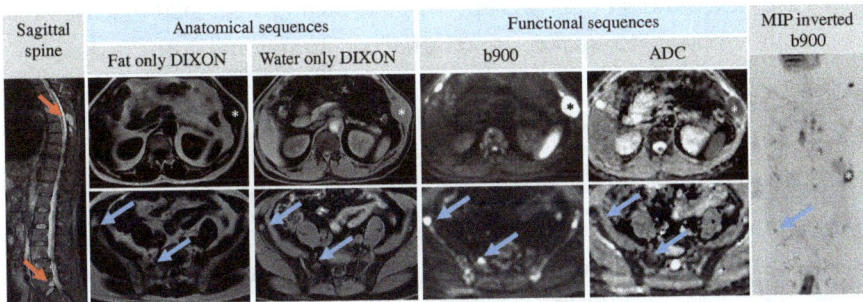

Fig. 10.4 Myeloma. Whole body diffusion MRI showing multiple sites of focal osseous disease on the anatomical sequences and diffusions weighted imaging (functional sequnces) which detects hypercellular lesions. Lesions include expansile left lower rib lesion (*), spine lesions (red arrows) and focal pelvic bone lesions (blue arrows). ADC, apparent diffusion coefficient; MIP, maximum intensity projection; MRI, magnetic resonance imaging. *Images courtesy of Prof Tara Barwick, Imperial College Healthcare NHS Trust.*

Clinical stages and risk stratification

The International Staging System (ISS) provides prognostic information for survival by utilising two simple clinical parameters, serum beta-2 microglobulin and serum albumin, to capture the disease burden and host factors, respectively. The Revised-ISS (R-ISS) incorporates disease biology and includes the high-risk cytogenetic abnormalities t(4;14), t(14;16), del 17p and elevated serum LDH levels. More than one high-risk cytogenetic abnormality, a scenario referred to as double-hit or triple-hit multiple myeloma, and early relapse from first-line treatment are also features of high-risk disease and are linked to poor outcomes.

Management of Multiple Myeloma

The treatment landscape for multiple myeloma has rapidly evolved over the past 25 years, offering outstanding overall response rates and prolonged periods of disease-free survival. Traditionally, multiple myeloma was viewed as an incurable malignancy which relapses after initial treatment and, over subsequent years, becomes a remitting–relapsing disease before evolving into a multi-refractory terminal cancer. However, recent advances in immunotherapy in combination with proteasome inhibitors (PI), immunomodulatory drugs (IMiD) and the new-generation cereblon E3 ligase modulators (CelMoD) produce deep and sustained disease control, long enough to make operational or functional cure a tangible objective for many patients.

Thalidomide was the first novel drug introduced to multiple myeloma treatment in the late 1990s for its presumed anti-angiogenic properties. Thalidomide revolutionised first-line treatment, replacing conventional cytotoxics, and it improved outcomes after autologous stem cell transplantation. Lenalidomide and pomalidomide are derivatives belonging to the same class, but with higher potency and more favourable toxicity profiles. Iberdomide and mezigdomide are newer CelMoDs that induce remarkable clinical responses in heavily treated, refractory multiple myeloma.

Bortezomib is a prototype PI that was introduced in 2003 for the treatment of relapsed multiple myeloma. Carfilzomib is more potent and effective in bortezomib-refractory disease, and ixazomib is an oral drug with a favourable safety profile. PI, IMiD and dexamethasone combinations exert strong clinical synergy and used to constitute the backbone of multiple myeloma therapy before the advent of immunotherapy.

The anti-CD38 monoclonal antibody daratumumab became the first clinically licensed immunotherapy for multiple myeloma in 2015. Daratumumab, in combination with bortezomib, thalidomide and dexamethasone (D-VTD), is the current induction therapy for autologous stem cell transplant-eligible patients. Other daratumumab combinations with PI and IMiD are approved for use in the relapsed setting. Isatuximab became the second approved anti-CD38 antibody for the treatment of relapsed multiple myeloma in combination with PI and/or IMiD.

B cell maturation antigen (BCMA) is a transmembrane receptor of the tumour necrosis factor superfamily, specifically expressed in normal and malignant plasma cells. BCMA expression beyond plasma cells is minimal, making it an ideal immunotherapeutic target.

Belantamab-mafadotin is an anti-BCMA antibody conjugate with the toxin monomethyl auristatin F, which exhibits efficacy in multi-refractory multiple myeloma. The main limiting toxicity is keratopathy, which has been observed to be ameliorated with appropriate treatment intervals and dose adjustments.

T-cell engagers (TCEs) are synthetic IgG-like or non-IgG-like molecules with specificity for both tumour targets and the CD3 molecule of T-cell receptors. TCEs facilitate the physical contact between T-cell effectors and tumour cells and activate T-cell cytotoxic killing in a co-stimulatory independent manner. Teclistamab and elranatamab are the first BCMAxCD3 TCEs approved for the treatment of relapsed and refractory multiple myeloma. Both demonstrated remarkable response rates of over 70%, including in patients with high-risk disease and extramedullary plasmacytomas. TCE immunotherapy is readily available and feasible even for unfit, elderly patients.

Idecabtagene vicleucel (ide-cel) and ciltacabtagene autoleucel (cilta-cel) are the first anti-BCMA CAR-T cells approved for the treatment of relapsed multiple myeloma. Ide-cel and cilta-cel produce unprecedented overall response rates for this patient population (71% and 84%, respectively) and MRD-negative complete responses in 20% and

60%, respectively. In one study the median PFS with ide-cel was 13.1 months, and with cilta-cel 78% of patients remained in remission at 12 months. Beyond BCMA, TCE and CAR-T cells in multiple myeloma are being developed against GPRC5D and the FcRL5 surface proteins.

Cytokine release syndrome (CRS) and immune effector cell-associated neurotoxicity syndrome (ICANS) are notable side effects of TCE and CAR-T cell therapy, and they mostly occur in the early days following treatment. CRS and ICANS are more frequent and severe with CAR-T cell therapy (see Chapter 14). Late toxicity of TCE and CAR-T cell therapy includes prolonged cytopenias and hypoglobulinaemia, leading to infections and delayed neurotoxicity, including parkinsonian-like and neurocognitive disorders.

The plethora of available drugs allows for several combinations to be used in newly diagnosed and relapsed patients. Current treatment algorithms are adjusted to a diverse clinical spectrum. Determinants of the treatment plan include: patient-related factors, such as age, performance status, frailty, organ function and comorbidities; biology, as defined by cytogenetics, extramedullary disease and early relapse; refractoriness and toxicities from previous treatments; and finally, patient preference, goals and expectations, along with other aspects impacting their quality of life.

Younger (usually <70 years) and fit patients at diagnosis are usually eligible for autologous stem cell transplantation (ASCT). Induction therapy with three or four cycles of D-VTD or a similar regimen is followed by peripheral blood stem cell mobilisation, high-dose melphalan-conditioned ASCT and consolidation with two cycles of D-VTD. The importance of long-term lenalidomide maintenance after ASCT has been demonstrated in several clinical trials, and maintenance is now considered integral to first-line treatment.

Patients not eligible for ASCT at diagnosis may be treated with daratumumab, lenalidomide and dexamethasone until progression. Alternative options include triplet or quadruplet combinations of anti-CD38, PI and oral low-dose alkylators. In recent years, frailty has been recognised as a crucial determinant of treatment choice in this population. Elderly patients may be classified as fit, unfit or frail, and treatment is tailored accordingly.

The remarkable efficacy of modern myeloma treatments has consequently shifted treatment objectives and expectations. MRD-negative CR is currently the optimal treatment outcome, and several studies demonstrate its importance for PFS and OS. Moreover, sustained MRD-negative status over >12 months represents a more stringent yet powerful predictor of outcomes.

Supportive therapy is as important as systemic chemotherapy in the management of multiple myeloma. The bisphosphonate zoledronic acid, along with vitamin D and calcium supplements, reduces bone pain and skeletal events and is recommended for all multiple myeloma patients at diagnosis for at least one year. Vertebroplasty, kyphoplasty and spinal bracing are used to stabilise the spine and reduce pain and fracture risk. Thromboprophylaxis is required during treatment with IMiD and CelMoD, especially when the disease burden is high. Vaccinations, anti-microbial prophylaxis, growth factors (G-CSF) and IVIg replacement are amalgamated into treatment protocols. Finally, radiotherapy can be used for pain palliation and to treat plasmacytomas, especially when they compromise organs.

Conclusions

Multiple myeloma is the second-most common blood cancer, with an increasing prevalence. MGUS and smouldering multiple myeloma are asymptomatic precursors but are occasionally linked to AL amyloidosis, MGRS and POEMS, which are rare but devastating conditions. Bone disease, kidney cast nephropathy, anaemia and infections are the clinical hallmarks of symptomatic multiple myeloma. Cord compression, hypercalcaemia and renal failure are notable emergencies. Patients with multiple myeloma have experienced dramatic improvements in their outcomes over the past 25 years. The recent addition of TCE and CAR-T cell therapy to the treatment arsenal offers deep and durable disease responses and prolongs survival in patients with relapsed disease. Although most patients eventually succumb to refractory disease, operational cure is increasingly achievable.

Test Case 10.1

A 67-year-old man has a six-month history of fatigue, backache and recurrent chest infections. Over a 48-hour period, he develops worsening back pain, weakness affecting his legs and difficulty passing urine. His GP arranges investigations: FBC shows WBC 7.8×10^9/l, Hb 95 g/l (normal range, NR: 118–148), MCV 106 fl (NR: 82–98) and platelet count 102×10^9/l; the ESR is 74 mm in one hour (NR: 0–20); serum calcium is 2.8 mmol/l (NR: 2.15–2.55); IgG is elevated at 35 g/l (NR: 6–16); other immunoglobulins (IgA and IgM) are reduced.

Questions

1. What further laboratory investigations are required?
2. Describe an initial management plan.

Write down your answers before checking the correct answer (page 407) or re-reading any relevant part of the chapter.

11

Platelets, Coagulation and Haemostasis

Andrew Godfrey

What Do You Need To Know?

☞ How haemostasis is initiated and propagated

☞ The function of the platelet

☞ How coagulation is controlled and blood clots are lysed

☞ The coagulation cascade *in vivo* and *in vitro*

☞ How to interpret coagulation screening tests

☞ Point-of-care testing in haemostasis

☞ The clinicopathological features and diagnosis of the most common inherited defects of coagulation

☞ The clinicopathological features and diagnosis of common acquired defects of coagulation

☞ The principles of treatment of coagulation abnormalities

☞ The causes, investigation and management of thrombocytopenia, including autoimmune thrombocytopenic purpura and thrombotic thrombocytopenic purpura

Overview of Haemostasis

There are many stimulants for haemostasis, including vessel wall damage, inflammation and turbulent flow within blood vessels. Although the primary physiological function of haemostasis is to prevent blood loss after vessel wall damage, the coagulation system has a role in both healing and immune function.

When a vessel wall is damaged or breached, the blood is exposed to molecules that initiate the process of haemostasis or coagulation, resulting in the formation of a stable clot that prevents death from haemorrhage. Once initiated, a clot will propagate by positive feedback until the damaged area in the vessel wall is closed. At the same time, processes that ultimately dissolve the clot are initiated and healing commences. Intricate anticoagulant mechanisms are also activated, which prevent the propagation of the clot away from the area of damage; obstruction of blood flow in other vessels is thus prevented. The haemostatic process can be usefully divided into primary and secondary haemostasis, although in fact they are initiated and progress more or less simultaneously.

When this process occurs outside of the context of vessel wall damage, the natural tendency of clots to propagate is the cause of thrombotic disorders, such as deep vein thrombosis and pulmonary embolism. A tendency to develop venous thromboembolism can occur under conditions that result in excess stimulation of the coagulation system (e.g. antiphospholipid syndrome), overactivity of the coagulation factors (e.g. factor V Leiden) or a deficiency in a natural anticoagulant system (e.g. protein S deficiency).

Primary haemostasis: Platelets

A breach of the vessel wall exposes collagen and other elements of the extracellular matrix to which plasma von Willebrand factor (vWF) and platelets will bind, a process enhanced by the shear stress of blood flow. vWF has multiple binding sites to other factors involved in the coagulation cascade and exists in multimeric form in the blood. Once vWF is bound to collagen, this facilitates the binding of more platelets. During the process of binding, platelets become activated through a number of different chemical signals within the blood and vessel walls. Once stimulated, the platelets undergo a conformational change, releasing adenosine diphosphate (ADP), thromboxane A2 and vWF so that additional platelets are captured and activated. The result is the formation of a primary platelet plug, which blocks further loss of blood.

There are additional roles in coagulation for the immune system, notably the neutrophils, which are stimulated by activated platelets to release neutrophil extracellular traps (NETs). These NETs play a primary role in the phagocytosis of bacteria but a secondary role in the recruitment of further activated platelets, binding to vWF and activation of factor XII.

Secondary haemostasis: Coagulation

Blood escaping from a damaged blood vessel is exposed to tissue factor, which is expressed at high levels on cells surrounding the vessel, forming what has been called a 'haemostatic envelope'. Tissue factor binds to factor VII in plasma, forming an activated complex, and thus blood coagulation is initiated. This is called the 'extrinsic pathway' because tissue factor is regarded as extrinsic to the blood. It is the physiological pathway for coagulation activation *in vivo*. The tissue factor–factor VII complex converts factor X into its active form (Xa) by proteolytic cleavage, and Xa is now able to convert a small amount of prothrombin (factor II) into thrombin, again by proteolytic cleavage (Fig. 11.1).

Thrombin generation is an important step in the common coagulation pathway, as thrombin has numerous positive feedback actions within the remainder of the coagulation pathway. A crucial action of this thrombin is to convert the two co-factors, factor V and factor VIII, into their active forms: factor VIIIa and factor Va are not enzymes but greatly increase the activity of the enzymes factor IXa (also activated by the tissue factor–factor VII complex) and factor Xa by approximately five orders of magnitude. The result is a major amplification of the original stimulus and an enormous burst of thrombin generation (Fig. 11.2).

Although we use laboratory tests, such as the activated partial thromboplastin time (APTT) and the prothrombin time (PT), to measure the coagulation system, measuring the thrombin generation potential offers a

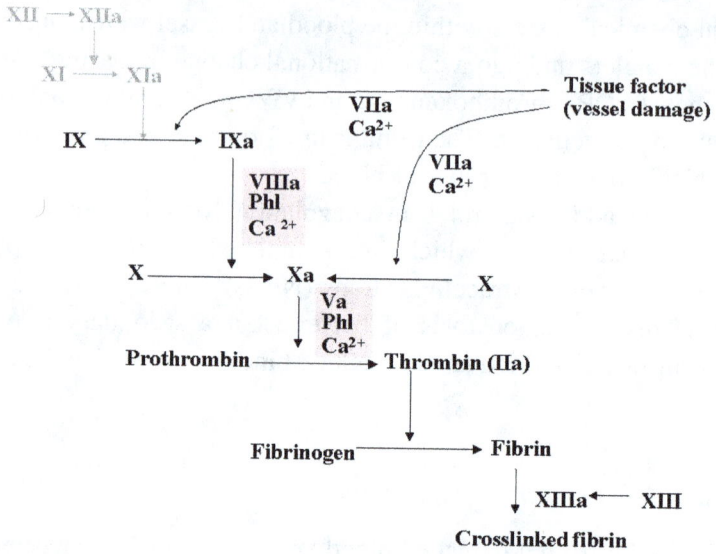

Fig. 11.1. The first steps of *in vivo* coagulation. Phl denotes phospholipid provided by activated platelets.

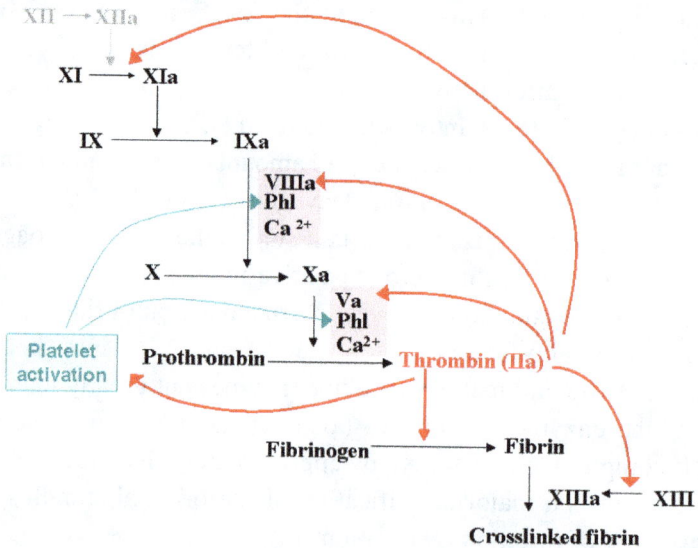

Fig. 11.2. Enhancement of *in vivo* coagulation by thrombin that is generated (red arrows) and by activated platelets (green arrows). It will be seen that factor XII has no role in *in vivo* coagulation.

significantly better way of assessing the potential of the coagulation cascade to form a thrombus. Although this test is difficult to conduct in large quantities in clinical scenarios, it is commonly quoted in the scientific literature.

The final stage is the thrombin-induced cleavage of fibrinopeptides A and B from fibrinogen to form fibrin monomers. These monomers form dimers and then polymers. The process is completed by the thrombin activation of factor XIII, which cross-links the fibrin monomers to form a stable clot. Soluble fibrinogen is thus converted into stable insoluble fibrin. Fibrin binds and stabilises the platelet plug, which is otherwise prone to disaggregation, so that, finally, there is a firm and insoluble clot composed of fibrin, platelets and other blood cells. In addition to leading to the formation of a clot, thrombin activates thrombin-activatable fibrinolysis inhibitor (TAFI), thus contributing to the maintenance of a stable clot.

Most of the coagulation factors are synthesised by hepatocytes. Exceptions are vWF, which is synthesised by endothelial cells and megakaryocytes, and factor VIII, which is also synthesised by endothelial cells.

Platelet structure and function: Platelet interaction with coagulation factors

Platelets are formed in the bone marrow by the fragmentation of megakaryocyte cytoplasm. They enter the circulating blood when they are shed into bone marrow sinusoids. Each megakaryocyte can produce about 4,000 platelets. Platelets survive in the circulation for about 10 days before being removed by splenic macrophages. A platelet has surface receptors and cytoplasmic granules that are crucial to its function (Fig. 11.3). Platelets are activated by ADP and thrombin and by adhesion to constituents of the extracellular matrix, all of which bind to specific receptors. Activated platelets become adherent, undergo a release reaction and form aggregates with other platelets. vWF is essential for normal platelet adhesion. Once activated, platelets release their granule contents, which include procoagulants and aggregants, such as ADP, vWF, factor V and fibrinogen. They also release serotonin, which causes smooth muscle contraction and thus arteriolar constriction. Fibrinogen, factor V and

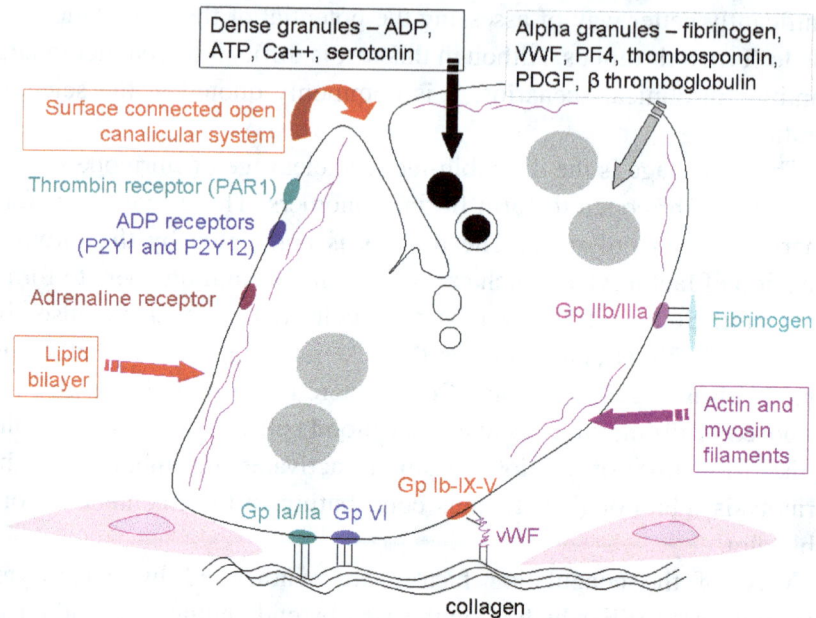

Fig. 11.3. A diagram of a platelet showing some of the components that are crucial for function. The platelet is enclosed by a lipid bilayer membrane, which when altered by platelet activation, provides phospholipid to interact with factors IXa, VIIIa and Ca^{++}, as well as with factors Xa, Va and Ca^{++}. The membrane lipid is also the source of arachidonic acid, which is converted by cyclo-oxygenase to thromboxane A2, a potent aggregant. Embedded in the membrane are various receptors: a thrombin receptor; several types of receptor for adenosine diphosphate (ADP); an adrenaline receptor; platelet glycoprotein (Gp) IIb/IIIa which, when its conformation is altered, is able to bind fibrinogen; GpIa/IIa and Gp VI, both of which can bind to exposed collagen; and Gp Ib-IX-V, which can bind to VWF and thus to collagen. Activated platelets are bound to each other by fibrinogen molecules, which bind to altered Gp IIb/IIIa on adjacent platelets. The platelet has various types of granules, among which are the dense bodies (containing ADP, adenosine triphosphate (ATP), serotonin (a vasoconstrictor) and Ca^{++}) and the α granules (containing fibrinogen, fibronectin, VWF, platelet factor 4 (PF4, a heparin antagonist), thrombospondin, platelet derived growth factor (PDGF) and β thromboglobulin). When platelets are activated, granule contents are discharged into the surface-connected canalicular system and are thus able to activate other platelets. Both thromboxane A2 and ADP enhance platelet aggregation induced by weak aggregants. Platelet shape is maintained by actin and myosin filaments, which are responsible for platelet contraction after activation.

serotonin have previously been taken up from plasma. Thromboxane A2, a vasoconstrictor and potent aggregant, is generated by cyclo-oxygenase from arachidonic acid, which is released from membrane phospholipids. Activation also causes the rearrangement of membrane phospholipids so that the negatively charged phosphatidyl serine is exposed and facilitates blood coagulation. Platelets become spherical and adhere to each other, forming a loose platelet plug, which also adheres to the site of tissue damage.

The assembly of enzyme–cofactor–substrate complexes by binding to negatively charged phospholipid surfaces provided by activated platelets is an important element of the coagulation pathway. The activation of the platelets is also completed by the action of thrombin; therefore, the primary and secondary coagulation mechanisms function together and are interdependent.

The vessel wall and haemostasis

A primary function of the vessel wall in health is to prevent thrombosis and to maintain the flow of blood. This is achieved by the surface expression of molecules with an anticoagulant function, such as tissue factor pathway inhibitor, thrombomodulin, heparans and the endothelial protein C receptor. The vessel wall also acts as a direct barrier to the collagen and factor VII expressed in the extravascular cellular space.

The endothelium also actively releases prostacyclin and nitric oxide (NO), which inhibit platelet activation. These processes can be downregulated in response to inflammation or injury, and in response to damage, a vasoconstrictor response will also act to reduce blood loss.

In Vitro Coagulation

Blood that is shed from the body forms a clot. Coagulation is initiated by contact with various negatively charged surfaces, including glass. This route, known as 'contact activation', is considered the 'intrinsic pathway' because it appears to be an intrinsic property of the blood. The contact

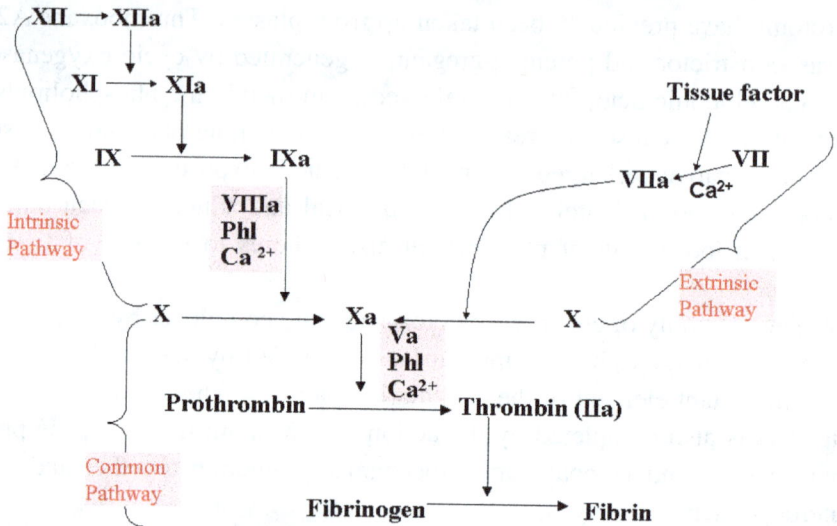

Fig. 11.4. Blood coagulation *in vitro*. The intrinsic and extrinsic systems are conceived as separate entities. It will be seen that, *in vitro*, factor XII has a significant role in contact activation and the intrinsic pathway.

pathway utilises factor XII (as well as prekallikrein and high-molecular-weight kininogen), but the initiation of coagulation by the contact pathway is not an important route for coagulation *in vivo*, and deficiencies of these factors do not result in an increased tendency to bleeding. The other components of the intrinsic pathway (e.g. factors IX and VIII) that are not directly stimulated by contact activation are important in secondary haemostasis, and deficiencies of these factors form the basis of the bleeding disorders haemophilia A (low factor VIII) and haemophilia B (low factor IX).

Understanding laboratory tests of coagulation requires knowledge of the intrinsic and extrinsic pathways as they operate *in vitro* (Fig. 11.4). This is somewhat different from the complex interactions that occur *in vivo*. The two pathways share a final common pathway.

Limitation of Coagulation and Fibrinolysis

Flowing blood does not clot in normal blood vessels since endothelial cells provide a barrier between the blood and procoagulant extracellular proteins, such as collagen and tissue factor. In addition, endothelial cells secrete NO and prostacyclin. Both of these dilate vessels and inhibit platelet aggregation. Endothelial cells also express thrombomodulin, which helps to limit coagulation. Normally, coagulation occurs only at the site of injury since that is where tissue factor is activated and where platelets are exposed to the subendothelial matrix; the platelet aggregates that form at that site tether the developing clot and help to limit it to that site.

The coagulation cascade leads to a rapid generation of procoagulant proteins so that haemostasis is achieved and blood loss is limited. However, if this process were not limited, extensive unwanted thrombosis would ensue. Uncontrolled thrombin generation would convert the entire circulatory system into a thrombus. Coagulation is normally localised to the site of injury and is controlled by a number of naturally occurring anticoagulant proteins, which are activated during haemostasis. These anticoagulants include protein S, protein C and antithrombin and will be discussed in Chapter 12.

Once haemostasis has been achieved and the vessel wall damage has healed, it is desirable for the blood clot to be lysed so that blood flow is restored to the previously damaged tissue. This is achieved by a process known as fibrinolysis. Fibrinolysis is initiated by the formation of the fibrin clot itself. The formation of fibrin exposes binding sites for tissue plasminogen activator and plasminogen, both of which are normally present in plasma but are now brought into close proximity. This greatly facilitates the conversion of plasminogen into the active fibrinolytic enzyme, plasmin, by the tissue plasminogen activator (Fig. 11.5). Thus, plasmin generation is usually limited to the region of the clot, and if plasmin diffuses into plasma, it is inactivated by the circulating plasmin inhibitor (also known as $\alpha 2$ antiplasmin). Plasmin cleaves fibrin to form fibrin degradation products (among which is D-dimer). There are also other physiological activators of plasminogen, but these are probably more important in extravascular tissues (Fig. 11.5). Plasmin has an extremely short half-life in the circulation — in the absence of fibrin, this is less than one second, and once bound to fibrin, it is around 10 seconds. This short half-life ensures that the effects of plasmin are localised to the thrombus *in situ* and do not affect the activity of the coagulation system elsewhere in the body.

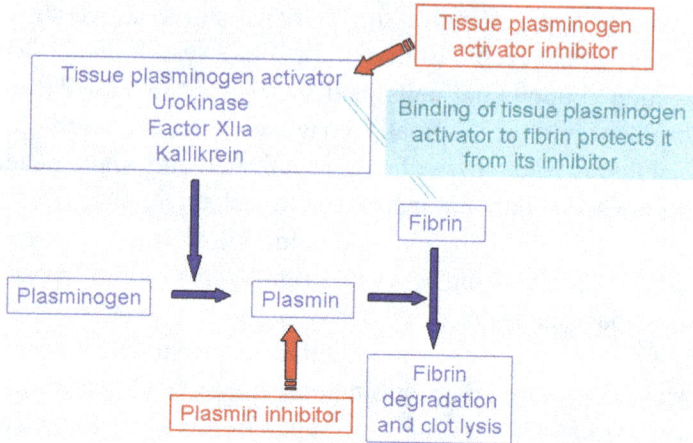

Fig. 11.5. A diagram illustrating fibrinolysis. Inhibitors are shown in red.

Box 11.1.
**Differences between bleeding due to platelet defects
and bleeding due to coagulation factor deficiency**

Bleeding due to thrombocytopenia or platelet functional defects is mainly into the skin and mucous membranes (epistaxis, bleeding gums and menorrhagia) and occurs immediately following injury.

Bleeding due to a coagulation factor deficiency is mainly into deep tissues, such as muscles and joints, and may be delayed.

Assessment of Coagulation Status

Assessment of coagulation status requires both a clinical assessment and laboratory tests. Depending on the clinical features, it may be necessary to assess both the adequacy of coagulation factors and platelet number and function (Box 11.1).

Clinical assessment of coagulation

A clinical assessment includes personal and family history, drug history and a physical examination. The clinical history includes that of the presenting complaint and of previous bleeding episodes, while also taking note of the patient's response to previous haemostatic challenges. The International Society for Thrombosis and Haemostasis has published a clinical scoring system, called the Bleeding Assessment Tool (BAT; Table 11.1), which includes questions relevant to haemostasis. Where a bleeding disorder is suspected, a BAT should be performed. The history is complex and includes spontaneous bleeding, physiological bleeding (such as menorrhagia) and provoked bleeding (after surgery or dental intervention). Mothers of

Table 11.1. The ISTH Bleeding Assessment Tool.

Epistaxis		Oral cavity bleeding	
None/trivial	0 Points	None/trivial	0 Points
>5/ year or >10 minutes	1 Point	>5/ year or >10 minutes	1 Point
Consultation only	2 Points	Consultation only	2 Points
Packing/cauterisation/antifibrinolytic agents	3 Points	Surgical haemostasis or antifibrinolytic agent	3 Points
Blood transfusion or replacement agents (- haemostatic components/ rVIIa) or desmopressin	4 Points	Blood transfusion or replacement agents or desmopressin	4 Points
Cutaneous bruising		**GI bleeding**	
None/trivial	0 Points	None/trivial	0 Points
5 or more (>1cm) in exposed areas	1 Point	Present — not associated with portal hypertension, ulcer, haemorrhoids or angiodysplasia	1 Point
Consultation only	2 Points	Consultation only	2 Points
Extensive	3 Points	Surgical haemostasis or antifibrinolytic agent	3 Points
Spontaneous requiring blood transfusion	4 Points	Blood transfusion or replacement agents or desmopressin	4 Points
Bleeding from minor wounds		**Haematuria**	
None/trivial	0 Points	None/trivial	0 Points
>5/ year or >10 minutes	1 Point	Present — macroscopic	1 Point

(*Continued*)

Table 11.1.   (*Continued*)

Consultation only	2 Points	Consultation only	2 Points
Surgical haemostasis	3 Points	Surgical haemostasis, iron therapy	3 Points
Blood transfusion or replacement agents or desmopressin	4 Points	blood transfusion or replacement agents or desmopressin	4 Points

Bleeding following dental extractions		**Menorrhagia**	
None/trivial or no extractions	0 Points	None/trivial	0 Points
Reported in ≤ 25% of procedures, no interventions	1 Point	Consultation only	1 Point
Reported in > 25% of procedures, no interventions	2 Points	Time off work/school >2 × year/minor therapy	2 Points
Surgical haemostasis or antifibrinolytic agent	3 Points	Requiring combined treatment with antifibrinolytic agents and hormonal therapy	3 Points
Blood transfusion or replacement agents or desmopressin	4 Points	Acute menorrhagia requiring hospital admission and emergency treatment	4 Points

Bleeding associated with surgery		**Post-partum haemorrhage**	
None/trivial or none done	0 Points	None/trivial or no deliveries	0 Points
Reported in ≤ 25% of procedures, no interventions	1 Point	Consultation only	1 Point
Reported in > 25% of procedures, no interventions	2 Points	Iron or fibrinolytic therapy	2 Points
Surgical haemostasis or antifibrinolytic agent	3 Points	Requiring blood transfusion, replacement agents, desmopressin	3 Points
Blood transfusion or replacement agents or desmopressin	4 Points	Any surgical intervention	4 Points

Muscle haematomas		**CNS bleeding**	
Never	0 Points	Never	0 points
Post-trauma, no therapy	1 Point	Subdural, any intervention	3 Points
Spontaneous, no therapy	2 Points	Intracerebral, any intervention	4 Points

Table 11.1.   *(Continued)*

Spontaneous or traumatic requiring desmopressin or replacement therapy	3 Points
Spontaneous or traumatic requiring surgical intervention or blood transfusion	4 Points

Haemarthrosis		Other bleeding problems	
Never	0 Points	None/trivial	0 Points
Post-trauma, no therapy	1 Point	Present	1 Point
Spontaneous no therapy	2 Points	Consultation only	2 Points
Spontaneous or traumatic requiring desmopressin or replacement therapy	3 Points	Surgical haemostasis or antifibrinolytic agent	3 Points
Spontaneous or traumatic requiring surgical intervention or blood transfusion	4 Points	Blood transfusion or replacement agents or desmopressin	4 Points
Normal total score for adult males	**0–3**		
Normal total score for adult females	**0–5**		
Normal total score for children (age <18)	**0–2**		

children should be asked if there was bleeding from the umbilical cord or following the circumcision of male infants. If there has been previous haemorrhage, the nature and severity must be assessed. It is diagnostically important to know if bleeding is characteristic of a platelet defect or of a coagulation factor deficiency (see Box 11.1). The severity of haemorrhage can be established by an assessment of the duration of bleeding, how much blood was lost and whether hospitalisation or blood transfusion was required. Family history should include not only parents and siblings but also male maternal relatives since some congenital coagulation factor deficiencies have an X-linked recessive inheritance. The drug history should include establishing if the patient is taking aspirin or a nonsteroidal anti-inflammatory agent which interferes with platelet function.

Table 11.2.   Some terminology used in coagulation.

Term	Meaning
Purpura	Bleeding into the skin and mucous membranes (can be thrombocytopenic or non-thrombocytopenic)
Petechia (plural petechiae)	Pinpoint cutaneous haemorrhages, a form of purpura
Ecchymosis (plural ecchymoses)	Large cutaneous haemorrhages, a form of purpura
Bruise	Bleeding into subcutaneous tissues

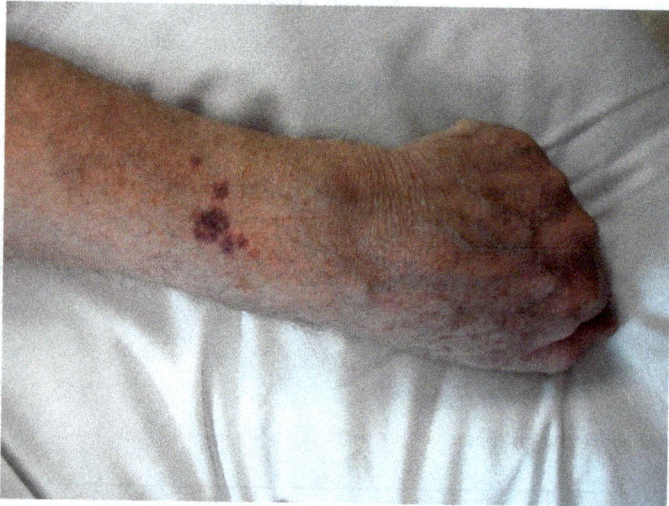

Fig. 11.6.   'Senile purpura' on the arm of an elderly man. This type of purpura occurs particularly on the hands and arms and is due to atrophy of soft tissues with ageing.

The ISTH bleeding assessment tool

Physical examination should look for evidence of haemorrhage, including the presence of petechiae, ecchymoses or bruises (see Table 11.2), bleeding from venepuncture sites and any systemic disease that could cause abnormal haemostasis, such as liver or renal disease. Evidence should be sought for any inherited or acquired blood vessel or connective tissue abnormality, such as 'senile purpura' (Fig. 11.6), scurvy (perifollicular haemorrhage and corkscrew hairs), abnormally large or delicate scars, hereditary haemorrhagic telangiectasia (telangiectasia on lips or tongue) or Ehlers–Danlos syndrome, which could cause haemorrhage.

A number of other systemic illnesses are associated with disorders in platelet function or thrombosis. These include inherited conditions such as occulocutaeous albinism (associated with various types of platelet function disorder) and acquired conditions, including autoimmune disorders such as systemic lupus erythematosus (SLE) or systemic vasculitis.

Laboratory assessment of coagulation

A 'coagulation screen' always includes a prothrombin time and an activated partial thromboplastin time. It may also include a thrombin time and an assay of fibrinogen. Coagulation tests are usually performed on platelet-poor plasma, i.e. plasma from blood that has been anticoagulated with sodium citrate and centrifuged to remove platelets. A platelet count should be performed, and a blood film should be examined since some congenital defects of platelet function are associated with large platelets or poorly granulated platelets (Fig. 11.7). It is important to note that the 'coagulation screen' tests only a very small portion of the entire haemostatic

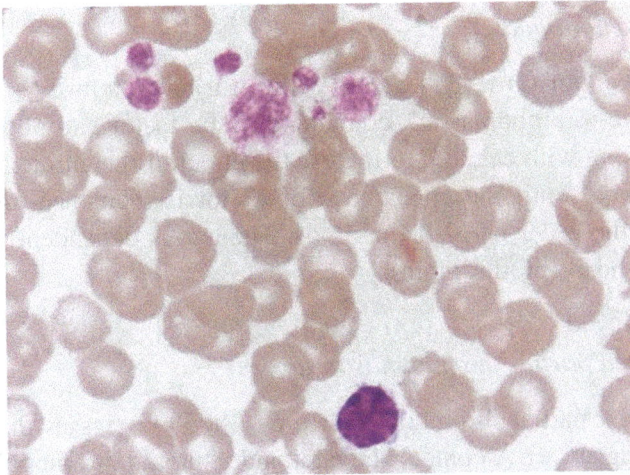

Fig. 11.7.   Blood film of one of two sisters with autosomal recessive thrombocytopenia with giant platelets and impaired platelet function (suspected Bernard–Soulier syndrome). May–Grünwald–Giemsa stain.

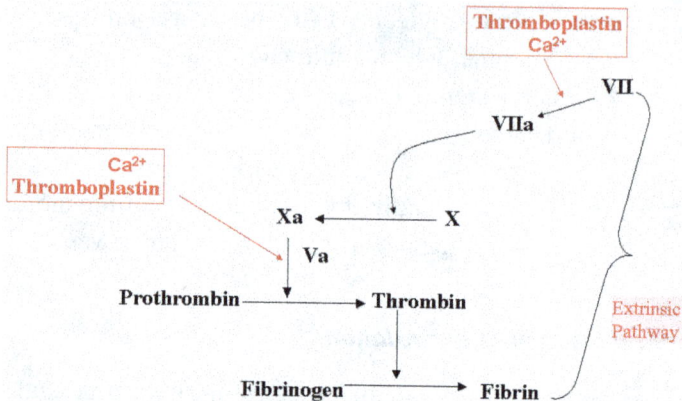

Fig. 11.8. A diagram of the prothrombin time. Factors that are added to the test tube containing the patient's platelet-poor plasma are shown in red. The extrinsic system is tested.

mechanism, and even this with limited sensitivity. In the presence of a suggestive clinical history, individual coagulation factors and platelet function may require specific assessments.

The prothrombin time

The prothrombin time (PT) assesses the extrinsic pathway (Fig. 11.8). A 'complete thromboplastin', containing tissue factor and phospholipid, is added along with calcium to reverse the effect of the citrate anticoagulant. The time until the appearance of a clot is then measured and is usually of the order of 12–14 seconds. The test is dependent on factors VII, X, V and II (prothrombin).

The activated partial thromboplastin time

The activated partial thromboplastin time (APTT) assesses the intrinsic pathway (Fig. 11.9). A contact activator and a 'partial thromboplastin' are added to the plasma; subsequently, calcium is added, and clotting is then timed. A partial thromboplastin does not activate the extrinsic pathway but replaces platelet phospholipid in the steps where it is required in the intrinsic and common pathway. The test is dependent on factors XII, XI,

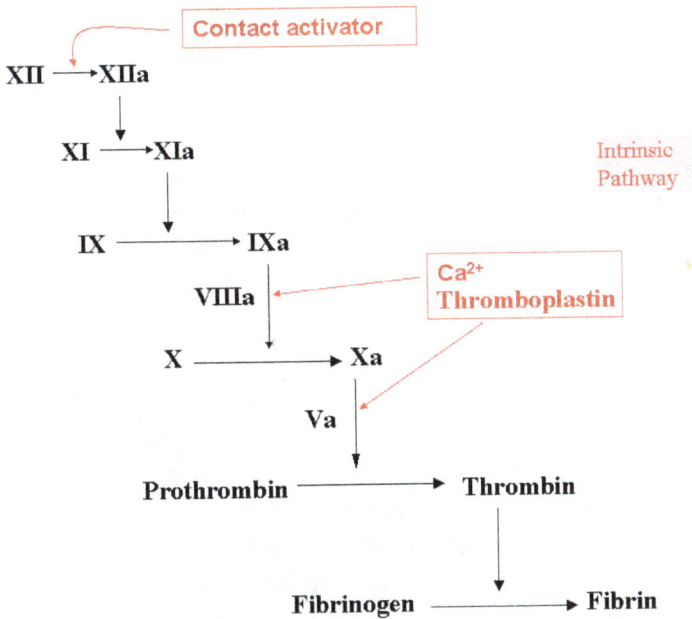

Fig. 11.9. A diagram of the activated partial thromboplastin time. Factors that are added to the test tube containing the patient's platelet-poor plasma are shown in red. The intrinsic system is tested.

IX, VIII, X, V and II. The normal range is usually of the order of 30–40 seconds but varies considerably according to the specific reagents used.

Fibrinogen assay

A coagulation screen should include a functional fibrinogen assay in addition to the PT and APTT. This test will detect abnormalities in both fibrinogen activity and level. A low fibrinogen level (<1.0 g/l) results in both an increased risk of bleeding *in vivo* and prolongation of the PT and APTT, as these tests have clot-based end points, and without sufficient fibrinogen, a clot cannot form.

The thrombin time

Where disorders of fibrinogen are suspected, a thrombin time (TT) can be useful. In the TT, thrombin is added to plasma, and the time taken for clotting to occur is recorded. A normal result is dependent on the presence of an adequate amount of normally functioning fibrinogen and on the absence of factors that might inhibit the conversion of fibrinogen to fibrin, such as exogenous heparin, thrombin-inhibiting drugs or endogenous fibrin degradation products. The concentration of thrombin added to the plasma sample is adjusted so that clotting usually occurs in 15–20 seconds.

Platelet function tests

Platelet function can be assessed by assays such as the PFA-100 and PFA-200, which aspirate a citrated blood sample at high shear rates through a capillary into a cartridge with a perforated membrane coated with either collagen plus adrenaline or collagen plus ADP. The time for occlusion of the aperture by a platelet aggregate is recorded (the closure time). This test requires normal platelet number and function as well as vWF but will not detect some milder forms of platelet defects. In platelet aggregation studies, various platelet aggregants, such as adrenaline, ADP, collagen or ristocetin, are added to platelet-rich plasma; the rate and completeness of platelet aggregation are studied by recording changes in optical density.

Platelet function can be more completely assessed using aggregometry — directly measuring the ability of platelets to aggregate in response to different stimuli — although this testing is often difficult to perform and reproduce.

Genetic testing for inherited platelet function disorders is now preferred, as the genetic basis for most of these conditions is well described and these tests are both highly sensitive and specific.

Viscoelastic haemostatic assays

Viscoelastic haemostatic assays (VHA), such as thromboelastrography (TEG) and rotational thromboelastrometry (ROTEM), are replacing the PFA-100, as these are point-of-care tests and are able to assess a wide range of coagulation parameters, including coagulation factor levels, fibrinogen activity, platelet number and function, inhibitory drugs and fibrinolysis.

VHA are primarily used in surgical situations, such as cardiac interventions and obstetrics, where rapid results are required. The testing is relatively expensive compared to standard laboratory assays, and the interpretation of the results is often complicated.

Other coagulation tests

Each individual coagulation factor can be assayed. There are numerous ways to assess the activity of clotting factors, including both direct measurements of activity where an artificial fluorescent substrate to the clotting factor is measured (chromogenic assays) and indirect measurements, such as the ability of the patient plasma to correct the abnormal coagulation time in specific factor-deficient laboratory plasma.

These tests should be discussed with a haematologist, as both their clinical utility and relevance are determined by the clinical scenario.

Inherited Coagulation Defects

All inherited defects of coagulation are uncommon or rare. Von Willebrand disease may have a prevalence of as high as 1%; however, many cases are mild or even asymptomatic. All other disorders are rare or very rare. Haemophilia A (factor VIII deficiency) has a birth incidence in males of about 1 in 5,000. Factor IX deficiency, also referred to as haemophilia B, is about a quarter as common as haemophilia A. Haemophilia C results from a deficiency of factor XI and is found to have a higher incidence among certain populations, such as Ashkenazi Jews. The overall prevalence of haemophilia C is around 1 in 100,000 people. All other inherited coagulation defects are extremely rare, with some having incidences so low that we cannot assess them accurately (<1 in 5 million).

Haemophilia A

Haemophilia A results from an X-linked inherited deficiency of factor VIII. Some cases are due to spontaneous mutations in the factor VIII gene, so not all patients have a positive family history. Factor VIII concentration may be less than 1%, leading to an extremely severe bleeding disorder (Fig. 11.10).

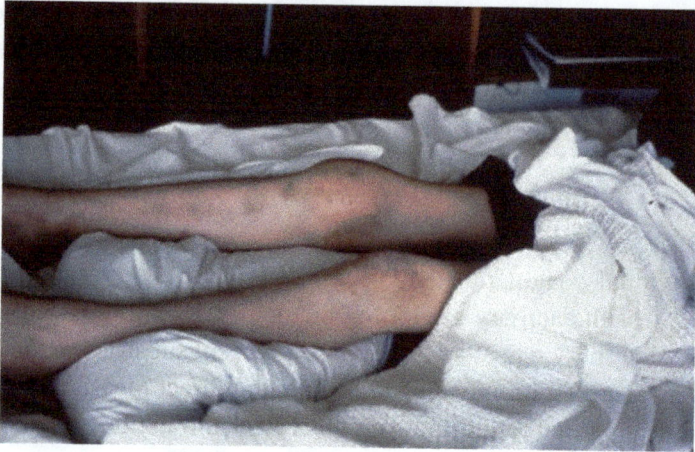

Fig. 11.10.   Bilateral knee haemarthroses in haemophilia. There are also some bruises.

There is spontaneous haemorrhage into joints and muscles, disproportionate bleeding following minor trauma or surgery and, sometimes, gastrointestinal haemorrhage, haematuria or intracranial haemorrhage. The PT and fibrinogen are normal, whereas the APTT is prolonged (study Figs. 11.4, 11.8 and 11.9 to understand why). Confirmation is achieved through an assay of factor VIII by both direct (chromogenic) and indirect (plasma mixing) methods. Both methods are required, as some patients exhibit discrepancies in the different functions of the factor VIII molecule. There is a reduction in factor VIII clotting activity, whereas the carrier molecule, vWF, remains normal.

Haemophilia A is ideally treated with recombinant human factor VIII or with alternatives that replace the function of factor VIII, such as emicizumab. We routinely use emicizumab, a humanised bispecific monoclonal antibody that is able to bridge factors IXa and Xa, to restore the function of the missing factor VIII. This has some benefits over direct factor VIII supplementation in terms of the frequency of administration and the risk of inhibitor formation.

In countries that cannot afford these products, treatment can involve plasma-derived factor VIII concentrate (which has had virucidal treatment) or cryoprecipitate, a blood product prepared by freezing and thawing plasma and isolating the cryoprecipitate, which is slowest to redissolve. Cryoprecipitate contains fibrinogen as well as factor VIII, so it can also be used for other purposes.

Ideally, parents and children should learn injection techniques since home treatment avoids any delay in treatment and thus lessens morbidity. The half-life of factor VIII is short (about 12 hours), but nevertheless it is possible to give prophylactic factor VIII on alternate days or three times weekly to children with severe haemophilia in order to prevent haemorrhage and thus avoid chronic joint and other tissue damage; the incidence of cerebral haemorrhage is also reduced by prophylaxis. Prophylaxis is now the standard of care for all patients with severe haemophilia A or those with an established bleeding history. The half-life of recombinant factor VIII can be improved by pegylation or other alterations of the protein so that injections can be less frequent. Humanised bispecific antibodies replacing factor VIII activity can be given weekly, which is a significant advantage.

Some 30% of patients with severe haemophilia develop antibodies that act as inhibitors of factor VIII. The initial approach is an attempt to eliminate the inhibitor by immune tolerance induction. In the presence of an inhibitor, alternative forms of treatment are needed. Acute bleeding events can be treated with bypassing agents — activated prothrombin complex concentrate or recombinant activated factor VII, a factor VIII derived from a non-human source (porcine factor VIII is most commonly used if the patient's inhibitor does not cross react with this). Prophylaxis in patients with inhibitors should include emicizumab.

Patients with mild haemophilia can be treated with desmopressin, which leads to the release of vWF-factor VIII from endothelial cells; it is often given together with an inhibitor of fibrinolysis, such as tranexamic acid, since its administration also leads to the release of tissue plasminogen activator.

Gene therapy is under development and is likely to be introduced into clinical practice in the near future.

When haemophilia is diagnosed in a child, it is necessary to consider the genetic as well as social implications for the family. Pedigree analysis and genetic testing of the mother to establish whether or not she is a carrier should be performed.

Haemophilia B

Haemophilia B, or factor IX deficiency, has similar clinical features to haemophilia A, including an X-linked recessive inheritance. It is also characterised by a normal PT and fibrinogen level and a prolonged APTT. Confirmation of the diagnosis is obtained by a factor IX assay.

Treatment is with recombinant factor IX, which can be given less frequently than factor VIII because its half-life is approximately 24 hours.

Pegylation or other alteration of the recombinant protein can extend the half-life considerably. Prophylaxis is preferred, rather than treating only when bleeding occurs. The development of a factor IX inhibitor is uncommon. Gene therapy with a high-specific-activity factor IX variant (FIX Padua) is under development and is likely to be introduced into clinical practice in the near future.

Similar to haemophilia A, genetic implications must be considered.

Von Willebrand disease

Von Willebrand disease (vWD) results from an inherited deficiency of vWF or the inheritance of a defective vWF molecule with reduced activity. vWF is synthesised in megakaryocytes and endothelial cells, although only the endothelium contributes to the levels measured in plasma. Deficiency of vWF, particularly if severe, can also result in deficiency of factor VIII since vWF transports and stabilises factor VIII. There are several types of vWD. Type 1 vWD is characterised by a reduced amount of vWF antigen, but the activity of vWF is normal. Type 2 vWD occurs when the antigen is both reduced and unable to perform its normal function. Type 3 vWD is rare and is characterised by a complete absence of the vWF antigen. Most cases are type 1 and are mild in both bleeding phenotype and laboratory assays.

Most cases show autosomal-dominant inheritance, with the severity of the disease varying greatly between families. Occasional severe cases have autosomal recessive inheritance. Since vWF is required for normal platelet function, patients with vWD experience bleeding from mucosal surfaces, and those with low levels of factor VIII experience deep-seated bleeding. The coagulation screen is frequently normal, but the APTT may be prolonged if the level of factor VIII is low. The bleeding time is prolonged in severe cases but often normal in milder forms of the disease, and except in a resource-poor setting, it is no longer used in diagnosis. The PFA-200 analysis can be used instead. vWF activity in plasma can be measured by the ability of the plasma to induce platelet aggregation in the presence of the antibiotic ristocetin; this is called ristocetin cofactor activity.

Treatment can include: intermediate-purity factor VIII concentrate, which contains vWF as well as factor VIII; high-purity vWF concentrate (supplemented with factor VIII concentrate if immediate efficacy is needed); or recombinant vWF. It is also possible to treat mild cases with tranexamic acid (to inhibit fibrinolysis) or with desmopressin (to cause the release of vWF from endothelial cells) plus tranexamic acid.

Other inherited coagulation factor deficiencies

Table 11.3 summarises the test results expected in inherited defects of coagulation factors and illustrates how coagulation tests can be interpreted.

Table 11.3. Laboratory tests results in inherited defects of coagulation factors.

Deficient factor	APTT	PT	TT
XII*	Prolonged	Normal	Normal
XI	Prolonged	Normal	Normal
IX	Prolonged	Normal	Normal
VIII	Prolonged	Normal	Normal
X	Prolonged	Prolonged	Normal
V	Prolonged	Prolonged	Normal
II (prothrombin)	Prolonged	Prolonged	Normal
I (hypofibrinogenaemia)	Prolonged	Prolonged	Prolonged
I (dysfibrinogenaemia)	Prolonged	Prolonged	Prolonged
VII	Normal	Prolonged	Normal
XIII†	Normal	Normal	Normal

*No clinical coagulation defect present.
†Alternative test assessing stability of clot is needed, such as a viscoelastic haemostatic assay (VHA).

Other than the conditions already discussed, inherited deficiencies in coagulation factors are quite rare.

Acquired Defects of Coagulation

Acquired defects of coagulation can result from: defective synthesis or increased utilisation of coagulation factors; dilution following transfusions for massive haemorrhage; the development of a coagulation factor inhibitor; or the presence of a drug, such as heparin, that inhibits coagulation. The two common causes of defective synthesis are liver disease and the administration of vitamin K antagonists for the prevention of thromboembolic disease.

Vitamin K deficiency or antagonism

The commonly used oral anticoagulants include vitamin K antagonists, which, by blocking the recycling of vitamin K, reduce the ability to perform the final step (γ-carboxylation) in the synthesis of factors II, VII, IX and X. Although the primary effect of vitamin K inhibitors is to reduce plasma factor levels, some of the anticoagulant factors, such as protein C and protein S, are also dependent on vitamin K for their metabolism. Deficiencies in the clotting factors interfere with the intrinsic (factor IX), extrinsic (factor VII) and common (factors X and II) pathways. As would be expected, both the PT and APTT are abnormal; however, in practice, the PT is relatively more prolonged. The fibrinogen and TT are normal. A similar coagulation abnormality can be seen in obstructive jaundice, when there is poor absorption of the fat-soluble vitamins, including vitamin K. Coeliac disease can also lead to a bleeding disorder due to malabsorption of vitamin K. Neonates are prone to vitamin K deficiency in the first week of life because vitamin K does not readily cross the placenta, although in most countries, this is prevented by the administration of prophylactic vitamin K, either orally or intramuscularly.

Bleeding resulting from a deficiency of vitamin K is readily treated by parenteral administration of the vitamin. There are several forms of vitamin K in the circulation, and the body has some ability to convert between these. However, it should be noted that oral vitamin K supplements usually contain vitamin K1 or K2, whereas the most active form for haemostasis is K4. When administering oral vitamin K, K1 or K2 may not be sufficient to correct the coagulopathy, and so vitamin K4 is recommended. Even with IV supplementation, correction of the coagulation defect may take 24 hours or longer; therefore, if rapid correction is needed, the missing factors are replaced using a blood product containing the vitamin K-dependent coagulation factors (termed prothrombin complex concentrate, or PCC) or, if this is not available, fresh frozen plasma (FFP). FFP only partially corrects the abnormality caused by vitamin K deficiency and can result in volume overload due to the quantity required. FFP should be reserved for use only when PCC is not available and vitamin K supplementation has not been effective or is not practical due to the emergency nature of the situation.

Liver disease

Since all coagulation factors, except vWF and factor VIII, are synthesised in the liver, liver disease can cause a reduction in most coagulation factors and a resultant prolongation of the PT and APTT.

As protein S, protein C and antithrombin are also synthesised in the liver, patients with mild to moderate liver disease are usually prothrombotic despite the deranged coagulation profile.

In severe liver disease, a reduced fibrinogen concentration may be encountered. Some forms of liver disease, particularly carcinoma, are associated with an acquired dysfibrinogenaemia, characterised by prolongation of the TT and elevation of the fibrinogen concentration. This is not necessarily associated with an increase in bleeding. If there is an obstructive element to the liver disease, a specific deficiency of vitamin K-dependent factors occurs, in addition to the generalised reduced rates of synthesis of all factors. There is impaired clearance of activated coagulation factors (making disseminated intravascular coagulation, or DIC, more likely) and of tissue plasminogen activator (leading to enhanced fibrinolysis). Thrombocytopenia as a result of hypersplenism can also be present.

Renal disease

Renal failure can lead to haemorrhage as a result of inhibition of platelet function.

Massive transfusion

During blood loss, replacement is initially done with reconstituted plasma-reduced red cells and colloid solutions. If it is clear that blood loss is going to be considerable, replacement should also include FFP and platelet concentrates. If replacement does not keep pace with loss, a global defect of clotting will occur, characterised by prolongation of the PT, APTT and TT, a reduced fibrinogen concentration and a low platelet count. The coagulation defect may be aggravated by DIC (which can be triggered by trauma, acidosis and hypoxia) and activation of fibrinolysis. Once a serious clotting defect has developed, management involves the transfusion of FFP (which contains all clotting factors), cryoprecipitate (supplying factor VIII, factor XIII and fibrinogen) and platelet concentrates.

Disseminated intravascular coagulation

DIC is a haemorrhagic disorder with disseminated activation of coagulation within the circulation, accompanied, when the process is acute, by increased fibrinolysis. Some of the causes are shown in Table 11.4.

DIC occurs *in vivo* in four distinct stages, with the first being prothrombotic with minimal derangement in coagulation tests and platelet count. By stages 3 and 4, there is a considerable reduction in the circulating coagulation factors, as these have been consumed by microvascular thrombotic events during stages 1 and 2.

Table 11.4. Some causes of disseminated intravascular coagulation.

Cause	Examples
Infection	Meningococcal septicaemia, other septicaemia
Tissue injury related to trauma, shock, hypoxia and acidosis	Trauma, hypotension due to acute blood loss including that due to injury and to obstetric misadventures, burns
Release of procoagulant substances into the circulation	Acute promyelocytic leukaemia, concealed antepartum haemorrhage, amniotic fluid embolism, disseminated carcinoma, incompatible blood transfusion

Clinical features of late-stage DIC are haemorrhage, including diffuse oozing from venipuncture sites and from small vessels in surgical wounds or at sites of trauma. There is also end-organ impairment related to intravascular fibrin deposition and ongoing microvascular thrombosis, affecting the lungs, kidneys and brain. Increased utilisation of coagulation factors leads to a global coagulation defect with prolongation of PT, APTT and TT, fibrinogen deficiency, the presence of fibrin degradation products and thrombocytopenia. Sometimes, the blood becomes incoagulable. The prolongation of the TT is due not only to fibrinogen deficiency but also to inhibition of the conversion of fibrinogen to fibrin by the anticoagulant action of fibrin degradation products. Haemorrhage may be aggravated by abnormal platelet function, for example if the patient has been on cardiopulmonary bypass, if the patient has been taking aspirin or other anti-platelet drugs or if there is renal failure. Tests indicated in suspected DIC are PT, APTT, TT, fibrinogen assay, measurement of fibrin degradation products and a full blood count, including a platelet count. A commonly used test for fibrin degradation products is a measurement of D-dimer, which is a breakdown product of fibrin that is formed only when there has been cross-linking of fibrin and subsequent fibrinolysis.

Management is by transfusion of red cells, platelets, FFP and cryoprecipitate. Vigorous efforts to correct the underlying cause as well as supportive care to try to correct hypotension, hypoxia and acidosis are also of considerable importance.

Coagulation inhibitors

Some coagulation inhibitors, developed as an autoimmune phenomenon, lead to the destruction of coagulation factors and serious bleeding. Others interfere with coagulation tests without causing bleeding. The clinical significance clearly differs.

Coagulation inhibitors that can lead to bleeding

Coagulation inhibitors that can aggravate or lead to bleeding can develop not only in patients with an inherited deficiency of a coagulation factor but also in previously healthy people, the latter as an autoimmune phenomenon. Sometimes, their occurrence is related to pregnancy or exposure to a drug (e.g. penicillin) or is associated with a known autoimmune disease (e.g. rheumatoid arthritis or systemic lupus erythematosus). Inhibitors directed at factor VIII are the most common, and this is termed acquired haemophilia A. Its management is somewhat different from that of congenital haemophilia, as the principle concern is to eliminate the production of the inhibitor while preserving haemostasis. Antibodies to other coagulation factors (IX, vWF, II and X) have been reported.

Coagulation tests are similar to those found in deficiency of a coagulation factor, but with the difference that, in deficiency, mixing of normal plasma with the patient's plasma corrects the defect, whereas in the presence of an inhibitor it does not. Treatment can be with high doses of the relevant coagulant factor or with coagulation factors designed to bypass the defect, for example, in the case of a factor VIII inhibitor, porcine factor VIII, prothrombin complex or activated prothrombin complex (containing factors II, IX and X as well as variable, often low, amounts of factor VII), or recombinant factor VIIa. In the longer term, immunosuppressive therapy may be useful. Management is difficult and there is significant mortality.

Lupus anticoagulant

This *in vitro* coagulation inhibitor develops both in patients with systemic lupus erythematosus and as a primary autoimmune disease. It is an antiphospholipid antibody that interferes with coagulation tests that require a phospholipid, particularly the APTT and is further discussed on page 272.

Thrombocytopenia

Thrombocytopenia may be inherited or acquired. Inherited thrombocytopenia is rare. It may involve associated giant platelets, abnormally staining platelets on a blood film (grey platelets) or platelet dysfunction. In some inherited thrombocytopenias, there are abnormal inclusions in leucocytes; their detection is important in alerting the haematologist to an inherited condition and avoiding misdiagnosis as autoimmune thrombocytopenia. Acquired thrombocytopenia is common. Some of the causes are shown in

Table 11.5. Some causes of acquired thrombocytopenia.

Mechanism	Examples
Decreased platelet production	Acute leukaemia, aplastic anaemia, administration of cytotoxic chemotherapy
Increased consumption	Disseminated intravascular coagulation, massive haemorrhage, thrombotic thrombocytopenic purpura
Increased destruction	Autoimmune thrombocytopenic purpura, alloimmune thrombocytopenia (e.g. in the fetus and neonate), drug-induced thrombocytopenia (including heparin-induced thrombocytopenia), post-infection thrombocytopenia, post-transfusion purpura
Pooling in an enlarged spleen*	Hypersplenism (e.g. in portal cirrhosis)

*Usually, about one-third of the body's platelets are found in the spleen, but in hypersplenism, it may be up to 90%.

Table 11.5. Drug-induced thrombocytopenia is usually the result of an antibody that recognises a drug (or metabolite) bound to a specific platelet glycoprotein, usually either glycoprotein II/IIIa or Ib/IX. It is usually severe. Heparin-induced thrombocytopenia (page 259) has different characteristics from other drug-induced thrombocytopenias.

Haemorrhage due either to thrombocytopenia or impaired platelet function can be treated by platelet transfusions. To some extent, the probability of haemorrhage can be predicted from the platelet count (Fig. 11.11). In some clinical circumstances, for example in treating patients with acute leukaemia, prophylactic platelet transfusions are given when the platelet count is very low to prevent haemorrhage occurring; this is usually done when the platelet count falls below $10–15 \times 10^9/l$. Associated inflammation will increase the tendency to bleed at any given platelet count.

Autoimmune thrombocytopenic purpura

Autoimmune thrombocytopenic purpura, previously known as idiopathic thrombocytopenic purpura (ITP), results from the production of an autoantibody directed at platelet antigens or, in some cases, from T-cell-mediated autoimmunity. This condition is often referred to as 'immune thrombocytopenic purpura,' but this term is less satisfactory since it also encompasses alloimmune and drug-induced immune thrombocytopenia. Splenic and

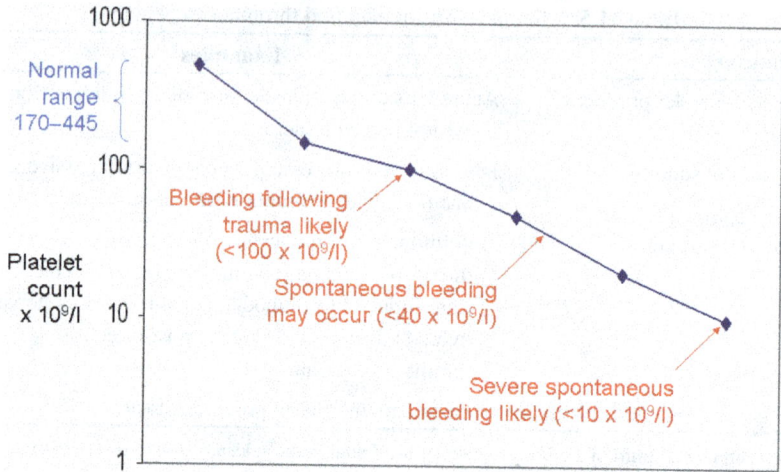

Fig. 11.11. A diagram of a falling platelet count, showing the points at which significant haemorrhage may occur or is likely to occur.

other macrophages have receptors for the Fc fragment of immunoglobulin G, enabling them to bind and phagocytose the platelet. The specific antigen on the platelets that the antibody binds to is often not identified. Autoimmune thrombocytopenia can occur as an isolated phenomenon or as a feature of an autoimmune disease. It can also occur as a complication of chronic lymphocytic leukaemia or lymphoma. Occasionally, it coexists with autoimmune haemolytic anaemia (Evans syndrome) or autoimmune neutropenia. Autoimmune thrombocytopenia also occurs with an increased incidence when there is infection by the hepatitis C virus, the human immunodeficiency virus (HIV) or *Helicobacter pylori*.

Autoimmune thrombocytopenia appears to manifest somewhat differently in children and adults. In children, the peak incidence is around the age of 5, and its frequency is the same in boys and girls. It often remits spontaneously. It is suspected that it is often triggered by an infection, and treatment is usually not needed. In adults, peak incidence is in young adults, and it is more common in women than in men. It is more likely to become chronic, and treatment is usually needed.

Clinical features

Presentation is usually with bruising, epistaxis or bleeding from mucosal surfaces. Cerebral haemorrhage is an uncommon complication. Physical

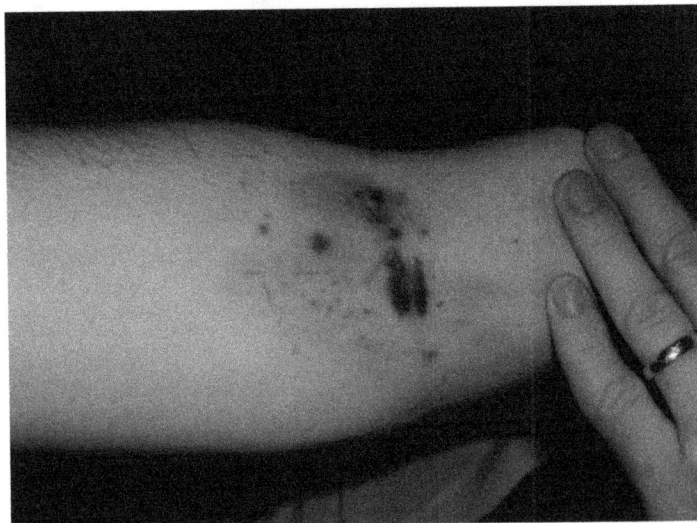

Fig. 11.12. The arm of a young man with autoimmune thrombocytopenic purpura showing petechiae and bleeding at venipuncture sites.

examination shows purpura (petechiae and ecchymoses) and bruises (Fig. 11.12). There may be blood blisters in the mouth. When the condition is a feature of an autoimmune disease, such as systemic lupus erythematosus or rheumatoid arthritis, there will be clinical features of the primary disease.

Laboratory features

The blood count and blood film confirm thrombocytopenia. If the condition is acute, the platelets are of normal size; however, if it is chronic, there may be some large platelets, which are haemostatically more effective.

Diagnosis and differential diagnosis

The blood count and film are important for the exclusion of other causes of thrombocytopenia, such as thrombotic thrombocytopenic purpura (page 262) and acute leukaemia. A coagulation screen is always performed in order to exclude DIC as an alternative cause of thrombocytopenia. The coagulation screen may also give evidence of a lupus anticoagulant.

Autoantibodies are tested for, including antinuclear factor, anti-DNA anti-bodies and anticardiolipin antibodies. However, testing for platelet autoantibodies is not useful because of the poor sensitivity and specificity of the available tests. In adults, a bone marrow aspirate is usually per-formed, megakaryocyte numbers are usually normal or increased. In children, this investigation can usually be avoided, as the clinical picture is very typical; however, if treatment with corticosteroids is considered to be indicated, then it may be performed (because of anxiety that thrombo-cytopenia may be the result of an otherwise unsuspected acute lymphoblastic leukaemia).

Management

Platelet transfusion is indicated only if there is a life-threatening haemor-rhage since the presence of an antiplatelet antibody means that transfused platelets survive only briefly in the circulation. Children are usually not actively treated. In adults, the immune process is initially treated with corticosteroids. High-dose intravenous immunoglobulin can be given if rapid elevation of the platelet count is required, but its use does not affect the underlying disease. The aim of treatment is to prevent bleeding rather than to raise the platelet count to a normal level; a platelet count of $20–50 \times 10^9/l$ may well be adequate. If the disease proves to be refractory to corticosteroids, other options include other immunosuppressive drugs, splenectomy (with appropriate prophylaxis against infection) and agents that mimic the action of thrombopoietin and increase platelet production. Aspirin and other drugs that either interfere with platelet function or increase the risk of gastrointestinal haemorrhage should be avoided.

Thrombotic thrombocytopenic purpura

Thrombotic thrombocytopenic purpura (TTP) results from platelet aggregation in small vessels and is characterised by five clinical and lab-oratory features — fever, neurological abnormalities, thrombocytopenia, microangiopathic haemolytic anaemia and renal impairment. This is con-sidered one of the haematological emergencies, and the management or diagnosis of any suspected case should be urgently discussed with a haematologist.

Of the features of TTP, thrombocytopenia is universal, and blood film examination demonstrates fragments of red cells. Both laboratory scientists and haematologists should be able to confirm or refute a suspected diagnosis of TTP based on a blood film examination, which is the initial investigation of choice.

TTP results from a deficiency of vWF-cleaving protease (ADAMTS13), usually as a result of the production of an autoantibody directed at this factor but inherited forms are also seen. As a result, ultra-large molecules of vWF are present, which bind spontaneously to platelets, trapping them on the endothelial surface. The platelet microthrombi cause the microangiopathic haemolytic anaemia. This results in the red cell fragmentation seen in the blood film. This condition is rare, but its diagnosis is nevertheless important since urgent treatment is needed and the case fatality without appropriate intervention is extremely high.

Clinical features

Presentation is usually with symptoms of anaemia, purpura, neurological impairment and fever.

Laboratory features

The blood count and film confirm thrombocytopenia and, in addition, show red cell fragments and polychromasia. Serum creatinine is elevated, and there is biochemical evidence of haemolysis.

Diagnosis and differential diagnosis

Diagnosis is based on the presence of all or most of the characteristic five clinical and laboratory features, with the demonstration of reduced ADAMTS13 and the presence of an ADAMTS13 inhibitor. The differential diagnosis includes other causes of thrombocytopenia and red cell fragmentation.

Management

Treatment involves plasmapheresis to remove the autoantibody and replace the ADAMTS13, often followed by immunosuppressive treatment. Pre-emptive treatment often needs to precede a definitive diagnosis in order to reduce early mortality. Other adjuncts to therapy include rituximab, a monoclonal antibody which reduces the B cell reservoir and the ability of the body to form antibodies, and caplacizumab, an antibody to vWF that prevents vWF from binding to platelets. Platelet transfusion is contraindicated since it may aggravate the microangiopathy and organ damage.

Defective Platelet Function

Defective platelet function may be inherited or acquired.

Inherited defects of platelet function

Inherited defects of platelet function are rare. Associated thrombocytopenia may sometimes occur. Platelet size may be increased, or there may be hypogranularity of platelets. Diagnosis is by blood count and film, platelet aggregation or other studies of platelet function. Deficiency of platelet glycoprotein can be assessed most readily through flow cytometry and platelet granule content through the measurement of platelet nucleotides (ADP and adenosine triphosphate, ATP). Management is by platelet transfusion if serious haemorrhage occurs or prophylactically if there is an urgent need for surgery. Mild defects may also respond to desmopressin.

Acquired defects of platelet function

The most common cause of acquired platelet dysfunction is exposure to drugs that interfere with platelet function. In addition to aspirin, many patients are prescribed dipyridamole or inhibitors of the ADP receptor, such as clopidogrel, to therapeutically reduce platelet function. Platelet inhibition also results from nonsteroidal anti-inflammatory drugs prescribed for other indications; these drugs can also be bought over the counter. In myelodysplastic syndromes and acute myeloid leukaemia, platelets may be intrinsically abnormal. Impaired function due to the accumulation of gua-nidinosuccinic acid is common in renal failure. Platelet dysfunction due to prior activation and granule release occurs following cardiopulmonary bypass and in DIC. In essential thrombocythaemia with very high counts, there can be paradoxical bleeding because of acquired vWD, which leads to platelet dysfunction (page 232).

Management of acquired defects of platelet function involves control of the primary condition, withdrawal of relevant drugs (if possible) and, if serious haemorrhage occurs, platelet transfusion. Following cardiopul-monary bypass and in DIC and myeloid neoplasms, platelet transfusions are indicated not only when the platelet count is low but also when there is bleeding at a platelet count that would normally be adequate for haemostasis.

Conclusions

Clinical history is the most important means of detecting abnormal coag-ulation or platelet function and often suggests whether there is any defect in the coagulation factors or platelets. A full blood count, film and a coag-ulation screen are indicated when clinical history suggests a possible defect. These basic investigations are supplemented by other tests when clinically indicated.

Test Case 11.1

A 64-year-old man with metastatic prostate cancer experiences epistaxis, widespread bruising and persistent oozing from cannula sites. The platelet count is 95×10^9/l, and the blood film reveals the presence of schistocytes (red cell fragments). The coagulation screen shows:

Prothrombin time 16 seconds (normal range (NR)): 12–14,
Activated partial thromboplastin time 42 seconds (NR: 30–40),
Thrombin time 24 seconds (control: 21 seconds), fibrinogen 1.3 g/l (NR: 1.8–3.6) and D-dimer 768 mg/l (NR: <50).

Questions

1. What is the haematological diagnosis?
2. Can you explain the pathophysiology of this condition?

Write down your answers before checking the correct answer (page 408) or re-reading any relevant part of the chapter.

Test Case 11.2

A 27-year-old previously healthy woman presents with a haematemesis. She has not suffered any indigestion and has not been taking aspirin or any other antiplatelet drugs. While an urgent gastroscopy is being arranged, the junior doctor records her full history and finds that she has suffered from recurrent nosebleeds and has always had heavy periods. She is aware that her mother also suffered from nosebleeds. A coagulation screen and subsequent assays show:

Prothrombin time 13 seconds (NR: 12–14),
Activated partial thromboplastin time 55 seconds (NR: 30–40),
Thrombin time 19 seconds (control: 21 seconds),
Factor VIII 25% (NR: 50–150) and vWF 17% (NR: 50–200).

Questions

1. What is the most likely cause of the bleeding disorder?
2. Do you think platelet function would be abnormal?
3. Why is the factor VIII low?

Write down your answers before checking the correct answer (page 408) or re-reading any relevant part of the chapter.

12

Thrombosis and Its Management: Anticoagulant, Antiplatelet and Thrombolytic Therapy

Andrew Godfrey

What Do You Need To Know?

☞ Why thrombosis occurs and how it can be prevented
☞ The nature of thrombophilia and how it is managed
☞ The clinical role and management of heparin therapy
☞ The clinical role and management of oral anticoagulants
☞ The clinical role and management of direct-acting oral anti-coagulants
☞ The clinical role of antiplatelet drugs
☞ The clinical role of thrombolytic therapy
☞ Reversal of anticoagulation, with or without bleeding

Haemostasis and Thrombosis

Haemostasis is essential to normal life, and the impairment of normal haemostasis seen in patients lacking coagulation factors (haemophilia A and B, see Chapter 11) highlights this. Normally, coagulation is limited

A. Godfrey

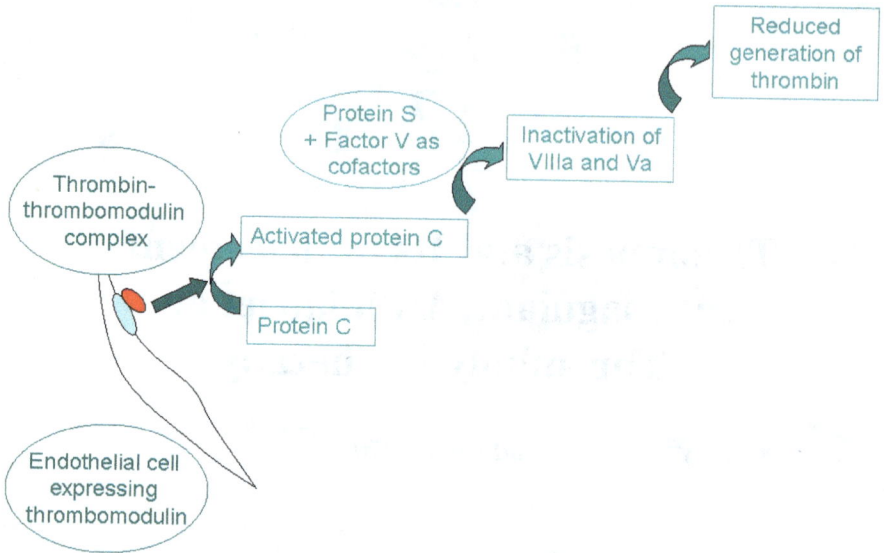

Fig. 12.1. The interaction of naturally occurring anticoagulants, protein S and protein C.

to sites of injury and inflammation. Generation of clots is also controlled by the action of a number of naturally occurring anticoagulants, including antithrombin, tissue factor pathway inhibitor (TFPI) and activated protein C, which are activated whenever blood coagulation occurs. Both protein C and protein S are vitamin K-dependent serine proteases. Protein C is activated by thrombin complexed to endothelial membrane thrombomodulin (Fig. 12.1). In turn, protein C, with protein S and factor V as cofactors, inactivates the activated forms of factor V and factor VIII, thus serving to control thrombin generation.

Perturbation of this physiological response to injury can lead to a pathological process known as thrombosis, in which clotting occurs in arteries, arterioles, capillaries, venules or veins, potentially leading to disability or death.

Due to the different vessel structures and pressures involved, thrombosis affecting arteries is different from that affecting veins. This is highly relevant in terms of the treatment of these events — arterial events are better treated with antiplatelet agents, whereas venous events are better treated with anticoagulants.

Atherosclerosis and arterial thrombosis are responsible for significant morbidity and mortality. As unhealthy diets, lack of exercise, obesity and cigarette smoking are increasingly common, this is becoming a global problem. A thrombus can narrow or totally block a coronary vessel, leading to myocardial ischaemia or infarction. When this occlusion occurs, it is often due to the rupture of an atherosclerotic plaque and the occlusion of downstream arterioles. Thrombosis in cerebral blood vessels can lead to infarction of part of the brain, recognised clinically as a stroke. Ischaemic (as opposed to haemorrhagic) stroke can also result from the embolism of a blood clot in the brain. A frequent underlying cause of this is atrial fibrillation, which is common in an ageing population. The ineffective and irregular contractions of the atrium lead to the formation of blood clots in the atrial appendage; these can embolise from the left atrium to the brain.

A further large burden of disease and a significant number of deaths result from venous thrombosis and pulmonary embolism. Venous thrombosis usually occurs in the deep veins of the legs and pelvis with part of the thrombus sometimes breaking free and embolising to the lung. Venous thromboembolism (VTE) is a common condition with an overall incidence of 1–3 per 1,000 per year. In developed countries, it accounts for 5–10% of deaths of hospitalised patients and 10–15% of deaths related to pregnancy and childbirth. In the United Kingdom, it remains a leading cause of maternal death, although the death rate has been reduced by risk assessment and increased use of thromboprophylaxis.

Morbidity and mortality can also result from the deposition of fibrin and aggregation of platelets within capillaries, leading to end-organ damage and thrombocytopenia.

Anticoagulant and antiplatelet therapies have been developed in an attempt to deal with the disease burden resulting from thrombosis.

Aetiology of thrombosis

Thrombosis in arteries is usually the result of atheroma, to which an individual is predisposed by hypertension, diabetes mellitus, hyperlipidaemia (including that related to obesity) and smoking. Atheroma leads to the aggregation of platelets on the atheromatous plaque and subsequent thrombosis. Increased concentration of certain coagulation factors can

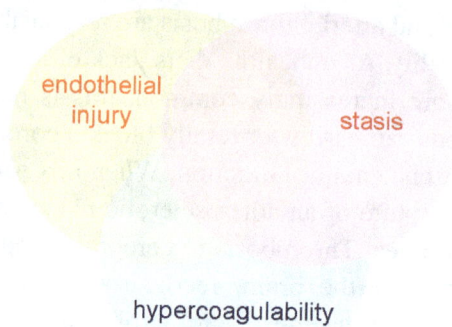

endothelial
injury

stasis

hypercoagulability

Fig. 12.2.   A diagram illustrating Virchow's triad.

predispose one to arterial occlusion, as can an increased platelet count and increased blood viscosity due to a high haematocrit. Polycythaemia vera and essential thrombocythaemia can thus predispose an individual to arterial thrombosis.

Venous thrombosis is related mainly to an increased concentration of coagulation factors, endothelial damage and stasis within vessels, including that due to partial obstruction by external pressure (as in pregnancy). A reduction in naturally occurring anticoagulants can also contribute. Virchow's triad summarises the contributing factors: hypercoagulability, stasis and endothelial injury or dysfunction, two or three of which may co-exist (Fig. 12.2). There are many other factors that increase the risk of venous thromboembolism, including pregnancy, childbirth, surgery, trauma, immobility (including long-distance travel), cancer, advancing age, a high haematocrit, oral contraceptives, hormone replacement therapy and administration of thalidomide or lenalidomide.

Thrombosis within the microcirculation can be the result of thrombocytosis, as in myeloproliferative neoplasms. It can also result from increased aggregability of platelets as a result of an increased concentration of ultra-large multimers of von Willebrand factor, as occurs in thrombotic thrombocytopenic purpura.

Management of thrombotic diseases requires not only pharmacological measures but also a consideration of the factors that contribute to atherosclerosis and increase the risk of thrombosis such as obesity, lack of exercise, hyperlipidaemia, hypertension, smoking and exposure to oral contraceptives or other hormones.

Thrombophilia

Some individuals have an increased risk of VTE due to inherited abnormalities of naturally occurring plasma proteins, either anticoagulant or coagulation proteins. This is referred to as thrombophilia. Although we have identified some genetic variants which increase the risk of developing thrombosis, whole genome sequencing has provided insights into the complexity of thrombosis and its regulation. There are a growing number of genetic variants which offer some predictive value in the risk of thrombosis; however, we rarely perform thrombophilia screening as the picture we gain from a handful of tests is incomplete and the clinical scenario is usually much more relevant to the management of the patient.

The incidence of these abnormalities varies widely. Some of these defects are uncommon but cause a marked increase in the risk of thrombosis. Others are very common but the degree of increase in risk is less. The inherited abnormalities for which we routinely screen are summarised in Table 12.1.

Some patients who develop VTE benefit from investigation for thrombophilia if this will inform management decisions regarding the optimal length of anticoagulation. Such investigation can reasonably be carried

Table 12.1.   Inherited thrombophilia.

Defect	Prevalence in Caucasian populations	Approximate increased risk of thrombosis in heterozygotes
Antithrombin deficiency[*]	1 in 2,000	20-fold
Protein C deficiency[*]	3 in 1,000	10-fold
Protein S deficiency[*]	1 in 700	8-fold
Factor V Leiden[†]	3–15%	4–8-fold (much higher if homozygous)
Factor II, *F2* 20210 mutation[†]	1–1.5%	About 5-fold

[*]Loss of function mutation in a gene for a naturally occurring anticoagulant.
[†]Gain of function in a coagulation factor gene.

out in patients who are young (less than 40 years of age) and who have a strong family history of thrombosis. Outside of these individuals, testing rarely influences management and should not be performed. Informed consent is required for thrombophilia screening and this is normally undertaken by a haematologist. There is no role for thrombophilia screening in the immediate phase after a thrombosis, as protein C and S levels are reduced in the presence of active thrombosis.

Thrombophilia can also be the result of an acquired abnormality. The most important of these is the presence of the so-called 'lupus anticoagulant' (see the following section), an anticardiolipin antibody or an anti-$\beta2$ glycoprotein I antibody, or any combination of these.

Inherited and acquired thrombophilic abnormalities are associated with an increased incidence of recurrent miscarriage and fetal loss. They can interact with other factors, such as surgery and immobility, that promote thrombosis in individuals who do not have thrombophilia.

Lupus anticoagulant and the antiphospholipid syndrome

The lupus anticoagulant is an autoantibody or an antiphospholipid antibody that inhibits coagulation in laboratory tests (hence its name) but in the patient can actually predispose to thrombosis. Although it shares a name and a patient group with systemic lupus erythematosis (SLE), the two are not synonymous and should not be confused with each other.

The presence of a lupus anticoagulant is a common finding amongst hospital inpatients and does not in itself confer a diagnosis of antiphospholipid syndrome. Most often, this is a transient finding whose main significance is that it complicates decisions around interventional procedures as medical teams will be concerned that the coagulation profile is abnormal.

The British Society for Haematology currently recommends that activated partial thromboplastin time (APTT) screening is routinely performed using reagents that are not sensitive to lupus anticoagulants for this reason. Strong lupus antibodies will affect even a lupus-insensitive reagent and may even affect the prothrombin time (PT).

Lupus anticoagulants can occur in individuals who are well, hospital inpatients, or as a feature of systemic lupus erythematosus. The screening tests for antiphospholipid syndrome also include associated anticardiolipin and anti-β2 glycoprotein I antibodies. In order to ensure that these are not transient abnormalities (such as those found in hospital inpatients with no evidence of thrombosis), it is essential to retest twelve weeks after the original sample.

Where this laboratory abnormality is persistent and is associated with clinical features of thrombotic events (venous, arterial and micro-vascular) or pregnancy complications, it has the clinical term of anti-phospholipid syndrome (APS). APS is a complex, heterogeneous disorder where some patients experience extensive thrombosis and microvascular organ impairment (catastrophic APS) and others have isolated arterial events or miscarriages without other features of the disease. Management is individualised, and the optimal anticoagulation strategy is hotly debated. There is some evidence that higher doses of anticoagulants such as vitamin K antagonists or a combination of antico-agulants with antiplatelet agents reduces the risk of thrombosis in such patients, but it can also significantly increases the risk of bleeding. The final decision on management is therefore usually left to a haematologist or rheumatologist.

The Need for Anticoagulant and Antiplatelet Therapy

The morbidity and mortality of vascular and venous thromboembolic dis-ease have led to new and successful attempts to treat or prevent thrombosis by interfering with blood clotting or platelet action.

Anticoagulant therapy is also needed to prevent blood clotting during haemodialysis and heart-lung bypass and may be needed to maintain patency of arterial stents (e.g. in coronary arteries), arterial grafts for peripheral vascular disease or arteriovenous shunts (e.g. those established for haemodialysis).

Arterial and venous thrombosis may be managed with a single agent but often requires the combination of more than one agent (see Table 12.5). Since therapy leads to an increased risk of haemorrhage, the use of such treatment requires a careful consideration of risks and benefits. Decisions on the choice of treatment should be evidence based and appropriate to the specific clinical features of individual patients. Randomised trials and meta-analyses of similar trials provide a sound basis for treatment decisions.

The important anticoagulants that are well established in clinical use are heparin (used parenterally), vitamin K antagonists (active orally) and the more commonly used oral direct thrombin and direct factor Xa inhibitors.

Non-Pharmacological Means of Reducing Venous Thromboembolism

Around a quarter of all venous thromboembolism occurs in hospitalised patients. In surgical and high-risk medical patients, the risk of thrombosis can be reduced by non-pharmacological means such as early ambulation, encouraging leg and foot exercises and the use of pneumatic compression devices. Graduated compression stockings have historically been used for post-surgical care but do little to reduce the risk of thrombosis in other scenarios. In pregnant women, avoiding an unnecessary caesarean section reduces the incidence of venous thromboembolism.

Parenteral Anticoagulants

Parenteral anticoagulants are summarised in Table 12.2. The most frequently used of this group of drugs is heparin, either unfractionated or low molecular weight.

Heparin

Heparin is a heterogeneous mixture of sulphated polysaccharides. It is a naturally occurring anticoagulant that is found in human and animal tissues. As a therapeutic product, it is extracted from animal tissues such as pig intestines. Heparin can be either unfractionated heparin, with a mean molecular weight of around 15,000 daltons, or low-molecular-weight heparin, which has been depolymerised and has a molecular weight of around 4,000–5,000 daltons. Heparin does not cross the placenta and is not secreted in breast milk. Hence, it may be the anticoagulant of choice in pregnant and breastfeeding women.

Low-molecular-weight heparins have a significantly longer half-life in circulation and can be administered effectively once or twice a day,

Table 12.2. Parenteral anticoagulants.

Agent		Uses
Heparin, unfractionated and LMWH (dalteparin, enoxaparin, tinzaparin)		Haemodialysis and maintenance of extracorporeal circuits; maintaining patency of cannulae; sometimes for treatment of venous thromboembolism, arterial thrombosis, myocardial infarction and acute coronary syndrome; LMWH for venous thromboembolism prophylaxis
Heparinoid: danaparoid (contains mainly depolymerised heparan sulphate and dermatan sulphate)		Management of heparin-induced thrombocytopenia
Direct factor Xa inhibitor: fondaparinux		Prophylaxis and treatment of venous thromboembolism; treatment of unstable angina and myocardial infarction; management of heparin-induced thrombocytopenia or allergy to LMWH formulations
Direct thrombin inhibitors	Argatroban	Management of heparin-induced thrombocytopenia
	Bivalirudin (a hirudin analogue)	Management of unstable angina and myocardial infarction

Note: LMWH, low-molecular-weight heparin.

whereas unfractionated heparin is usually given three times a day or as a continuous infusion, making it unsuitable for long-term use.

Heparin has an anticoagulant effect when complexed in the circulation with antithrombin. The heparin–antithrombin complex inhibits factor XIa, factor IXa, factor Xa and thrombin (Fig. 12.3).

The main unwanted effect is haemorrhage. Less common are cutaneous reactions and heparin-induced thrombocytopenia (see page 277). Long-term administration of heparin can lead to osteoporosis.

Unfractionated heparin

Unfractionated heparin can be administered intravenously, with a loading dose being followed by a continuous infusion, or subcutaneously

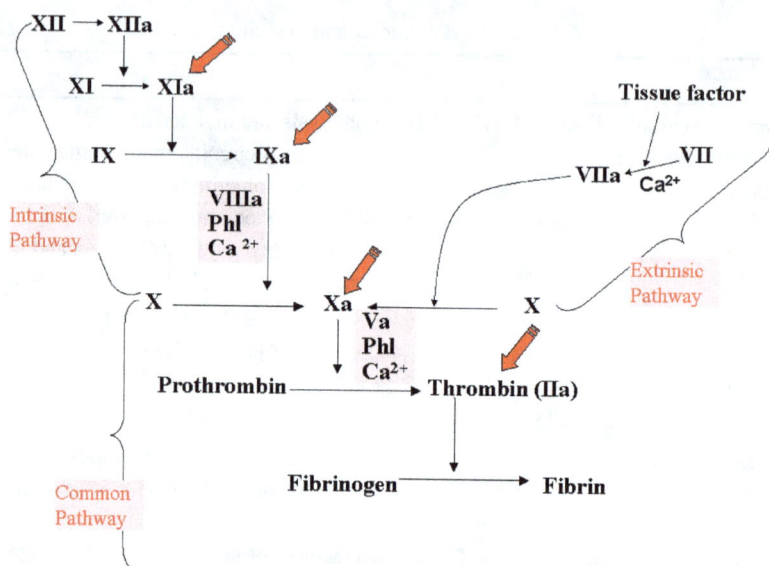

Fig. 12.3. The sites of action of the heparin–antithrombin complex (red arrows). Note that an activated partial thromboplastin time will be affected by all four of these interactions.

twice or three times a day. If given intravenously, the anticoagulant effect is immediate. The effect largely disappears 6 hours after cessation of therapy, but if necessary, it can be reversed rapidly by the administration of protamine sulphate (see Table 12.6). Unfractionated heparin is indicated whenever immediately effective anticoagulation is required or in a clinically unstable patient in whom cessation or reversal of therapy may become necessary. It is used during cardiopulmonary bypass and reversed at the end of the procedure. It is the heparin of choice in end-stage renal disease and can be used during haemodialysis, although low-molecular-weight heparin is an alternative. Unfractionated heparin is indicated in patients with acute coronary syndromes, in whom it reduces the risk of myocardial infarction and death. This type of heparin is excreted by the liver. Therapy requires monitoring and dose adjustment based on the APTT.

Low-molecular-weight heparin

In comparison with unfractionated heparin, low-molecular-weight heparins, such as enoxaparin and tinzaparin, have enhanced anti-Xa activity in relation to their antithrombin activity. They have a longer duration of action and can be administered subcutaneously once or twice daily. They do not usually require monitoring but, when monitoring is considered necessary (e.g. during pregnancy or progressive thrombosis), an anti-Xa assay can be used. Low-molecular-weight heparins are effective in venous thromboembolism prophylaxis and treatment and in acute coronary syndrome. They are less effectively neutralised by protamine sulphate than unfractionated heparin. Other neutralising agents are under development. Low-molecular-weight heparin does not cross the placenta and is not secreted in breast milk and is an option if anticoagulation is needed during specific, vulnerable periods of pregnancy or during lactation. Low-molecular-weight heparins are mainly excreted by the kidney so avoidance or appropriate dose reduction is required if there is renal impairment.

Heparin-induced thrombocytopenia

In a minority of patients, heparin (mainly unfractionated heparin) induces immune thrombocytopenia, usually between 5 and 10 days from the start of therapy. In these cases, patients develop an antibody to the heparin–platelet factor 4 complex. Thrombocytopenia is not very severe (median platelet count at nadir 60×10^9/l) but is of considerable clinical importance because of its association with paradoxical arterial and venous thrombosis. It is managed by immediate cessation of heparin and replacement by another immediate-acting anticoagulant (see Table 12.2).

Other parenteral anticoagulants

Other parenteral anticoagulants are used in specific circumstances but this should only be done with specialist guidance from a haematologist (see Table 12.2).

Oral anticoagulant therapy

Traditional oral anticoagulants are direct factor Xa inhibitors, direct thrombin inhibitors or vitamin K antagonists (VKAs). The oral anti-Xa and thrombin inhibitors are often referred to as DOACs — direct (or direct-acting) oral anticoagulants. They are summarised in Table 12.3. DOACs have a much shorter duration of action than vitamin K antagonists and a significantly better bleeding profile compared to VKAs. This allows for rapid institution and interruption of therapy as needed. However, it does mean that compliance is important since missing doses can lead to a rapid loss of the anticoagulant effect.

Direct factor Xa inhibitors

Orally active direct factor Xa inhibitors, such as rivaroxaban, apixaban and edoxaban, are the primary anticoagulants used in the UK. Clinical trials have shown that these are both more effective and safer than warfarin (Table 12.4) and are more convenient for patients as they require fewer dietary restrictions.

Rivaroxaban or edoxaban are often preferred for the acute treatment of VTE as these drugs have a once-daily dosing regimen. There is little head-to-head data comparing DOACs to each other, and clinically they are considered similar in terms of efficacy. Edoxaban is preferred in patients who may be taking other drugs such as anti-cancer or anti-HIV medication as it has relatively few drug interactions.

Apixaban is given twice daily, but in some patients may be a superior anticoagulant.

Table 12.3. Orally active anticoagulants.

Class	Agent	Used
Vitamin K antagonists — coumarins (e.g. warfarin) and indanediones (e.g. phenindione)		Venous thromboembolism, arterial thrombosis, atrial fibrillation, prosthetic cardiac valves
Direct oral anticoagulants (DOACs)	Direct thrombin inhibitor (e.g. dabigatran)	Venous thromboembolism, atrial fibrillation
	Direct factor Xa inhibitors (e.g. rivaroxaban, apixaban, edoxaban and betrixaban)	Prophylaxis and treatment of venous thromboembolism; stroke prevention in atrial fibrillation

Table 12.4.   Studies comparing warfarin and DOAC.

	Trial	Scenario	Outcome
Rivaroxaban versus warfarin	EINSTEIN-DVT	Acute DVT	Breakthrough thrombosis 2.1% on rivaroxaban versus 3% on warfarin Bleeding 0.8% on rivaroxaban versus 1.2% on warfarin
	EINSTEIN-PE	Acute pulmonary embolism	Breakthrough thrombosis 2.1% on rivaroxaban versus 1.8% on warfarin Bleeding 1.1% on rivaroxaban versus 2.2% on warfarin
Dabigatran versus warfarin	RE-COVER	Symptomatic VTE	Breakthrough thrombosis 2.4% on dabigatran versus 2.1% on warfarin Bleeding 1.6% on dabigatran versus 1.9% on warfarin
Apixaban versus warfarin	AMPLIFY	Deep vein thrombosis	Breakthrough thrombosis 2.3% on apixaban versus 2.7% on warfarin Bleeding 0.6% on apixaban versus 1.8% on warfarin

DOACs can be used long term with excellent safety data. For apixaban and rivaroxaban, a dose reduction is recommended after 6 months to reduce the risk of bleeding. For apixaban, the risk of being on long-term low-dose apixaban appears to be extremely low in terms of bleeding, and therefore it is often used for patients requiring long-term anticoagulation.

Monitoring of DOACs is not generally required, although we sometimes do this in patients with significant renal or hepatic impairment, extremes of body weight or suspected drug interactions.

If a patient has a breakthrough thrombosis on a DOAC, then compliance must be assessed. If the patient has been taking the drug appropriately (rivaroxaban *must* be taken after food, for example), then a switch to an alternative DOAC can be considered, but most often treatment with LMWH or a VKA is recommended.

The effects of DOACs can be selectively reversed with andexanet alpha or overcome through the use of a low dose of prothrombin complex concentrate (PCC); however some patients then suffer a thrombotic event (see Table 12.6).

Vitamin K antagonists

The vitamin K antagonists fall into two drug groups, the coumarins and the indanediones such as phenindione (Table 12.3). The vitamin K antagonist most used in the United Kingdom is warfarin, which is one of the coumarins. Vitamin K is needed for the final step in the conversion of precursors of the vitamin K-dependent coagulation factors (factors II, VII, IX and X) into their active forms; they similarly affect the naturally occurring anticoagulants protein C and protein S. This final step, γ-carboxylation, is blocked when vitamin K deficiency or a vitamin K antagonist prevents vitamin K from being converted to its active form. The vitamin K-dependent factors are needed for both the intrinsic and the extrinsic pathways of coagulation (Fig. 12.4). However, they have a greater effect

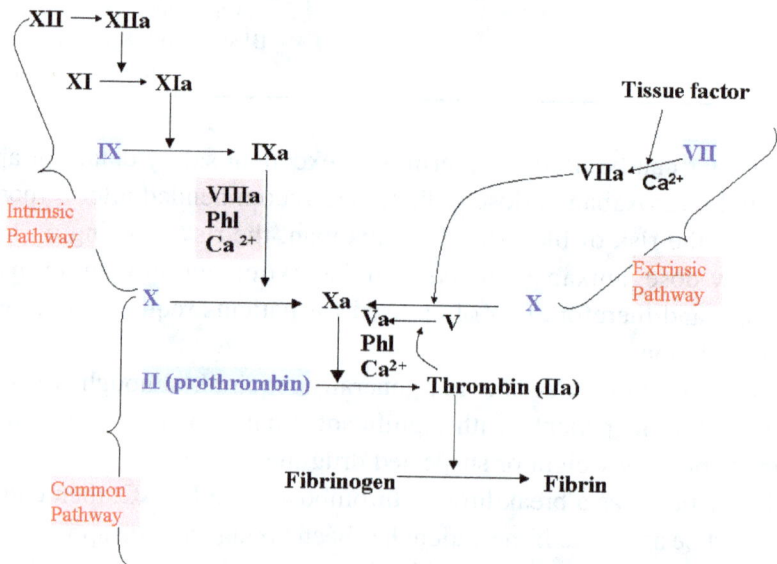

Fig. 12.4.   Coagulation factors, the synthesis of which is affected by vitamin K-dependent factors (blue). Note that the prothrombin time will be affected by concentrations of three of these four factors.

on the extrinsic than the intrinsic pathway so a modification of the prothrombin time (PT) is used for monitoring. The half-life of factor VII (4–6 hours) is much shorter than factor II (72 hours), IX (24 hours) or X (36 hours), so the PT is much more sensitive to immediate dose changes. As the PT reference range can change depending on the laboratory reagents used and to ensure that results between laboratories are comparable, a calculation is applied to the PT to give a separate result, which is the international normalised ratio (INR). This takes account of the difference in prothrombin times measured with different thromboplastins. Each batch of thromboplastin produced by a manufacturer is compared with an international reference thromboplastin and is assigned an International Sensitivity Index (ISI). The INR is then calculated as the ratio of the patient's prothrombin time to the prothrombin time of pooled normal plasma, raised to the power of the ISI:

$$INR = \left(\frac{\text{Patient's prothrombin time}}{\text{Mean normal prothrombin time}} \right)^{ISI}$$

The time for vitamin K antagonists to have an effect depends on the plasma half-life of the various vitamin K-dependent factors. However, for the PT is at least a number of days because it is the level of factor II, which has a long half-life, that is the most important factor determining the anticoagulant effect. When there is a need for immediately effective anticoagulation, it is necessary to use heparin initially and continue it for at least 5 days; there should also be a 3-day overlap of the oral anticoagulant and heparin, often called bridging. In hospitalised patients, the INR is measured daily during this period until it is in the therapeutic range, and it should be in the therapeutic range for at least 2 days before stopping heparin.

Vitamin K antagonists have a narrow therapeutic window. To reduce the risk of bleeding their effect must be carefully monitored throughout therapy and a therapeutic range appropriate to the degree of thrombotic risk must be selected. For example, an INR of 2.0–3.0 is sufficient for a patient being treated after initial heparinisation for a venous thrombosis or a pulmonary embolus, whereas for a patient with a prosthetic cardiac valve, an INR of 2.5–4.0 is usually selected. Many patients can self-test and monitor their own therapy.

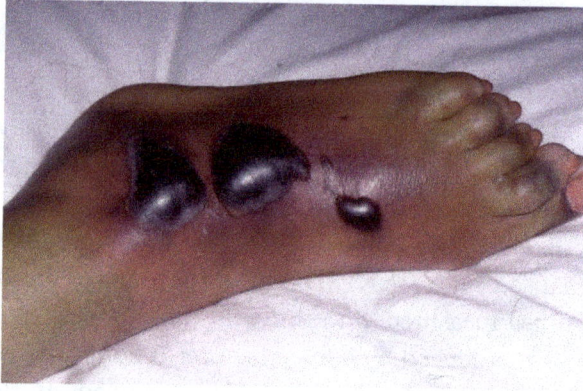

Fig. 12.5. Haemorrhage as a result of tripping on a footpath in a patient taking warfarin for a prosthetic cardiac valve.

The effect of vitamin K antagonists can be unpredictable, being influenced, for example, by diet, alcohol and the intake of drugs that interfere with the metabolism of the oral anticoagulant. Drug interactions are common and it is prudent to check the British National Formulary before commencing any new drug in an anticoagulated patient. Dosage requirement is lower in the elderly and in those with congestive cardiac failure or liver disease. It is therefore necessary to check the INR at least every four to six weeks even in a patient who is usually stable. Patients whose anticoagulant control is unstable need monitoring much more frequently.

The most frequent adverse effect of oral anticoagulant therapy is haemorrhage (Fig. 12.5). The effect on the coagulation system can be reversed by the administration of vitamin K1 either orally or intravenously (see Table 12.6). This takes several hours to be effective since coagulation factor precursors must be γ-carboxylated. More rapid reversal can be achieved with infusion of prothrombin complex concentrate (which contains factors II, IX and X and variable, often low, amounts of VII) or by transfusion of fresh frozen plasma if the concentrate is not available.

Coumarin anticoagulants cross the placenta and are teratogenic; they should not be administered during the first trimester of pregnancy. They are also better avoided after 36 weeks of gestation because of the risk of maternal and fetal haemorrhage.

Direct thrombin inhibitors

Orally active direct thrombin inhibitors can be used in a similar manner to warfarin but in a fixed dose and without the need for monitoring. One of these drugs, dabigatran, has shown similar efficacy and safety to warfarin in atrial fibrillation, treatment of acute VTE and prevention of VTE after high-risk orthopaedic surgery including total hip and knee arthroplasty.

It should be avoided, or the dose reduced, in patients with end-stage renal disease or on haemodialysis, and the dose should be reduced in patients with an estimated glomerular filtration rate of 15–30 ml/min/ 1.73 m^2 or less. Its effect can be reversed by idarucizumab, a monoclonal antibody (see Table 12.6).

Dabigatran is the anticoagulant which is least likely to cause abnormal uterine bleeding (menorrhagia) in young women, and is the drug of choice for the management of thrombosis in this population. It cannot be given while pregnant or breastfeeding.

Antiplatelet Agents

Various drugs interfere with platelet aggregation and can be used as antithrombotic agents. Their sites of action are shown in Fig. 12.6. Antiplatelet drugs with different mechanisms of action are synergistic.

Aspirin

Arachidonic acid in the platelet membrane is converted to the aggregating agent thromboxane A2 by the consecutive actions of cyclo-oxygenase and thromboxane synthase. Aspirin acetylates and irreversibly inactivates cyclo-oxygenase. It thus causes an impairment of platelet function that persists for the lifespan of the platelet. In higher doses, aspirin interferes with the synthesis of endothelial cell prostacyclin, and therefore when it is used as an antithrombotic agent it is used in low doses, e.g. 75 or 100 mg daily. Aspirin is indicated in patients with acute coronary syndromes and should be continued indefinitely. Its long-term use is also indicated following myocardial infarction and ischaemic stroke, and to maintain patency following stenting of coronary arteries. Aspirin is

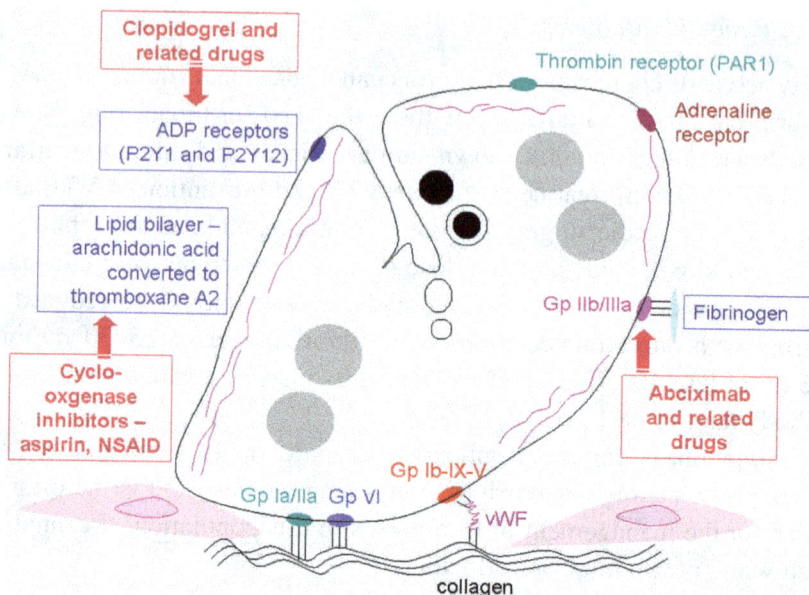

Fig. 12.6. Sites of action of different classes of antiplatelet drugs (bold red). For an explanation of other parts of the diagram, see Fig. 11.3. NSAID, non-steroidal anti-inflammatory drug.

administered to patients at risk of thrombosis because of polycythaemia vera and essential thrombocythaemia. Non-steroidal anti-inflammatory drugs (NSAIDs) also inhibit cyclo-oxygenase but the effect is reversible.

Aspirin therapy is associated with an increased risk of haemorrhage, particularly gastrointestinal haemorrhage. Because platelet function is impaired for the lifespan of the platelet, serious haemorrhage may require platelet transfusion.

Platelet phosphodiesterase inhibitors

Platelet phosphodiesterase inhibitors increase platelet cyclic adenosine monophosphate and thus inhibit platelet aggregation. They include dipyridamole, which is used for its antithrombotic effect, and anagrelide, which reduces platelet production from megakaryocytes in addition to inhibiting platelet function.

ADP receptor antagonists

Drugs of this group, or their active metabolites, antagonise platelet function by binding to the platelet adenosine diphosphate (ADP) receptor (known as P2Y12). The most frequently used drug of this group is clopidogrel. Both clopidogrel and prasugrel are prodrugs, which are converted to an active metabolite, whereas ticagrelor and cangrelor are themselves active drugs. ADP receptor antagonists are indicated, together with aspirin, in patients who are at acute risk of thrombosis following percutaneous coronary angioplasty (stent insertion) for an acute coronary syndrome. These drugs can also be used in other circumstances when aspirin therapy would be indicated but cannot be tolerated by the patient. The effects of clopidogrel and prasugrel are irreversible, whereas the effects of ticagrelor and cangrelor are reversible.

Platelet glycoprotein IIb/IIIa fibrinogen receptor inhibitors

This group of drugs binds to the platelet fibrinogen receptor, platelet glycoprotein IIb/IIIa. The group includes eptifibatide, tirofiban and abciximab (a human–mouse chimaeric monoclonal antibody). They are indicated as a supplement to aspirin and clopidogrel in some patients with acute coronary syndromes and, briefly, following percutaneous coronary intervention. In a small percentage of patients (0.5–1%), first exposure to these drugs can lead to the sudden onset of severe thrombocytopenia. The use of these drugs would normally be under the direct supervision of a cardiologist to balance the risks and benefits.

Epoprostenol

Epoprostenol (prostacyclin) is a potent parenteral vasodilator and inhibitor of platelet aggregation. Its main use is in refractory pulmonary hypertension.

Thrombolytic Therapy

Patients who have suffered thrombosis but do not yet have irreversible tissue injury may benefit from therapeutic thrombolysis. Such patients include those with recent coronary occlusion and actual or impending myocardial infarction and those presenting with a cerebrovascular accident and found to have cerebral thrombosis or embolism. Thrombolytic therapy should be given speedily, e.g. within 12 hours of the onset of symptoms of coronary occlusion. Thrombolytic therapy is also indicated in patients with clinically serious or massive pulmonary embolism, and the use of local (catheter-directed) thrombolysis is emerging as a safer alternative in patients with significant but less life-threatening thrombotic events.

Patients with both arterial thrombosis (MI/CVA) and venous thrombosis (extensive DVT and PE) can also be offered thrombectomy, where an interventional radiologist removes the thrombus using a capture device. This technique has proven benefits in the short term for reducing the immediate mortality of thrombotic events, but outside of stroke medicine, the long-term benefits are currently unclear.

In patients with primary myocardial infarction, percutaneous coronary intervention with the insertion of a stent is the preferred procedure, supplemented by aspirin, clopidogrel (or a related drug) and sometimes a platelet IIb/IIIa inhibitor such as abciximab. When this cannot be achieved within 90 minutes, thrombolytic therapy becomes the preferred option.

In patients with ischaemic stroke, thrombolytic therapy is indicated if there are no contraindications and if it can be given within 3 hours of the event. Treatment can even sometimes be effacious up to 4.5–6 hours after the event.

In patients with thrombosed indwelling catheters, cannulae or shunts (e.g. arteriovenous shunts to permit haemodialysis), thrombolytic therapy, which can be administered at the site of thrombosis, may restore patency. Regional thrombolysis, using catheter delivery, can also be of benefit for arterial thrombosis causing critical ischaemia and venous thrombosis causing arterial compromise.

Agents that can be employed for thrombolysis include recombinant human proteins and streptokinase, which is of bacterial origin. Human products that are available include recombinant tissue plasminogen activator (alteplase) and urokinase. Complications include bleeding (especially intracranial), hypotension and allergic reactions.

Diagnosis of Venous Thromboembolism

There are hazards associated with anticoagulant and thrombolytic therapy and diagnoses must therefore be firmly based. An algorithm showing how the diagnosis of deep vein thrombosis in the leg can be approached is shown in Fig. 12.7. The Wells score establishes the pre-test probability of a venous thrombosis measured from 0 to 9.

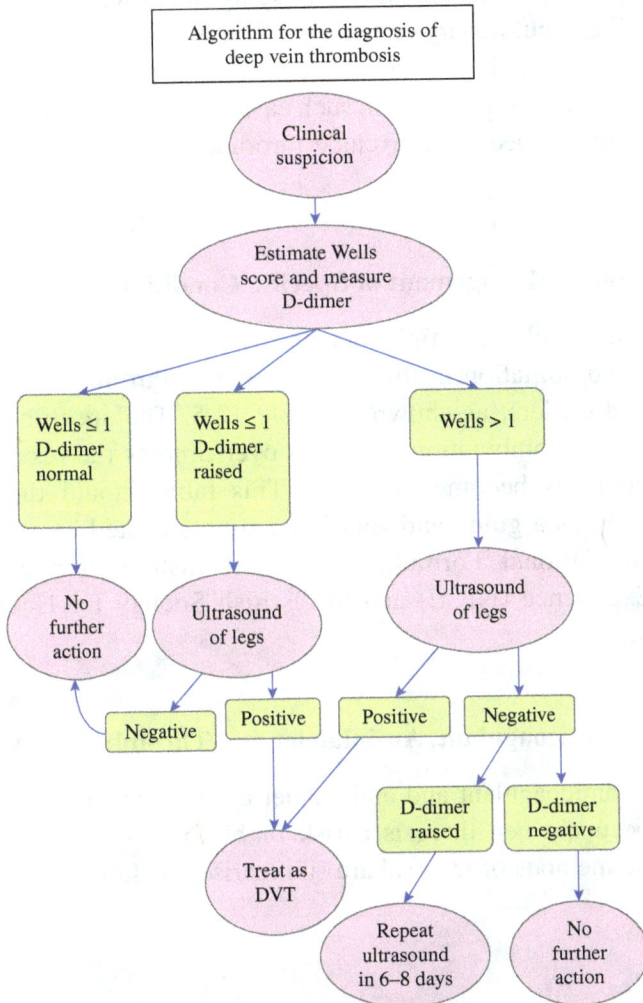

Fig. 12.7. An algorithm showing how the diagnosis of deep vein thrombosis in the leg can be approached.

The diagnosis of a pulmonary embolism can be confirmed with a ventilation–perfusion (VQ) scan (lung distal to an embolus is ventilated but not perfused) or computed tomography pulmonary angiography (CTPA). Although the techniques have different sensitivities and specificities for small versus large and acute versus chronic thrombosis, CTPA is usually the preferred imaging modality due to accessibility and capacity. VQ scanning requires dedicated radioisotopes which are in relatively short supply. The need for diagnostic imaging can be reduced by the application of a Wells pulmonary embolism score; if it is 4 or less and D-dimer is not increased, imaging is not needed as thrombosis is unlikely to be the cause of the current symptoms. In such cases, alternative causes should be sought before proceeding to exclude thrombosis as the aetiology of the current symptoms.

Antithrombotic Management of Specific Conditions

Various anticoagulant, antiplatelet and thrombolytic agents are used alone or in combination in the management of thrombotic and thromboembolic disorders, as shown in Table 12.5. The specific choice of drugs and drug combinations changes over time as the results of new randomised trials become available. This table should therefore be regarded only as a guide and should be supplemented by reference to the British National Formulary, National Institute for Health and Clinical Excellence (NICE) and the British Society for Haematology guidelines.

Reversal of Anticoagulant, Antiplatelet and Thrombolytic Agents

Reversal of anticoagulant and antiplatelet agents may be required when bleeding occurs, when there is a risk of bleeding or when surgery is needed. The methods of reversal are summarised in Table 12.6.

Table 12.5. The integration of anticoagulant, antiplatelet and thrombolytic therapy in the management of thrombotic disorders.

Conditions	Agents that are indicated
Prevention of venous thromboembolism in high-risk surgical patients	LMWH or possibly a direct thrombin inhibitor (dabigatran orally) or a factor Xa inhibitor (fondaparinux parenterally or rivaroxaban orally)
Treatment of deep vein thrombosis or pulmonary embolism without circulatory compromise	LMWH (or unfractionated heparin if there is a high risk of bleeding) + continuing warfarin (target INR 2.0–3.0) or possibly plus dabigatran; alternatively, rivaroxaban or apixaban without LMWH
Treatment of pulmonary embolism with compromised circulation	Thrombolytic therapy (alteplase, streptokinase or urokinase) followed by heparin and then continuing warfarin
Acute coronary syndrome (without ST segment elevation)	Aspirin + clopidogrel + an antiplatelet glycoprotein IIb/IIIa inhibitor; aspirin and clopidogrel continued for 12 months
Myocardial infarction, percutaneous coronary intervention possible within 90 minutes	Aspirin + clopidogrel + antiplatelet glycoprotein IIb/IIIa inhibitor (abciximab) + 8 days of LMWH; long-term aspirin + clopidogrel
Myocardial infarction, percutaneous coronary intervention not possible within 90 minutes	Thrombolytic therapy (e.g. streptokinase, alteplase, reteplase or tenecteplase) + 8 days of LMWH; long-term aspirin + clopidogrel
Acute ischaemic stroke	Thrombolytic therapy with alteplase within 3 hours (possibly useful up to 6 hours); long-term aspirin + modified-release dipyridamole
Transient ischaemic attack	Long-term aspirin + modified-release dipyridamole
Cardiopulmonary bypass	Unfractionated heparin
Haemodialysis	LMWH or unfractionated heparin
Prosthetic heart valve	Lifelong warfarin (target INR 2.5–4.0); dipyridamole can be used as an adjunct
Tissue valve	Warfarin for three months (target INR 2.0–3.0)
Atrial fibrillation	Warfarin (target INR 2.0–3.0) or dabigatran or factor Xa inhibitors such as rivaroxaban

Note: INR, international normalised ratio; LMWH, low-molecular-weight heparin.

Table 12.6. Reversal agents for antithrombotic agents.

Agent	Reversal agent	Additional information	Guide dose
Unfractionated heparin	Protamine sulphate	Full reversal is achievable	1 mg of protamine sulphate for every 100 units of heparin
Low-molecular-weight heparin	Protamine sulphate	Full reversal is not achievable	1 mg of protamine sulphate for every 100 anti-Xa units
Vitamin K antagonists	Vitamin K	Takes 8–24 hours; suitable if reversal is required in 12–24 hours	2 mg vitamin K1 orally
	Prothrombin complex concentrate (PCC)	Suitable for immediate reversal in life-threatening bleeding or emergency surgery in addition to vitamin K1 5 mg given slowly IV	20–50 units/kg, depending on INR
Direct thrombin inhibitor, dabigatran	Idarucizumab	Immediate reversal with 2 consecutive infusions	Risk of thrombotic complications
Direct Xa inhibitors: rivaroxaban, apixaban, edoxaban	Andexanet	Immediate reversal	Risk of thrombotic complications
Thrombolytic therapy	Tranexamic acid, (antifibrinolytic agent)	Thrombolytic agents have a very short half-life	1,000 mg IV stat
Antiplatelet agents	Platelet transfusion	May not be effective due to persistent antiplatelet effect in patient circulation	1 pool given at a time

Note: INR, international normalised ratio; IV, intravenous; LMWH, low-molecular-weight heparin.

Conclusions

Thrombotic disease is a major problem globally. It is the cause of significant mortality and morbidity. All antithrombotic and thrombolytic therapy requires a balancing of potential benefits and potential harm. A great variety of drugs based on different principles are available. The drugs that are chosen for an individual patient should be based on the best evidence available, which is likely to change with time.

Test Case 12.1

A 27-year-old woman presents with swelling and tenderness of the left calf. A Doppler examination shows a left deep vein thrombosis with some extension into the thigh. The patient is not taking the oral contraceptive and there are no obvious precipitating factors for a venous thrombosis. She has not visited her GP for some time but on specific questioning, she admits to intermittent joint swelling. An FBC and a coagulation screen performed prior to the planned anticoagulant therapy show the following:

WBC $3.4 \times 10^9/l$,
Neutrophil count $1.2 \times 10^9/l$,
Hb 129 g/l,
Platelet count $72 \times 10^9/l$,
Prothrombin time 14 seconds (normal range 12–14),
Activated partial thromboplastin time 67 seconds (normal range 30–40), thrombin time 20 seconds (control 21 seconds).

Questions

1. What do you suspect?
2. If your suspicions are correct, what treatment is indicated?
3. Are any further investigations indicated?

Write down your answers before checking the correct answer (page 408) and re-reading any relevant part of the chapter.

13

Blood Transfusion

Fateha Chowdhury

What Do You Need to Know?

☞ Blood provision and usage
☞ How donors are recruited, screened and tested
☞ The types of blood components and blood products that are used for transfusion
☞ The major blood group systems
☞ ABO and Rh blood group systems
☞ Haemolytic disease of the fetus and newborn
☞ The principles of tests done in a blood transfusion laboratory
☞ The indications for the use of blood and blood products
☞ How blood transfusions can be made safer
☞ Prescribing and setting up transfusions
☞ Risks in transfusions
☞ Management of transfusion reactions

Blood Provision and Usage

Improvements in blood-sparing techniques, such as laparoscopic surgery, advancements in interventional radiological procedures, cell salvage, identification and treatment of anaemia preoperatively and improved peri-operative management of anticoagulant and antiplatelet drugs, have resulted in better patient blood management. Consequently, blood usage has decreased over the past decade, although transfusion continues to play a crucial role in replacement following major surgery and after delivery or trauma. It also remains a cornerstone for the effective treatment of inherited and acquired bleeding disorders and malignant diseases such as leukaemia, lymphoma and other cancers needing surgery and/or chemotherapy.

The UK has four national blood services, which are required to be licensed as blood establishments. England's blood service, NHS Blood and Transplant (NHSBT), is the largest.

Hospital blood banks and blood establishments have key requirements, which are defined in the Blood Safety and Quality Regulations.[1] These are enforced through regular inspections by the Medicines and Healthcare Products Regulatory Agency (MHRA). The MHRA requires 100% 'vein to vein' traceability of all blood components and products, i.e. from donor to patient. An overview of the transfusion process is given in Fig. 13.1.

Blood Donor Recruitment and Screening

Blood donation eligibility

A potential donor must be fit and healthy, possess suitable veins and be able to meet all donor eligibility criteria. These are checked before every donation. People with chronic medical conditions, such as heart conditions, high blood pressure, diabetes, previous organ transplants, autoimmune disorders and cancers, are not eligible to donate. All UK donors are altruistic volunteers. The essential eligibility criteria is as follows:

- Unpaid volunteer
- Completion of medical questionnaire (lifestyle, travel history, medical history and medications)
- Pass mandatory and discretionary tests
- Has not received blood transfusion or tissue/organ transplant since 1980
- Age:
  - 17–65 for first-time donors
  - No upper age limit for regular donors (provided annual health check is passed)

---

[1] https://www.legislation.gov.uk/uksi/2005/50/contents/made.

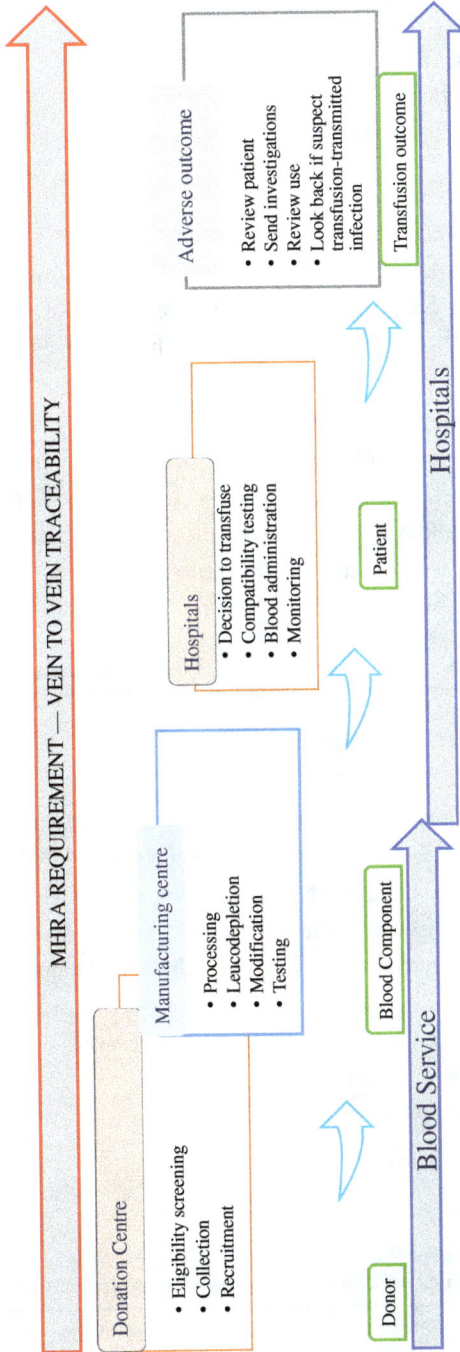

Fig. 13.1. Diagram of the transfusion process from donor to patient.

Note: Donations are sent to manufacturing sites, samples for mandatory tests (grouping, infection screen) are sent to testing sites. The end components will only be released to hospitals providing all the screening tests are satisfactory. Before blood components can be transfused, patients will need compatibility testing. During administration of blood component, the patient will need to be monitored by a qualified healthcare person for adverse reactions.

- Weight: 50–158 kg
- Haemoglobin estimation:
  - Male donors > 135 g/l
  - Female donors > 125 g/l

Donation safety check

All donors must meet all the criteria set out in the Donor Selection Guidelines and Donation Safety Check. These relate to lifestyle, travel, occupations and medical and sexual histories. There are certain professions and travel histories which may prevent donors/donations from being accepted either permanently or temporarily.

Donations are never accepted from individuals who have received transfusions (blood, plasma, platelets or any other blood products or tissue/organ) after 1 January 1980. This reduces the risk of variant Creutzfeldt–Jakob (vCJD) transmission. Table 13.1 details situations where donations may not be accepted.

Table 13.1.   List of situations where blood donation will not be accepted.

Donations are not accepted from people who:
- have tested positive for HIV
- are a carrier for hepatitis B or C
- have injected non-prescribed drugs including body-building and injectable tanning agents
- have a recent travel history that poses a risk, *e.g. malaria, T. cruzi and West Nile virus.*

Potential donors may be asked to wait up to three months before donating if:
- they have had anal sex with a new partner in the last three months
- have finished taking Pre-Exposure Prophylaxis or Post-Exposure Prophylaxis in the last three months

Or in the last three months have had sexual contact with a partner who:
- is HIV (human immunodeficiency virus) positive
- is HTLV (human T-cell lymphotropic virus) 1 or 2 positive
- is a hepatitis B carrier
- is a hepatitis C carrier
- is syphilis positive
- has received money or drugs for sex
- has injected non-prescribed drugs including body-building and injectable tanning agents

Note: Donations are not accepted from people who are undergoing investigations for a medical condition and who have recently got a tattoo or piercing. Pregnancy is a contraindication for donation; generally women must wait at least six months post pregnancy before being eligible.

Consent

All donors must grant their consent to allow the NHSBT to use their donations in the most appropriate way and are also required to agree to be informed should they fail any of the required mandatory tests.

How is blood donated?

Donors are usually required to make an appointment at a donation centre; however, occasionally, donors are accepted as walk-ins, depending on several factors, including location and stock levels nationally.

There are two ways of donating: whole blood donation (the most common) (Fig. 13.2) or by apheresis; the latter process allows the donation of a particular blood component.

Whole blood donation

Blood is obtained via venesection into one of two main pack types; this is determined by donor-related factors (such as blood group, gender and

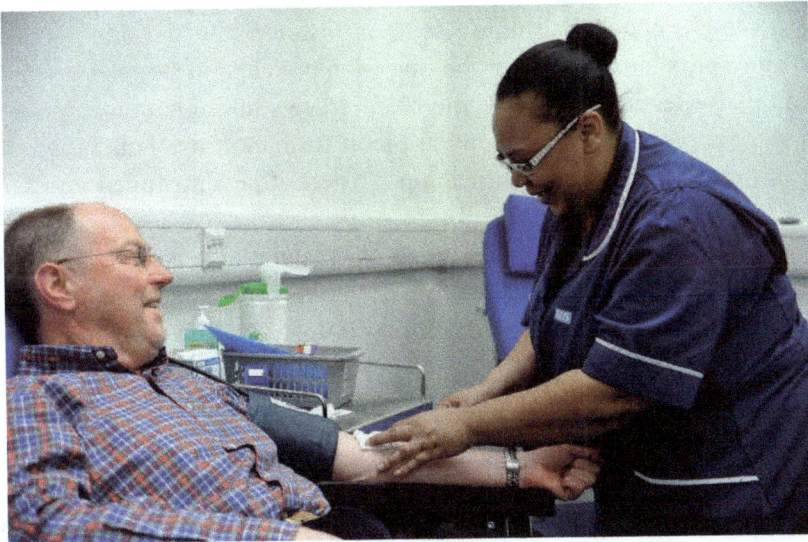

Fig. 13.2. Whole-blood donation at a transfusion centre. The donor is looked after by a donor carer throughout the process. Post-donation, donors are given tea and biscuits; this not only makes the donor feel cared for but also gives the donor carers the opportunity to observe the donor for adverse effects.

time of venepuncture) and the blood component required, which is driven by other factors, the main ones being demand and stock levels. This process is quick and inexpensive.

The first 20 ml of venesected blood is drawn into a sample pouch. Several samples are taken from the pouch into tubes containing EDTA (an anticoagulant which prevents the blood from clotting). Approximately 470 ml (±10%) is collected into a plastic bag containing citrate-phosphate-dextrose (CPD), which prevents the blood in the bag from clotting. The needle and sample pouch are cut away using a heat sealer and discarded safely after the session. The rest of the packs are sent to the NHSBT manufacturing site, while the samples are sent to the testing centre.

Apheresis donation

This procedure allows the collection of a specific blood component. It involves the donor being attached to a cell separator machine by two intravenous lines.

Similarly to whole blood donation, the first 20 ml of blood is drawn into a sample pouch. A single needle is inserted into the donor's arms. The tube splits into three after the diversion pouch, and samples are taken from this for testing. As the whole blood travels through a tube, citrate is added via a second tube to stop the blood from clotting. This blood then passes into the cell separator machine, where it is centrifuged and separated into its components.

Apheresis is often used for preparing platelet concentrates, allowing patients to receive platelets from a single donor. Using this method, up to three adult platelet doses or 12 paediatric doses can be obtained from a single procedure.

Apheresis donations of platelets and plasma can be collected more frequently than whole-blood donation, as the process allows red cells to be returned to the donor; this prevents the donor from becoming anaemic. The disadvantage of this procedure is that it is expensive and time-consuming for both the donor and the collection staff. An important advantage is that platelets can be matched to patients with specific needs or antibodies.

Frequency of donations

Before every donation, donors are screened for anaemia using a copper sulphate test to ensure that the haemoglobin level is above 135 g/l for males and above 125 g/l for females before proceeding.

Since men have higher iron stores than women, they can donate at shorter intervals, i.e. every 12 weeks. For women, the minimum donation interval is set at 16 weeks, not only because of their lower iron stores but also because of the regular menstrual blood loss they experience.

Platelet and plasma donations can be given every two weeks, i.e. 24 donations or up to a maximum of 15 litres per year.

Genetic haemochromatosis

Genetic haemochromatosis is an iron-loading condition. Donations are accepted from individuals with this condition, provided that all other criteria are met and the donor is under the care of a medical specialist. In addition, if the copper sulphate test is passed, donations can be given more frequently.

Tests on donation

Approximately 7,000 donations are tested daily by two testing laboratories in England. All donations undergo the mandatory tests listed in Table 13.2.

Table 13.2. Screening required for blood donations.

Mandatory tests	Travel history-dependant additional tests
HIV 1 and 2	Malarial
Hepatitis B	West Nile virus (WNV)
Hepatitis C	*Trypanosoma cruzi*
Hepatitis E	
HTLV 1 and 2	
Syphilis	

Depending on the donor's lifestyle or travel history, additional or discretionary testing may be undertaken.

Blood groups and antibodies

Every donation is tested for the ABO and D groups on red cells. The plasma is screened to detect the most common blood group antibodies which may be clinically significant, i.e. potentially causing a problem in the recipient of the transfusion. Some donations undergo extended phenotyping to allow closer matching. This is of particular importance for patients who need long-term red cell transfusion support, e.g. patients with haemoglobinopathies such as sickle cell disease.

Some group O donations are screened for high levels of anti-A and anti-B antibodies. When group O components containing a large amount of plasma (i.e. platelets) are transfused to group A, B or AB patients, it is important that they receive components with low anti-A and anti-B titres; this reduces the risk of haemolytic reactions. This is especially important for intrauterine/neonatal exchange transfusions and large-volume transfusions.

A percentage of donations are tested for cytomegalovirus (CMV) antibodies to ensure they are available for patients with certain immune deficiency states, pregnant women, intrauterine transfusions and neonates.

Testing for infectious diseases

Mandatory and discretionary tests (Table 13.2) must be passed for the donation to be deemed suitable for transfusion; this minimises the risk of transfusion-transmitted infections. Different methods of testing are undertaken; recently, all new donors have been tested for anti-HBV core antigen.

Where there is uncertainty about contact with an infectious agent, in certain situations, nucleic acid testing (NAT), which is more sensitive and able to detect positive results during the pre-serology window period, may be undertaken as a precautionary measure (Table 13.3).

All donations that exhibit a positive screening test are discarded; the donor is informed, counselled if further testing is needed and referred to

Table 13.3. Window period: Nucleic acid testing (NAT) vs. serology.

Infection	Days to detect		Difference (in days)
	NAT	**Serology (Ag/Ab)**	
HIV	12	17–22	5
HBV	28–31	35–44	12
HCV	10	70	60

Note: The benefit of NAT in identifying potential infections during the window period of any viral illness compared to serological tests is shown as the difference in the number of days required for obtaining test results. NAT allows earlier detection of positive results.

for treatment as required. Any donor with discrepant or inconclusive results will be withdrawn from donating until this is resolved through additional testing.

Reduction of bacterial contamination of blood components

Several measures are undertaken to reduce the risk of bacterial contamination. A significant reduction has been found by:

1. improved donor arm cleansing, which minimises bacterial skin contaminants in the collection bag;
2. diverting the first 20–30 ml of the blood into a pouch, which is used for mandatory and other tests;
3. using a closed bag system of multiple bags prepared in sterile facilities at manufacturing sites;
4. screening platelet components by culturing a sample using an automated microbial detection system, which continuously monitors the incubated culture bottles for 5–7 days, allowing the immediate identification of contaminated and associated units.

Transfusion transmission of prion-associated diseases

Since November 1999, all allogeneic blood components, except granulocytes, produced in the UK have been subjected to a leucocyte depletion process, leaving $<1 \times 10^6$ leucocytes in the pack. Leucodepletion reduces the risk of transmission of vCJD and makes transmission of CMV less likely. At-risk groups who are permanently deferred from donating as a precaution to prevent the transmission of prion-associated diseases are:

1. Individuals who may have been exposed to vCJD through the use of contaminated surgical instruments (from infected individuals), transfusion or transplant of tissues or organs.
2. Individuals who have been notified that a recipient of their blood/tissue/organ has developed a prion-related condition.
3. Individuals who have received: a tissue/organ transplant or blood transfusion since 1980, human pituitary-derived hormones, grafts of human dura mater or cornea, sclera or other ocular tissue.
4. Family members at risk of inherited prion disease.

Blood Components and Products

There are four main components of blood: plasma, red blood cells, white blood cells and platelets. Any therapeutic substance derived from blood is called a blood product.

At the manufacturing site, blood is processed and separated into different components through centrifugation. Fractionation of plasma is undertaken to produce products such as cryoprecipitate, albumin and immunoglobulins (Fig 13.3). During the COVID-19 pandemic, convalescent plasma was produced for use in several clinical trials.

Red cells

A specialised device compresses the bag of blood between two plates, squeezing the plasma out at the top and red cells at the bottom; this leaves the buffy coat which contains the granulocytes and platelets. Once plasma has been removed from the red cells, saline, adenine, glucose and mannitol (SAGM) are added to improve their survival *in vitro*. However, for neonatal components, SAGM are not used, as mannitol is a mild diuretic and can affect the kidneys and brains of infants. Instead, an anticoagulant

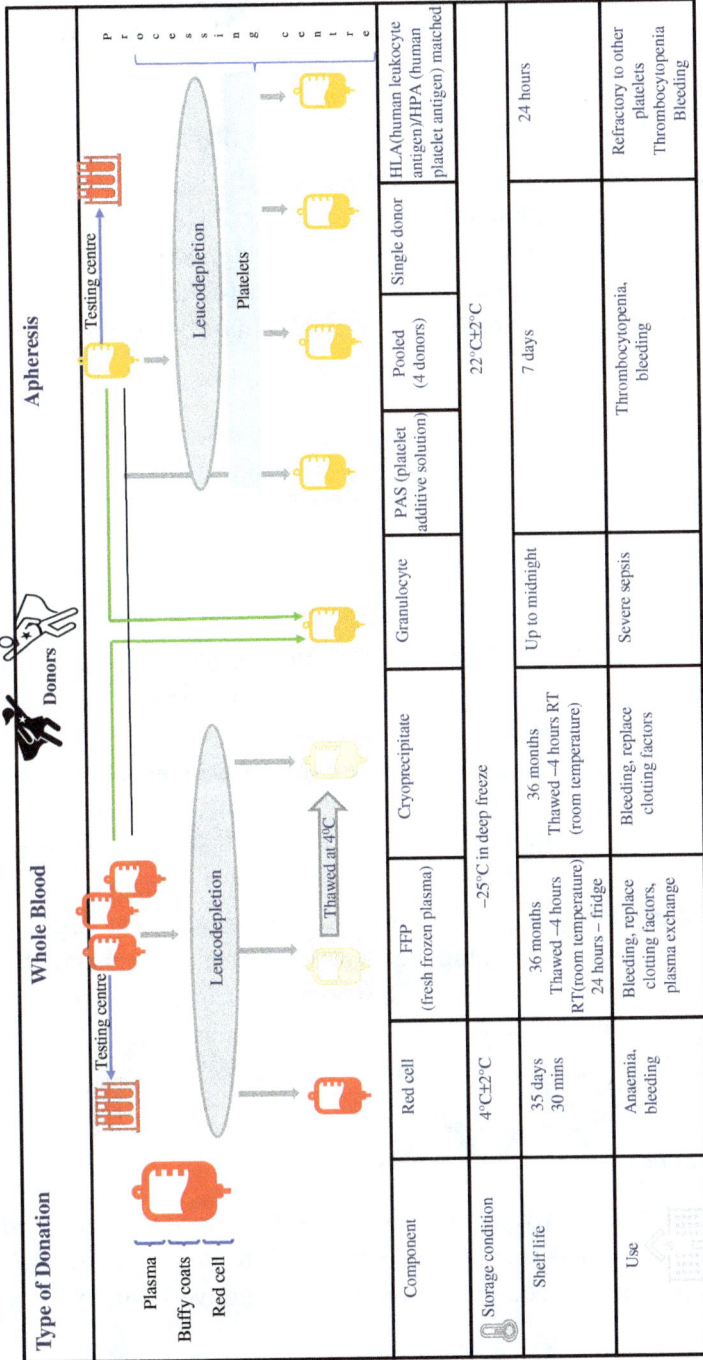

Component	Red cell	FFP (fresh frozen plasma)	Cryoprecipitate	Granulocyte	PAS (platelet additive solution)	Pooled (4 donors)	Single donor	HLA(human leukocyte antigen)/HPA (human platelet antigen) matched
Storage condition	4°C±2°C	−25°C in deep freeze			22°C±2°C			
Shelf life	35 days 30 mins	36 months Thawed −4 hours RT(room temperature) 24 hours – fridge	36 months Thawed −4 hours RT (room temperature)	Up to midnight		7 days		24 hours
Use	Anaemia, bleeding	Bleeding, replace clotting factors, plasma exchange	Bleeding, replace clotting factors	Severe sepsis		Thrombocytopenia, bleeding		Refractory to other platelets Thrombocytopenia Bleeding

Fig. 13.3. Production of blood components and storage conditions and usage.

solution containing CPD and adenine is used. This extends red cell survival by providing adenine, which is needed for the maintenance of red cell adenosine triphosphate (ATP) levels.

Red cells are stored in a temperature-controlled fridge; once removed, if not transfused, a unit must be returned to the fridge within 30 minutes to allow the core temperature to return to $4 \pm 2°C$, before being issued again. Units which are not returned to the fridge within this timeframe must be discarded. If red cells are being transfused, this must be completed within four hours; otherwise, the units must be discarded.

Whole blood

Military services transfuse whole blood, but this is not a routine medical practice in the UK. Whole blood is only available for use in clinical trials.

Platelets

Platelets possess ABO antigens on their surface. Ideally, platelets should be matched for ABO and Rh D groups to achieve the best response; this also reduces alloimmunisation.

Anti-A or anti-B antibodies in the plasma of platelet components may rarely cause haemolysis of the recipient's red cells, especially in infants and young children. High titre-negative platelets are only needed if there is a need to substitute across ABO groups. Group O platelets should ideally only be given to group O patients. Platelets are stored at $22 \pm 2°C$ (i.e. room temperature) and should be kept in motion on an agitator; this ensures their effectiveness. The shelf life of platelets has been extended to seven days since the introduction of screening for bacterial growth. There are several different types of platelet concentrates.

Pooled platelets

Pooled platelets are derived from whole blood obtained from four individual donations, pooled into a single bag and resuspended in a mix of plasma from a male blood donor and platelet additive solution (PAS).

Apheresis platelets

Apheresis platelets are often referred to as 'single donor platelets'. Approximately 48% of the platelets supplied to hospitals are apheresis platelets. All apheresis platelets are tested for CMV status, and approximately 60% of units are CMV negative.

Platelets in PAS

PAS platelets are often recommended if patients have had allergic reactions to pooled or apheresis platelets. PAS is a crystalloid nutrient medium used to enable the volume of stored plasma to be reduced by approximately 60–70%; it is the proteins in the plasma which are often responsible for allergic reactions. The washing process allows the removal of all the plasma, which can take 4–6 hours; therefore, this type of platelet concentrate needs to be ordered well in advance from the blood service.

HLA/HPA-matched platelets

Platelets express antigens which are shared with other cells, such as ABO and human leucocyte antigens (HLAs), but they also have platelet-specific antigens, i.e. human platelet antigens (HPAs), which can stimulate the production of antibodies once exposed to foreign platelets carrying different antigens.

Patients who are regularly transfused with platelets may develop antibodies, usually to HLA. If this is confirmed, HLA-matched platelets should be transfused. A repeat full blood count should be taken within 60 minutes after the completion of transfusion to assess the response. This ensures that the best HLA-matched platelets can be provided for subsequent transfusions. HPA antibodies are rare; they are identified in approximately 2% of patients, and HPA-matched platelets are available.

Patients with inherited platelet disorders should be transfused with HLA-matched platelets whenever possible to prevent antibody formation.

The blood service needs to be notified at least 24 hours in advance to source and manufacture these specialised platelets. All HLA/HPA platelets

Table 13.4.   Causes of platelet refractoriness.

Immune	Non-Immune (most common)

Platelet alloantibodies
    HLA or HPA
	Infections & treatments
	    Antibiotics (e.g. penicillin, teicoplanin)
	    Antifungals (e.g. ambisome)

Other antibodies
    Platelet autoantibodies
    Drug-dependant platelet antibodies
	Splenomegaly

Immune complexes	Bleeding
	Disseminated intravascular coagulation (DIC)

Note: Non-immune causes are the most common cause of refractoriness.

are irradiated, which prevents transfusion-associated graft-versus-host disease (TAGvHD).

In an emergency, such as a patient with major bleeding, transfusion should not be delayed in order to provide HLA/HPA-matched or washed platelets.

Platelet refractoriness

Platelet refractoriness, or a failure to respond to platelet transfusion, can be subdivided into immune mechanisms, most importantly HLA alloimmunisation, and non-immune platelet consumption. The response to a prophylactic platelet transfusion can be assessed by measuring the platelet count after the transfusion, ideally within 60 minutes of its completion. If a patient's platelet count fails to increase by at least 20×10^9/l, this indicates refractoriness. It is important to identify the underlying causes listed in Table 13.4 to ensure that the patient is managed appropriately.

Fresh frozen plasma

Plasma can be obtained by whole-blood donation or apheresis. Only plasma from male donors is used. This reduces the risk of transfusion-associated lung injury (TRALI). Plasma is frozen within 24 hours of collection to maintain the activity of blood-clotting factors.

For many years, the UK Department of Health recommended that patients born on or after 1 January 1996 should only receive plasma imported from countries with a low risk of vCJD. This decision was reversed in 2019. Now, everyone receives UK-sourced plasma. For neonates and infants, plasma is sourced from regular donors, not first-time donors. Commercially available fresh frozen plasma (FFP), prepared from large donor pools, is treated with solvent–detergents to reduce the risk of virus transmission and is tested for HIV, hepatitis B, C and E, hepatitis A and parvovirus B19.

FFP is used to treat many conditions that require plasma exchange, but its most common use is to replace clotting factors in bleeding patients. In a massive haemorrhage, FFP should be transfused in a 1:1 ratio (i.e. equal volumes) with red cells to prevent the development of coagulopathy.

Further fractionation of plasma pooled from large numbers of donors leads to the production of blood products such as cryoprecipitate, albumin, immunoglobulin, clotting factor concentrates and prothrombin complex concentrates. The therapeutic role of blood products is summarised in Table 13.5.

Table 13.5. Available blood products and indications for use.

Product	Indication
Cryoprecipitate	Massive haemorrhage,* to replace clotting factors, especially fibrinogen
Anti-D immunoglobulin (Ig) for obstetrics use	Pregnancy Routine antenatal anti-D prophylaxis for D-negative women Sensitising events during pregnancy
Immunoglobulin (Ig)	Correction of deficiency; in high doses, for autoimmune diseases, e.g. autoimmune thrombocytopenic purpura (ITP)
Human albumin solution	Hypoproteinaemia (e.g. liver disease, burns) or plasma exchange
Plasma-derived clotting factors (FVIII, FIX, FXI, FX)	Inherited bleeding disorders to cover surgery/bleeding episodes

(Continued)

Table 13.5.   (*Continued*)

Product	Indication
Prothrombin complex concentrate (Octaplex®)	Reversal of anticoagulants (warfarin or the direct-acting oral anticoagulants)
Fibrinogen concentrate	Inherited fibrinogen disorders and massive haemorrhage* where fibrinogen is low

Note: *Massive blood loss can be defined as blood loss equalling or exceeding one blood volume in 24 hours, with the normal adult blood volume being approximately 7% of ideal body weight; alternative definitions include loss of 50% of blood volume within 3 hours or, for an adult, blood loss at a rate exceeding 150 ml/minute.

Cryoprecipitate

Cryoprecipitate is a fraction of plasma obtained by freezing leucodepleted plasma and then thawing at $4 \pm 2°C$. The cryoprecipitate is the residue that does not redissolve upon slow thawing. For storage, it is rapidly frozen (within two hours of preparation) to a core temperature of below $-25°C$. Cryoprecipitate contains factor VIII, von Willebrand factor, factor XIII, fibrinogen and fibronectin. It is useful for treating patients with disseminated intravascular coagulation or specific coagulation abnormalities and is used as part of the management of massive haemorrhage.

Granulocytes

Granulocyte concentrates are prepared from buffy coats derived from whole-blood donations or can be collected through apheresis. The latter procedure requires the donor to be pre-treated with corticosteroids and/or granulocyte colony-stimulating factor (G-CSF) and is only used for specific recipients.

Granulocytes are used to treat life-threatening infections in severely immunosuppressed patients. All granulocytes are irradiated before issue to prevent TA-GvHD. Granulocytes contain significant numbers of red cells, and they must be ABO and D compatible and cross-matched.

Labelling of blood components

The label applied by the blood transfusion service is very specific; every label is barcoded. The label shows the component's name, producer's name, donation number, pack lot number and the ABO and Rh D groups. Every

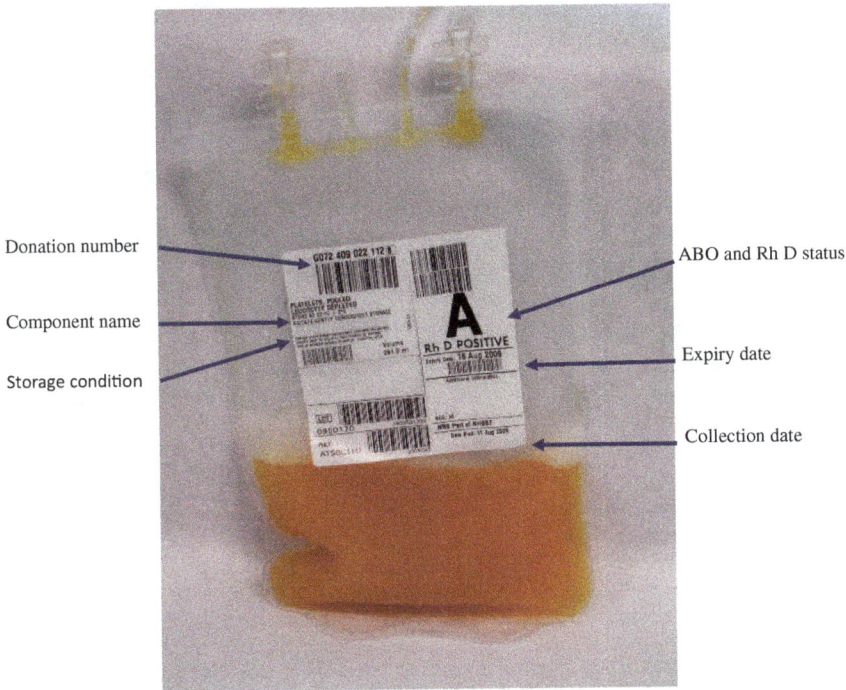

Donation number

Component name

Storage condition

ABO and Rh D status

Expiry date

Collection date

Fig. 13.4. A pooled platelet concentrate. Ideally platelets should be ABO identical with the intended recipient since anti-A and anti-B in platelet concentrates can cause haemolysis unless they are high titre-negative units. Due to small numbers of contaminating red cells, platelets should also be Rh D matched, particularly if given to people of childbearing potential.

unit also has the name, composition and volume of anticoagulant solution, the date of collection, storage temperature and expiration date on the label (Figs. 13.4 and 13.5).

Traceability

Traceability is "the ability to trace each individual unit of blood or blood component from the donor to its final destination and from its final destination back to the donor." Records of each stage of the component journey must be kept for 30 years (BSQR 2005).[2] Transfusion laboratories document all missing units and must submit this information to the MHRA annually. The traceability of blood components can also be reviewed at any time during an MHRA inspection.

---

[2] https://www.legislation.gov.uk/uksi/2005/50/contents/made.

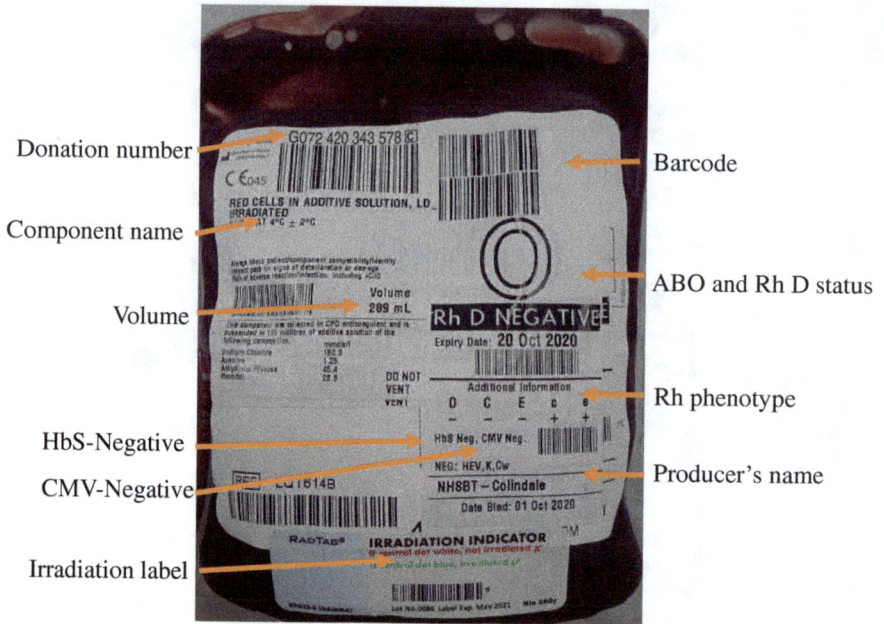

Fig. 13.5. Red cell unit. This red cell unit has been tested negative for the presence of haemoglobin S and CMV. The unit has been irradiated. This bag of blood has not yet been cross-matched. Once this is done another label is applied showing the recipient's full name, date of birth, gender and hospital or NHS number. This second label is cross-checked with the patient's self-identification, with the wrist band and with the request form for the blood at the bedside prior to transfusion.

Major Blood Group Systems

Antigens and antibodies

Over 400 red cell antigens have been identified; they may be carbohydrates (chains of sugars, e.g. ABO), proteins (e.g. Rh) or glycoproteins (e.g. Kell and Duffy). Most antigens have been organised into blood group systems by the International Society of Blood Transfusion (ISBT).

A blood group system consists of one or more antigens, controlled by one gene locus, such as the ABO gene, or two or more closely linked, similar genes, such as the Rh system, which has both the *RHD* and *RHCE* genes (Fig. 13.6). Inherited genetic variation results in differences in the protein structures, leading to different antigens arising within a system. Transfused red cells will appear foreign if they contain antigens that are not found in the patient's red cells, so if a patient is identified as having an antibody, it is important to ensure antigen-negative blood is provided for transfusion. Immunoglobulin (Ig)M antibodies can bind complement but are too big to cross the placenta and so do not cause haemolytic disease of the fetus and newborn (HDFN), whereas IgG antibodies, being much smaller, are able to cross the placenta. Anyone of childbearing potential should be given ABO-, D- and Kell-matched red cells. Kidd antibodies can often be difficult to detect, as they rapidly fall to below detectable levels and are hence missed in pre-transfusion testing. The most important antigens are those able to generate an alloantibody, e.g. anti-D. Table 13.6 lists all the most important, clinically significant antibodies.

While there are nine major blood group systems, the ABO system is the most important in transfusions.

Table 13.6. Blood group systems that generate clinically significant antibodies.

System	Antibody class	Haemolytic transfusion reaction	Haemolytic disease of fetus and newborn (HDFN)
ABO	Mostly IgM	Yes, severe immediate	Yes, mild
Rh	Usually, IgG	Yes, delayed	Yes, anti D & anti c and can be severe
Kell	Usually Ig G, sometimes IgM	Yes	Yes, suppresses erythropoiesis
Duffy	IgG	Yes, immediate and delayed	Yes
Kidd	IgG, many IgG + IgM, IgM	Yes, commonly causes delayed severe reaction	Yes, only a few cases have been reported
MNS	IgG and IgM	Yes	Yes
Lewis	IgM more frequent than IgG	Unlikely (but possible)	No
Lutheran	Often IgM, sometimes IgG	Yes	No
P1PK	IgM (IgG rare)	No (usually)	No

ABO & Rh System

ABO system

The ABO system was first discovered by Landsteiner, who deduced that individuals lacking the A or B antigen on their red cells would produce the corresponding antibodies in their plasma. He discovered groups A, B and O, and a year later, the group AB was discovered by Decastello and Sturli. The A and B antigens are formed from the precursor H substance by glycosyltransferases encoded by the A and B genes, respectively; the O allele does not encode a glycosyltransferase, so the H substance is unaltered.

The ABO antigens are encoded by a single genetic locus on chromosome 9. There are three alternative (allelic) forms — A, B and O. The A and B genes are co-dominant, and the O gene is amorphic and does not produce an antigen. To be group O, both O alleles must be inherited; it is therefore recessive. The distribution of ABO groups in the UK population is shown in Table 13.7.

ABO antibodies are naturally occurring, i.e. they develop without exposure to red blood cells expressing the corresponding antigens and are mostly IgM with a wide thermal amplitude, reactive at 37°C and able to activate complement. They are absent at birth but develop following exposure to environmental antigens. Some individuals also have IgG antibodies, particularly if they have received certain vaccinations.

Table 13.7   The Distribution of ABO blood groups and antibodies.

Red cell type	Antigen	Antibody in plasma	Phenotype-ABO group	Genotype (allele inherited)	UK blood donors
O	None	Anti-A	0	OO	47%
		Anti-B			
		Anti-A, B			
A	A	Anti-B	A	AA or AO	42%
B	B	Anti-A	B	BB or BO	8%
AB	A and B	No antibodies	AB	AB	3%

Note: The ABO group depends on the genes inherited from both parents. There are four blood groups (phenotype) but six possible genotypes. Group O, followed by group A are the most common in the UK population, this reflected in the percentage of donors. Group AB is the rarest group and subsequently the fewest donors.

IgM ABO antibodies can cause severe, immediate haemolytic transfusion reactions. If ABO-incompatible blood is given, intravascular haemolysis can be life-threatening.

ABO is the most immunogenic of all the blood group antigens. The most common cause of death from a blood transfusion is a clerical error in which an incompatible type of ABO blood is transfused.

Rh system

After ABO, Rh is the second-most important blood group system, and Rh antigens are highly immunogenic. Although there are currently 50 defined Rh antigens, only five are clinically significant, primarily in obstetrics. Rh blood group antigens are encoded by highly polymorphic genes. The two genes, *RHD* and *RHCE*, are closely linked and located on chromosome 1 (Fig. 13.6).

Eighty-five percent of the UK population are D-positive (also referred to as Rh positive), and the rest are D-negative. Women who do not produce the D antigen will produce alloantibody D (anti-D) if they are transfused with D antigen-positive red cells or exposed to D antigen-positive fetal red cells during pregnancy, through transplacental transfer; this can cause HDFN in future pregnancies.

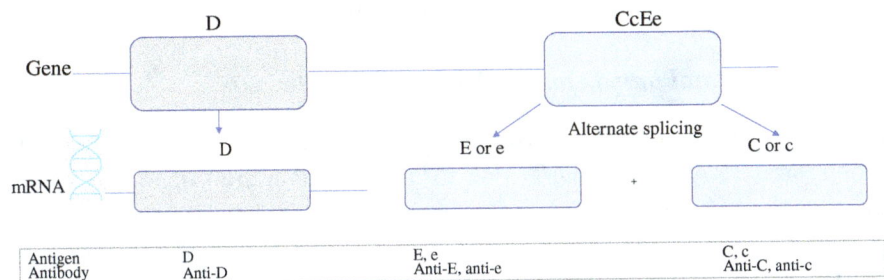

	D		E, e	C, c
Antigen	D		E, e	C, c
Antibody	Anti-D		Anti-E, anti-e	Anti-C, anti-c

Fig. 13.6. Molecular genetics of Rh system. RHD and RHCE genes are closely linked and located on chromosome 1. The D antigen is dominant, so a D positive individual may be DD or Dd, but d is not an antigen, it designates the absence of a gene encoding D at one or both allelic loci. D negative individuals are dd. Antibodies to D and c are the most common cause of HDFN. Antibodies against C, c, E, and e can be formed but these are less often a problem and generally blood for transfusion is selected without considering these antigens. Compatible ABO D blood should always be given.

Rh antibodies are usually IgG and are thus able to cross the placenta to cause HDFN, with anti-D and anti-c being the most common cause. Rh antibodies can also cause haemolytic transfusion reactions, leading to extravascular haemolysis.

It is therefore important that the Rh status is routinely determined in blood donors, transfusion recipients and during pregnancy. D-negative individuals who have previously been exposed to D-positive red cells can develop a delayed transfusion reaction because the antibody level is boosted from undetectable to clinically significant levels by the transfusion, which triggers extravascular haemolysis.

Haemolytic Disease of the Fetus/Newborn

HDFN is the consequence of maternal IgG antibodies crossing the placenta and binding to antigens on fetal red cells, causing destruction in the liver or spleen (reticuloendothelial system). If not correctly managed, this can cause serious HDFN, which can lead to death *in utero* or soon after birth due to anaemia-induced hydrops fetalis (Fig. 13.7).

Following birth, brain damage can occur if the plasma bilirubin is permitted to rise above a safe level; this condition is known as kernicterus and results from the binding of bilirubin to the basal ganglia. Due to the serious consequences of HDFN, management during pregnancy and after birth should be undertaken in specialist centres.

Routine antenatal anti-D immunoglobulin prophylaxis

Before the introduction of routine antenatal anti-D immunoglobulin prophylaxis (RAADP), HDFN due to anti-D was a significant cause of morbidity and mortality. Since the introduction of RAADP in the third trimester, i.e. 28 weeks, mortality has fallen to 0.2%.[3] RAADP (1,500 iu) can be given at 28–30 weeks of gestation or as a split dose, i.e. 500 iu at 28 weeks and another 500 iu at 34 weeks of gestation. After delivery, a dose of at least 500 iu is given, and further doses are determined by conducting a fetal maternal haemorrhage (FMH) test, also commonly known as the Kleihauer test.

Anti-D Ig should be administered after sensitising events (Table 13.8) to prevent the formation of immune anti-D, ideally within 72 hours of the

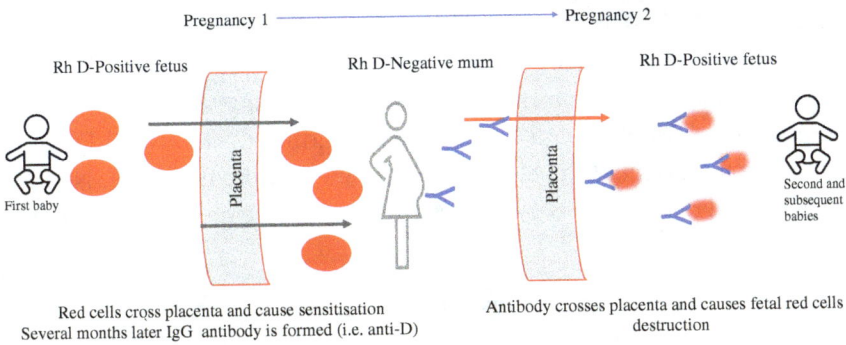

Fig. 13.7. Pathophysiology of HDFN.

In a D-negative mother, the first pregnancy with D-positive fetus results in fetal red cells crossing the placenta (during sensitising events but mainly delivery), this results in sensitisation to red cell antigens. Several months later an alloantibody can be detected in the mother; anti-D. In subsequent pregnancy with D-positive fetus, anti-D can cross the placenta and cause the fetal red cells in the liver and spleen to lyse. This results in fetal anaemia, which needs close monitoring by specialist in fetal maternal units.

Table 13.8. Sensitising events.

Events	Invasive procedures
Miscarriage	Amniocentesis
Fall or abdominal trauma	Chorionic villus biopsy
Ectopic pregnancy*	Cordocentesis
	In utero therapeutic interventions • Transfusion, • Surgery, • Insertion of shunts, etc.
Antepartum haemorrhage	Therapeutic termination*
Vaginal bleeding in pregnancy*	Evacuation of molar pregnancy*
External cephalic version	Instrumentation of uterus
Intrauterine death and stillbirth	
Labour	
Intraoperative cell salvage	

Note: *Minimum dose of 250 iu anti-D Ig if within 12 weeks of gestation.

event, although there is some benefit if anti-D Ig is given up to 10 days later. For sensitising events after 20 weeks of gestation, a minimum anti-D Ig dose of 500 iu should be administered within 72 h, and a test for fetal maternal haemorrhage (FMH) should be conducted. Further doses of anti-D Ig will depend on the extent of the bleed, as determined by the FMH test. No FMH test is needed before 20 weeks of gestation, and a dose of 250 iu is sufficient.

Monitoring of pregnancy to prevent HDFN

All pregnant women should have ABO and D groups and antibody screen undertaken at booking and again at 28 weeks of gestation.[4] D-negative women should be monitored more frequently if a clinically significant antibody is identified (Table 13.6). High-risk antibodies (anti-D, anti-c and anti-K) are associated with risks of mild to life-threatening anaemia/ jaundice in the fetus or neonate; this is dependent on antibody titre, which should be monitored monthly up to 28 weeks and thereafter every two weeks until delivery.[4] Anti-K does not cause haemolytic anaemia, but it suppresses the bone marrow synthesis of red cells.

If the titre of the antibodies reaches significant levels, the mother should be referred to fetal maternal specialists for non-invasive middle cerebral artery monitoring to detect and monitor fetal anaemia. Depending on the severity of the clinical picture, management may be complex and range from intrauterine transfusions and exchange transfusions at delivery for severe cases to phototherapy for milder cases. Phototherapy leads to the control of bilirubin through isomerisation, thereby enhancing its clearance without the need for conjugation.

It is now possible to predict the fetal *RHD*, *RHCE* and *KEL*01* genotypes using cell-free fetal DNA (cffDNA). This can be done simply by taking a blood sample from the mother at 16 weeks of gestation. If the fetus is predicted to be D-negative, RAADP will not be needed. Before cffDNA was available, when potentially clinically significant maternal antibodies were identified, paternal samples were often requested for testing to predict the risk to the fetus.

If a group O mother has a group A or B fetus, IgG antibodies can cross the placenta and cause ABO HDFN mainly in the newborn; this is usually mild and can be treated by phototherapy.

All women with a history of a baby affected by HDFN should be referred before the 20th week of gestation to a fetal medicine specialist for assessment in subsequent pregnancies.

Sampling and Testing in Blood Transfusion

Before ABO and D group-matched blood can be issued, the patient's blood group needs to be confirmed.

ABO and D grouping are the most important part of pretransfusion testing. If the patient has a historical ABO and D grouping, then only one sample is needed to confirm the ABO and D groups and exclude the formation of any new antibodies. Should verification checks against historical results reveal a discrepancy, a further sample must be obtained and tested immediately.

A second sample is recommended, prior to transfusion, for confirmation of the ABO and D groups in a patient who has not previously been tested.

Blood samples: Correct and safe practice

It is vital to identify patients before taking a sample for blood transfusion by asking them to state their name and date of birth and ensuring that these details match those in the patient's wristband. This should contain their full name, date of birth, unique hospital number and/or NHS number — this is called *positive patient identification*.

The blood sample must be labelled with the following essential patient information:

- patient's full name (first name and surname),
- date of birth,
- unique hospital or NHS number,
- date and time,
- signature/initials of the person taking the sample.

The person taking the sample **must label it at the patient's bedside**; this prevents clerical errors and reduces the risk of wrong blood in tubes (WBIT). A WBIT error can occur if a sample is taken from the wrong patient and is labelled with the intended patient's details (miscollection) or taken from the intended patient but labelled with another patient's details (mislabelling).

Errors in patient identification and sample labelling can lead to a potentially fatal ABO-incompatible transfusion; therefore, in addition to positive patient identification, accurate and complete labelling are absolute prerequisites of blood sampling. If followed correctly, this group-check rule prevents errors due to patient misidentification and potential death resulting from an ABO-incompatible transfusion.

All transfusion laboratories have a zero-tolerance policy and will reject inadequately labelled, mislabelled or underfilled samples.

In an emergency, if a transfusion is required before samples can be taken or processed, to avoid delays, standard emergency blood components will be issued if the laboratory is verbally informed or the Major Haemorrhage Protocol (MHP) is activated.

Sample validity

Group and screen samples remain valid for 72 hours if the patient has received a transfusion within the preceding three months. This ensures the detection of any new antibodies prior to issuing further units of blood. Samples from patients who have not received a transfusion in the previous three months remain valid for seven days.

Blood group testing

Historically, manual techniques including tiles, tubes and microplates were used for ABO grouping; however, column agglutination techniques are now routinely used in most hospital transfusion laboratories. It is standard practice to undertake blood grouping and antibody screening using automated analysers. This is safer because they are interfaced with laboratory information management systems (LIMS), in which all results are transmitted electronically to eliminate human errors. Column agglutination (see Fig 13.8) is performed at room temperature, taking about 10 minutes. Forward group — known anti-A and anti-B and anti-D reagents are put up against patient's red cells. Reverse group — known A and B group red cells are placed against patient's plasma (IgM antibodies) — internal control. Positive result — agglutination (clumping) at the top of the

Agglutination with anti-B and A₁ cells
No reaction with anti-A and anti-D or
with B cells

Blood Group = B RhD negative

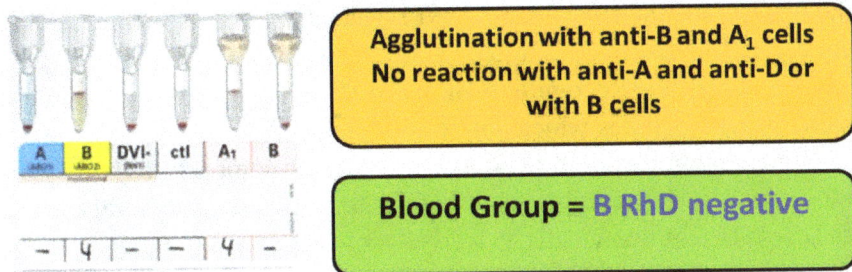

Fig. 13.8. Column agglutination technology.

The phenotype of the individual panel cells.

Rh	D	C	c	E	e	Cw	M	N	S	s	P1	Lua	K	k	Kpa	Lea	Leb	Fya	Fyb	Jka	Jkb	IAT	ENZ
R1wR1	+	+	0	0	+	+	+	+	+	0	3	0	+	+	0	0	+	0	+	0	+	4	5
R1R1	+	+	0	0	+	0	+	0	+	+	5	0	0	+	0	+	0	+	0	0	+	4	5
R2R2	+	0	+	+	0	0	0	+	+	0	0	0	+	+	0	0	+	0	+	+	0	4	5
r'r	0	+	+	0	+	0	0	+	0	+	4	0	0	+	0	0	+	+	0	+	0	0	0
r"r	0	0	+	+	+	0	+	0	+	0	4	0	0	+	0	+	0	+	0	+	+	0	0
rr	0	0	+	0	+	0	+	+	0	+	0	0	0	+	0	0	+	+	+	0	0	0	0
rr	0	0	+	0	+	0	0	+	0	+	0	0	0	+	0	0	0	0	+	0	+	0	0
rr	0	0	+	0	+	0	0	0	+	0	3	0	+	+	0	+	0	+	0	+	0	0	0
rr	0	0	+	0	+	0	0	+	0	+	4	+	0	+	+	+	0	0	+	0	+	0	0
rr	0	0	+	0	+	+	+	+	0	+	0	0	0	+	0	+	0	+	0	+	0	0	0
Auto																						0	

The results of testing showing anti-D.

10-cell panel to identify RBC antibodies

Fig. 13.9. An antibody panel showing a positive result. panel courtesy of Mrs Sally Procter.

column, negative result — red cells stay suspended and upon centrifugation form a small pellet at the bottom of the column.

Patients must have their samples taken for ABO and D groups and antibody screening before every transfusion. Antibody screening is performed on the plasma using a small panel of red cells expressing antigens for the clinically important antibodies one wishes to detect. This is usually a three-cell screen.

Should the antibody screen show a positive result, further investigation is undertaken with a larger panel of cells showing known antigen expression to allow the determination of the specification of the antibody or antibodies. More than one panel of cells may be required, and laboratories also use different techniques to aid identification (Fig. 13.9). So, one or more panels of red cells of a known phenotype is used and tested with an indirect antiglobulin test (IAT) reagent. Enzyme treating the reagent cells can enhance the antigen : antibody interaction for some antigens (e.g. Rh antigens). Recognition of the pattern of positive and negative reactions demonstrates which antibody is present.

For antibodies to high-incidence antigens or complex antibody mixtures, it may be necessary to send samples to a reference laboratory which has access to additional cells as well as more advanced techniques.

Serological testing

Antiglobulin test

The antiglobulin (previously called Coombs) test (Fig. 13.10) is widely used for blood group serology. Antihuman globulin (AHG) reagent is added to red cells coated with immunoglobulin or complement to aid the agglutination of red cells. The antiglobulin reagent can be specific for antibody (IgM, IgG or IgA) or complement or be broad spectrum. Red cells are mixed with plasma and incubated. If an antibody binds to the red cell antigen this is known as sensitisation. These sensitised red cells are exposed to anti-human globulin (AHG) which binds to the IgG antibody coating the red cells. The AHG will cross link the IgG antibodies onto the red cells and therefore cause the red cells to agglutinate. Agglutination indicates a positive result. This technique must be used in the absence of a functioning, validated information technology system or when an electronic issue is contra-indicated.

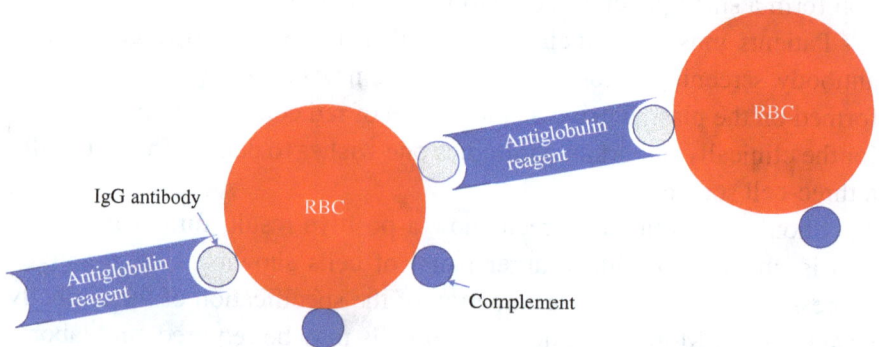

Fig. 13.10.   The antiglobulin test for antibody or complement.

The sensitivity of this test can be increased by adding colloid, proteolytic enzyme-treated red cells or low-ionic-strength saline (LISS).

Indirect antiglobulin test

This is used to detect antibodies coating red cells *in vitro*. It is a two-stage process: the first stage involves the incubation of red cells with plasma, and the second step involves washing the red cells and the addition of AHG. Agglutination implies that the original antibody was present in the plasma and has coated the red cells *in vitro*. The indirect antiglobulin test is the gold-standard test used routinely to identify clinically significant IgG antibodies.

Direct antiglobulin test

This is used to detect antibody or complement on the red cell surface, where sensitisation has occurred *in vivo*. If there is agglutination of washed red cells when AHG is added, this indicates a positive result. This is often the case in haemolytic transfusion reactions, HDFN and autoimmune or drug-induced immune haemolytic anaemia.

Saline agglutination

This detects IgM antibodies, usually both at room temperature and at 4°C. This can be used if a rapid manual ABO grouping is needed in an emergency.

Electronic issue

This is a safe and rapid technique which allows the issue of blood if the patient's ABO and D groups have been established and the antibody screen is negative. This enables the laboratory's computer algorithm to identify all compatible units without the need for further serological tests, thereby preventing the need to cross-match (Table 13.9).

However, an electronic issue cannot be used if the patient is known to have pre-existing antibodies or if the latest antibody screen is positive.

Table 13.9. Transfusion compatibility chart.

Patient ABO blood group	Compatible components		
	Red cells	Fresh frozen plasma/ octaplas /cryoprecipitate	Platelets
Unknown	O**	AB, A*, B*	AB, A*, B*
O	O**	O, A, B, AB	O, A, B, AB
A	A, O	A, AB, B*	A, AB, B*O*
B	B, O	B, AB, A*	B, AB, A*, O*
AB	AB, A, B, O	AB, A*, B*	AB, A*, B*, O*
Patient Rh D group			
Positive	Positive or negative	Not applicable	Positive or negative
Negative	Negative	Not applicable	Negative

Note: Group O red cells are known as flying-squad blood; this group is given for emergency transfusions of red cells. Group AB plasma is in short supply; high titre-negative A plasma is recommended for emergency use where the group of patients is unknown. *High titre-negative. **O-negative red cells should be given to patients of child-bearing potential (to prevent HDFN); O-positive red cells can be given to males and anyone who does not have child-bearing potential.

Consequently, a final cross-match step using saved patient serum and donated unit red cells is performed before issue. The other situations where an electronic issue is not possible include the presence of auto- or alloantibodies, following ABO-incompatible transplants (solid organ and stem cell) and in fetal/neonatal transfusions where the mother has IgG antibodies.

Molecular testing

In the past few years, molecular genotyping has become a standard practice. This is performed in reference laboratories to accurately determine blood groups when serological testing gives inconclusive results. However, the time required to process samples is such that this technique is likely to completely replace serological techniques in the near future. In addition, it allows patients to receive blood specifically matched to their genotype, thereby reducing the risk of sensitisation and antibody formation. In May 2023, a new project was launched by the NHSBT with the aim of determining the blood group genotype of all patients with sickle cell disease, thalassaemia and rare anaemias.

Indications for Transfusion

Red cell transfusion is indicated in anaemia or where there is active bleeding.

Platelet transfusions are usually needed when a patient's platelet count falls below the transfusion trigger or if the platelets are not functional due to drugs (such as antiplatelet agents) or an inherited platelet disorder (Table 13.10). They can be given as regular prophylaxis or used to cover procedures/high-risk surgeries to prevent bleeding.[5]

Plasma (FFP and cryoprecipitate) is given to correct abnormal clotting results in the presence of active bleeding or where invasive procedures may cause bleeding. FFP is also used for plasma exchange procedures.

Safe and Appropriate Use of Blood Components

The Blood Components app[6] has been developed to help guide healthcare professionals in decision-making regarding whether a transfusion is indicated or not. The app is based on national guidelines and indication codes. All individuals who authorise or prescribe blood components must undergo appropriate training and be assessed for competency at least every three years.

Consenting patients

The SaBTO report from 2020 recommends that healthcare professionals obtain and document valid consent for blood transfusions. If this is not possible before transfusion (e.g. for trauma victims or in the event of major haemorrhage), the patients should be informed prior to discharge and provided with relevant information. For patients on long-term transfusion support, a modified consent form should be used.

Special (or specific) requirements

There are a number of situations where patients are more vulnerable to complications from the transfusion of blood components. The main special requirements are listed in Table 13.11.

Table 13.10.   Platelet transfusion triggers.

Indication for prophylactic use — no bleeding	Threshold ($\times 10^9/l$)
Reversible bone marrow failure, including allogeneic/autologous stem cell transplant (considering no prophylaxis in autologous stem cell transplant); critical illness	10
Chronic bone marrow failure, on intensive chemotherapy	Count variable
Chronic bone marrow failure	*
Abnormal platelet function	
Platelet consumption/destruction (DIC, TTP*) or immune thrombocytopenia (ITP*, HIT, PTP)	
Indication for prophylactic use — in the presence of bleeding risk factors	**Threshold**
Sepsis	10–20
Abnormal haemostasis	
Reversible/chronic bone marrow failure/critical care	
Abnormal platelet function	*
Platelet consumption/destruction (DIC, TTP) or immune thrombocytopenia (ITP, HIT, PTP)	
Pre-procedure / Therapeutic use	**Threshold**
Central venous catheter (excluding PICC line)	20
Lumbar puncture	40
Percutaneous liver biopsy	50
Major surgery	
Severe bleeding	
Epidural anaesthesia (insertion and removal)	80
Neurosurgery or ophthalmic surgery, multiple trauma	100
Spontaneous intracerebral haemorrhage	
Non-severe bleeding	30
DIC — use pre-procedure threshold	Count variable

Note: As recommended by the BSH guidelines for the use of platelet transfusions. Disseminated intravascular coagulation (DIC), peripherally inserted central catheter (PICC), thrombotic thrombocytopenic purpura (TTP), autoimmune thrombocytopenia (ITP), heparin-induced thrombocytopenia (HIT), post-transfusion purpura (PTP). *Not indicated unless life-threatening bleeding.

Cytomegalovirus negative

A CMV infection can cause a potentially life-threatening infection in patients who are unable to mount an effective immune response. It is a major concern during pregnancy for the fetus if a mother becomes infected

Table 13.11. Situations where special (specific) requirements are required.

Irradiated units*	Hb S-negative red cells	Washed red cells/ platelets	CMV negative
Prevention of TAGvHD	**Prevention of sickling**	**Removal of plasma proteins**	**Prevention of CMV disease**
Conditions Hodgkin lymphoma Di George syndrome Stem cell transplant recipient	Sickle cell disease	Severe allergic/ anaphylactic reaction Ig A deficiency	Transfusion in pregnancy Neonates
Neonates who received intra uterine transfusion	Neonates		
Drugs Purine analogues ATG Bendamustine CAMPATH (in haematology patients only)			
Components** HLA/HPA-matched platelets Granulocytes			

Note: Neonates: <3 months of age. *RBC, granulocytes and platelets; **irrespective of the intended recipient, these components are always irradiated.

while pregnant. CMV-negative blood components for transfusion are recommended during pregnancy (but not during labour or delivery), for intrauterine transfusion and for the transfusion of neonates up to 28 days after the expected date of delivery.

Irradiated cellular components

Gamma irradiation of cellular components with a minimum of 25 Gy is recommended for at-risk patients to prevent TA-GvHD, which is the result of engraftment and proliferation of alloreactive donor lymphocytes in transfusion recipients. T-cells recognise allo-antigens in the recipient; activation leads to cytokine production and lymphocyte proliferation. Inflammation and tissue damage follow. Two factors allow the response to develop: the sharing of HLA-haplotypes between donor and recipient and defective recipient cell-mediated immunity.

Washed components

Washing red cells or platelets removes plasma proteins, which are the cause of allergic/anaphylactic reactions potentially seen in patients being transfused.

Hb S-negative red cells

Sickle cell disease patients are transfused (either a top up or an exchange) with the aim of lowering the Hb S percentage to alleviate symptoms related to sickling. It is important that Hb S negative red cells are given to anyone at risk of sickling.

Patient blood management

Patient blood management (PBM) was launched in England in 2012 by the National Blood Transfusion Committee to address the problems of anaemia, blood loss and coagulopathy. It is a patient-centred, systematic, evidence-based approach to improving patient outcomes and safety; this has been adopted by the WHO.[8] It aims to improve the patient's own blood count through diagnosis and aetiology-specific treatment of anaemia, preserve the patient's blood by minimising blood loss and promote patient empowerment by placing patients at the heart of decision-making. PBM follows international and national initiatives and promotes the use of alternative treatment options; this enables a tailored plan of care to be created. There are three pillars of PBM, which can be individualised according to the patient's needs, as shown in Fig. 13.11.

NICE quality standards for transfusion

The National Institute for Health and Care Excellence (NICE), which provides national guidance and advice to improve health and social care, issued guidance on transfusion quality standards in 2015.[9] There are four quality standards in transfusion: two relating to all patients and two relating to elective surgery. Iron deficiency anaemia should be treated before and after surgery with iron supplements, and the use of tranexamic acid is advised if moderate blood loss (>500 ml) is expected during surgery.

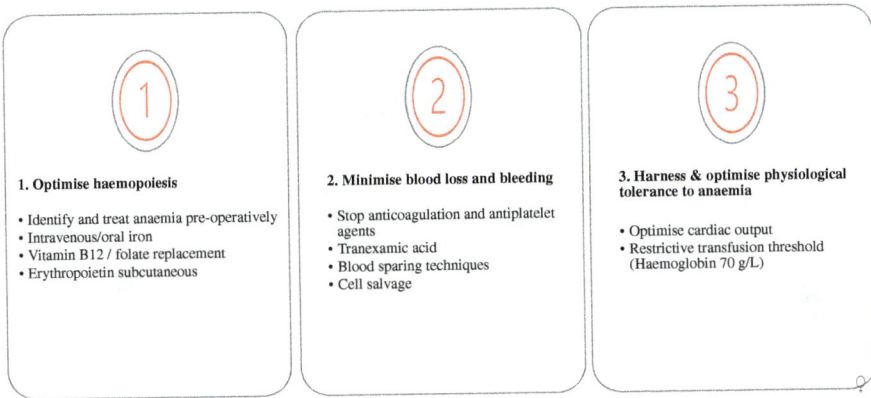

Fig. 13.11. The three pillars of patient blood management (PBM).

All patients should be given verbal and written information about the transfusion, and they should be reassessed clinically and/or have their haemoglobin concentration checked after each unit of red cells, unless they are bleeding or are on a chronic transfusion programme.

Authorising, Prescribing and Setting Up a Transfusion

Prescriptions

Prescriptions must be written and signed by trained healthcare professionals — usually doctors but this also includes other healthcare professionals who have received appropriate training. The accuracy and appropriateness of the prescription are the responsibility of the prescriber. All patients should be risk assessed for transfusion-associated circulatory overload (TACO) risk before the prescription is written (Fig. 13.12), especially if they are less than 50 kg and are very young or elderly, as mitigating actions may need to be taken, and alternatives to transfusion should be considered. The prescription must contain the patient's minimum identifiers and specify the component, dose/ volume, rate of transfusion and any special requirements. It should remain a permanent part of the clinical record. Consent from the patient should be obtained, and the indication for transfusion must be clearly documented in the medical records. When authorising transfusions, all of the above must be taken into consideration.

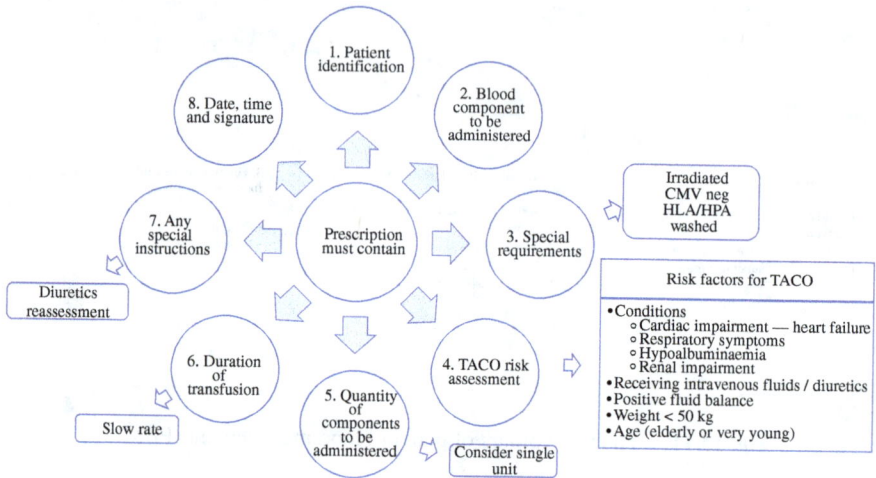

Fig. 13.12.   Information on transfusion prescriptions.

Setting up a transfusion

The patient must be brought to an area where close monitoring is possible and easily observable by qualified staff. The patient must remain in the clinical area while they receive the transfusion so that any reactions can be treated promptly. Temperature, pulse rate, respiration rate and blood pressure must be recorded and documented immediately before the transfusion is commenced and again after the first 15 minutes. Special attention must be paid to the patient during the first 15 minutes of a transfusion. The baseline and first set of observations must be conducted by qualified staff; subsequent observations can be conducted by healthcare support workers under the supervision of qualified staff.

In the absence of electronic equipment capable of reading barcodes on the patient's wristband and the blood component, the final bedside checks (Fig. 13.13) must be performed by two competent registered staff members, *independently* of each other, next to the patient's bedside or chair. All patients undergoing a transfusion must be wearing an identification wristband. The first step is to check the prescription, then the component and finally the patient. All these steps must be undertaken by the patient's bedside. Where electronic devices are available, these final

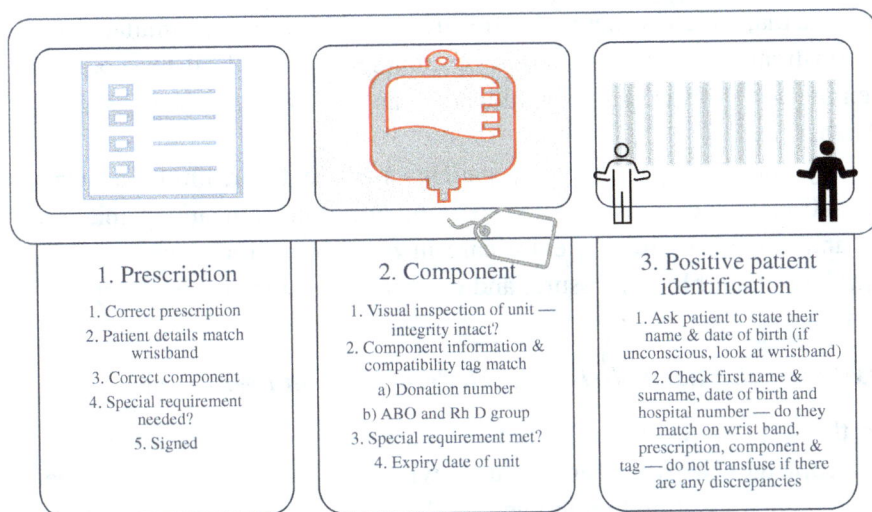

1. Prescription	2. Component	3. Positive patient identification
1. Correct prescription	1. Visual inspection of unit — integrity intact?	1. Ask patient to state their name & date of birth (if unconscious, look at wristband)
2. Patient details match wristband	2. Component information & compatibility tag match	2. Check first name & surname, date of birth and hospital number — do they match on wrist band, prescription, component & tag — do not transfuse if there are any discrepancies
3. Correct component	a) Donation number	
4. Special requirement needed?	b) ABO and Rh D group	
5. Signed	3. Special requirement met?	
	4. Expiry date of unit	

Fig. 13.13.   Final bedside checks.

bedside checks can be performed by one competent registered staff member. The start and finish times of each unit must be recorded clearly (as they are important for investigating transfusion reactions).

Clinical observations should be documented hourly and repeated at the end of the transfusion episode.

Risks in Transfusion

Intravascular haemolysis

In intravascular haemolysis, red cells are destroyed directly in the blood stream. This is immediate and is mainly due to ABO-incompatible transfusion, which is usually caused by a clerical/technical error and may be induced by as little as 20 ml of incompatible blood having been transfused.

Reactions are usually due to an IgM antibody or when two closely bound IgG antibodies interact with a foreign antigen on a red cell surface, activating complement via the classical pathway. A series of proteins in the blood and tissues are activated sequentially in an enzymatic cascade, which continues to the final stage of a membrane attack complex and ends with lysis and the destruction of red cells. This releases haemoglobin into the plasma, which is excreted in the urine, and bilirubin accumulates in the bloodstream. Massive activation of complement can lead to shock, disseminated intravascular coagulopathy and, in the worst-case scenario, death.

Symptoms experienced by patients include fever, chills, a burning sensation at the infusion site, chest and/or loin pain and palpitations. In anaesthetised patients, extra care in monitoring for signs, symptoms and heart rate, blood pressure, and oxygen saturations is necessary.

Extravascular haemolysis: red cell destruction in liver or spleen

In this type of haemolysis, red cells are removed by spleen and liver macrophages as they are coated with antibodies. When red cells have complement and antibodies on their surface, they are cleared more quickly than those coated only with antibodies. Extravascular haemolysis is slower, and the main symptoms are fever or chills with increased bilirubin production. Rh antibodies frequently cause extravascular haemolysis.

Classification of transfusion reactions

An acute transfusion reaction occurs within 24 hours; those which present after 24 hours are classified as delayed. Table 13.12 compares the differences, and Table 13.13 describes the causes, symptoms and management.

Metabolic and haemostatic effects

Metabolic and haemostatic abnormalities most commonly occur in massive transfusions.

Citrate toxicity

This can occur when large volumes of blood are transfused quickly. Units contain citrate, which chelates calcium irons; this can cause hypocalcaemia and its associated symptoms (including tingling in the hands and feet, numbness around the mouth, muscle cramps and confusion). Citrate toxicity is most commonly seen in patients undergoing red cell exchange or

Table 13.12. Classification of transfusion reactions: acute or delayed.

	Acute	Delayed
Timing	Within 24 hours	Approximately 1–14 days
Haemolysis type	Intravascular	Extravascular
Symptoms and signs	Rise in temperature or pulse rate or fall in blood pressure even before patient feels unwell. Features depend on the cause: depend on the cause but can include fever, rigors, flushing, vomiting, dyspnoea, pain at transfusion site, loin pain/chest pain, urticaria, itching, headache, collapse and a feeling of impending doom	Depend on cause (see Table 13.13)
Severity and complications	Severe DIC, renal failure, irreversible shock, death	Usually less severe. Jaundice, anaemia (occasional fever, renal failure, death) (Often missed if patient sent home)
Implicated antibodies	Most likely with ABO antibodies	Rh antibodies Kidd antibodies
Method for detection	Incompatible cross-match Free Hb (blood and urine)	Incompatible cross-match Reactive indirect antiglobulin test at 37°C
Blood results	↓Haemoglobin & haptoglobin ↑Bilirubin & lactate dehydrogenase Direct antiglobulin test positive Eluate positive	↓Haemoglobin & haptoglobin ↑Bilirubin & lactate dehydrogenase Direct antiglobulin test positive Eluate positive

those receiving a massive transfusion. Treatment involves the replacement of calcium.

Hyperkalaemia

As red cells age, potassium leaks out from them, so older units of red cells have higher extracellular potassium. The process of irradiation increases leakage and units have a higher potassium burden. Transfusion-associated

Table 13.13. Transfusion reactions, causes, symptoms and management.

Reaction	Cause	Symptom	Management
ABO-INCOMPATIBLE TRANSFUSION	Failure of bedside check Wrongly labelled blood sample Laboratory error	Restless, chest/loin pain, fever, vomiting, flushing, collapse ↓BP & ↑HR (shock), ↑temperature, haemoglobinuria (later)	1. Stop transfusion — check patient/component. 2. Take samples for FBC, biochemistry, coagulation, repeat cross-match and DAT. Monitor patient for DIC, renal impairment and ensure urine output maintained > 30 ml/min. 3. Return component to laboratory. Laboratory reports to the MHRA.
ANAPHYLAXIS	IgE antibodies in patient cause mast cell release of granules & vasoactive substances Can be severe in IgA deficiency	"Severe, life-threatening reaction soon after start of transfusion" ↓BP & ↑HR (shock), very breathless with wheeze, often laryngeal &/or facial oedema	1. Stop transfusion and treat with adrenaline 1 mg at IM (1:1,000) concentration. 2. Return component to laboratory.
BACTERIAL CONTAMINATION	Bacterial growth can cause endotoxin production, which causes immediate collapse From the donor (low grade GI, dental, skin infection) Introduced during processing (environmental or skin) Platelets > red cells > frozen components (storage temperature)	Restless, fever, vomiting, flushing, collapse ↓BP & ↑HR (shock), ↑temperature	1. Stop transfusion — check patient/component. 2. Take samples for blood cultures and start broad spectrum antibiotics. 3. Return component to blood service for culture. Laboratory/blood service reports to the MHRA.

Reaction	Cause	Clinical features	Management
FEBRILE NON-HAEMOLYTIC TRANSFUSION REACTION (FNHTR)	White cells release cytokines during storage	*Rise in temperature of 1°C, chills, rigors	Stop or slow transfusion, and treat with paracetamol
ALLERGIC	Allergy to a plasma protein in donor	Mild urticarial or itchy rash sometimes with a wheeze	Stop or slow transfusion, and treat with antihistamine
TRANSFUSION-ASSOCIATED CIRCULATORY OVERLOAD (TACO)	Patient not assessed for risk factors**	Clinical features: SOB, ↓SAO2, ↑HR, ↑BP. CXR — fluid overload/cardiac failure	TACO: Stop transfusion, and prescribe diuretics.
TRANSFUSION-RELATED ACUTE LUNG INJURY (TRALI)	Anti-leucocyte antibodies (HLA or neutrophil); neutrophils aggregate, get stuck in pulmonary capillaries → release neutrophil proteolytic enzymes & toxic O_2 metabolites → lung damage	Shortness of breath, ↓SAO2, ↑HR, ↑BP CXR: bilateral pulmonary infiltrates during/within 6 hr of transfusion	TRALI: Stop transfusion; if not responding to diuretics, begin supportive care on ITU, and send samples for testing for antibodies.
TAD (TRANSFUSION-ASSOCIATED DYSPNOEA)		Symptoms and signs do not fit TACO or TRALI	TAD: Stop transfusion, and begin supportive care.

Note: Eluate is produced by chemically cleaving antibodies from the red cell membrane. *Haemolysis screen: haemoglobin (Hb), haptoglobin ↓, bilirubin, lactate dehydrogenase (LDH), reticulocytes ↑, direct antiglobulin tests (DAT) positive, indirect antiglobulin test (IAT), intravenous immunoglobulin (IVIG), heart rate (HR), blood pressure (BP), oxygen saturations (SAO2), shortness of breath (SOB). **Risk factors: cardiac failure, respiratory disease, renal impairment, hypoalbuminaemia, positive fluid balance, <50 kg.

hyperkalaemia can occur during massive transfusions. Close monitoring of potassium levels via blood gases and prompt corrective measures are required. Patients at risk of developing symptoms associated with high potassium, such as renally impaired patients, should be given fresher red cells.

Hypothermia

Blood is kept at 4°C in the fridge; if large volumes are given quickly, e.g. for massive haemorrhage, this may lower the patient's core temperature and cause arrhythmias. Hypothermia can impair platelet and clotting factor function and hence cause further bleeding. In trauma, it is standard practice to transfuse blood through a blood warmer to prevent this.

Coagulopathy

Coagulopathy is often seen in massive transfusions/trauma victims who have lost more than 1–2 blood volumes and have only received red cells and fluids which causes a dilution of platelets and clotting factors. To prevent this, it is standard practice to transfuse red cells and FFP in a 1:1 ratio in major haemorrhage scenarios such that the FFP replaces the clotting factors; this is known as damage control resuscitation.

Air embolism

This is very rare now but should be considered in patients with central venous catheters. Air can enter catheters through the blood administration set as blood component bags are being changed or infused under pressure in an open system.

Management of Transfusion Reactions

All patients receiving a transfusion must be monitored closely for adverse effects. Where there is concern that a patient is having an adverse reaction, the transfusion must be stopped immediately, and the patient *must be assessed immediately* by a qualified healthcare individual (Fig. 13.14). It is important to exclude the transfusion of an ABO-incompatible unit,

Fever, chills, rigors, tachycardia, hyper or hypotension, collapse, urticaria, pain (chest, abdominal, muscle, bone), respiratory distress, nausea, vomiting, general malaise

STOP TRANSFUSION
Undertake rapid clinic assessment
Check patient identification/blood component compatibility
Visually assess blood component
Evidence of:
Life threatening Airway, Breathing or Circulatory problems and/or wrong component given and/or evidence of contaminated unit

Inform medical staff

YES   **NO**

SEVERE LIFE THREATENING
Call for urgent help
Initiate resuscitation ABCD
If haemorrhage excluded as cause of hypotension, discontinue transfusion
Maintain venous access
Monitor patient blood pressure, pulse, temperature, oxygen saturations, urine output – use this to guide fluid resuscitation
If likely anaphylaxis/allergy – follow anaphylaxis pathway
If bacterial contamination likely – take cultures & start broad spectrum antibiotics (Unit to be returned to blood service)
Inform hospital transfusion team
Return unit with administration set to transfusion laboratory
Perform appropriate investigations i.e. CXR

Document in notes

Review by transfusion team/committee
Report to SHOT/MHRA

MODERATE
Temperature ≥ 39°C and rise of 1-2°C and/or other symptoms/signs

Consider bacterial contamination
Review patients underlying condition & transfusion history
Monitor patient blood pressure, pulse, temperature, oxygen saturations, urine output

If not consistent with condition/history, discontinue/discard implicated unit
Perform appropriate investigations

Transfusion related

If consistent with condition/history, consider continuation of transfusion at slower rate with symptomatic treatment

Transfusion unrelated

MILD
Isolated temperature 38°C and rise of 1-2°C and/or pruritis/rash

Continue transfusion
Consider symptomatic treatment
Monitor more frequently
If symptoms/signs worsen manage as moderate/severe

Document in notes
No review needed by transfusion team
No SHOT report needed

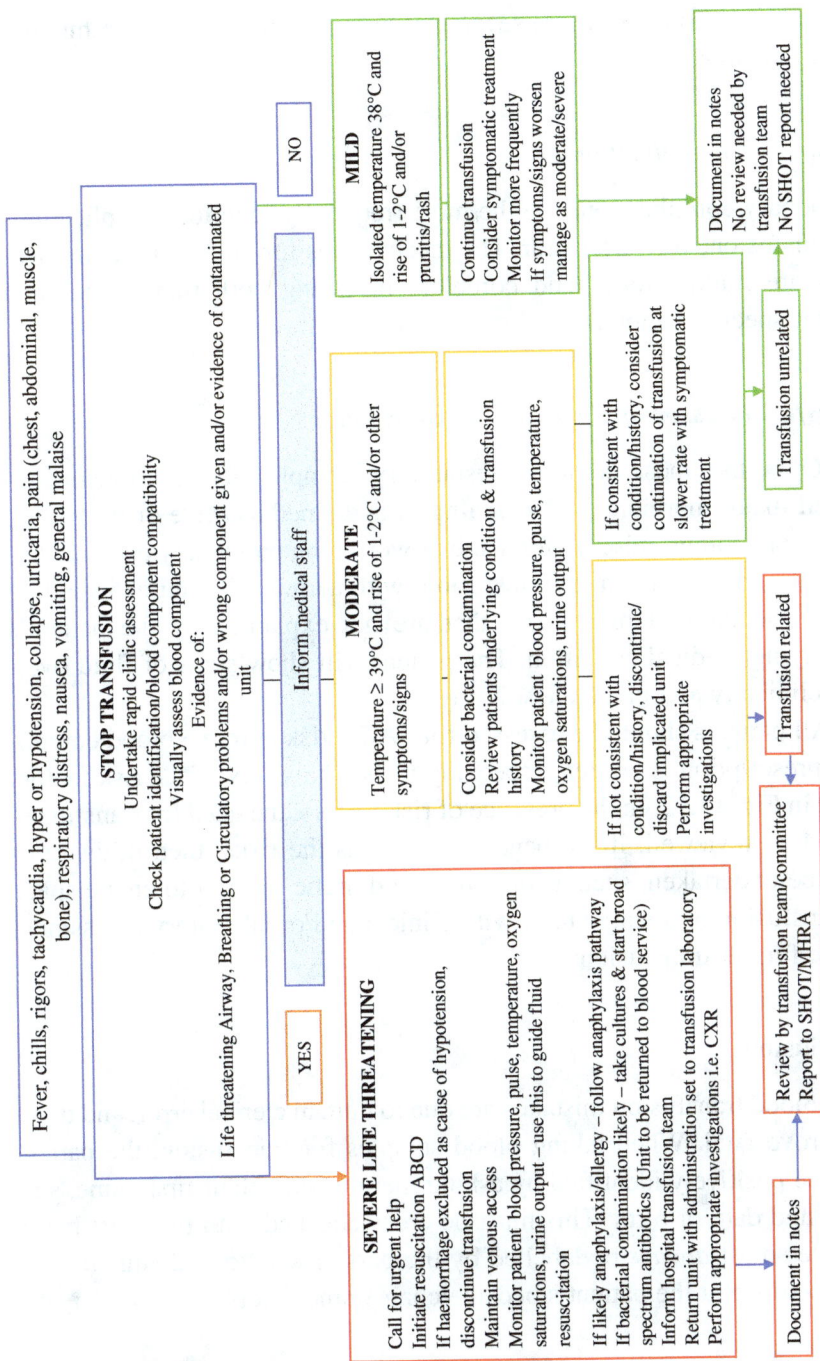

Fig. 13.14. How to manage an acute transfusion reaction.

particularly if symptoms are severe and occur within the first 15 minutes of the transfusion.

Pulmonary complications

Pulmonary complications are the most frequently reported complications of transfusion, year after year. The mechanisms for pulmonary complications are multifactorial and complex, involving both transfusion- and patient-specific factors.

Transfusion-associated circulatory overload

TACO is the most common respiratory complication of transfusion-related major morbidity and mortality. It is defined as acute or worsening respiratory compromise and/or acute or worsening pulmonary oedema during or up to 12 hours after transfusion, with additional features including cardiovascular system changes that are not explained by the patient's underlying medical condition. The patient will show signs of fluid overload clinically and in the chest X-ray.

All patients should be assessed for TACO risk before a blood component prescription is written, especially if they have any of the risk factors listed in Fig. 13.12. In the presence of risk factors, the need for transfusion should be reviewed; if the benefit outweighs the risks, then mitigations must be undertaken, such as pre-emptive diuretic therapy to create space or transfusion of a single unit, with clinical and/or laboratory assessment before further transfusions.

Conclusion

Most blood transfusion mistakes are due to human clerical error, and these can prove fatal. When taking blood samples for transfusion, the patient *must* be positively identified by asking them to state their first name, surname and date of birth. This must be cross-checked with the wrist band. Samples must *always* be labelled by the person who took them, and this *must* be done at the patient's bedside/chair immediately.

It is important to administer blood components in accordance with the national guidelines for usage and when there is no other alternative (e.g. iron infusion).

When setting up a transfusion, it is important to positively identify the patient and the unit; this is the last opportunity in the transfusion process to prevent a potentially fatal error. If there are any concerns about the transfusion, seek the advice and guidance of the hospital transfusion medical and laboratory staff.

Test Case 13.1

A 64-year-old woman with myelodysplastic syndrome has not responded to erythropoietin therapy and is now receiving a transfusion of two units of red cells every three weeks. This procedure is being performed in a daycare ward. On the day in question, she received one unit of red cells uneventfully with a furosemide injection to prevent volume overload. Fifteen minutes after the start of the transfusion of the second bag, she complains of suddenly feeling unwell and experiences chest tightness and loin pain. Her blood pressure is found to have dropped, and she has tachycardia.

Question

What do you think is happening, and what should be done?
Write down your answers before checking the correct answer (page 409) or re-reading any relevant part of the chapter.

14

Haemopoietic Stem Cell Transplantation and CAR-T Cell Therapy

Edward J. Bataillard

What Do You Need To Know?

☞ The principles of haemopoietic stem cell transplantation, its benefits and its possible adverse effects

☞ The principles and adverse effects of CAR-T cell therapy

Introduction

A number of haematological and non-haematological conditions can be treated by the transplantation of haemopoietic stem cells. Traditionally, these cells are harvested directly from bone marrow (hence the interchangeable term 'bone marrow transplantation'). This is done under a general anaesthetic with a large needle and syringe, aspirating from sites that contain red marrow, usually from multiple sites on both iliac bones. More frequently, however, haemopoietic progenitor cells are collected from peripheral blood on a cell separator (see Fig. 14.1), which is made possible by the prior injection of granulocyte colony-stimulating factor (G-CSF) or other agents that mobilise stem cells from the marrow. Occasionally, other sources of haemopoietic stem cells are used, such as

339

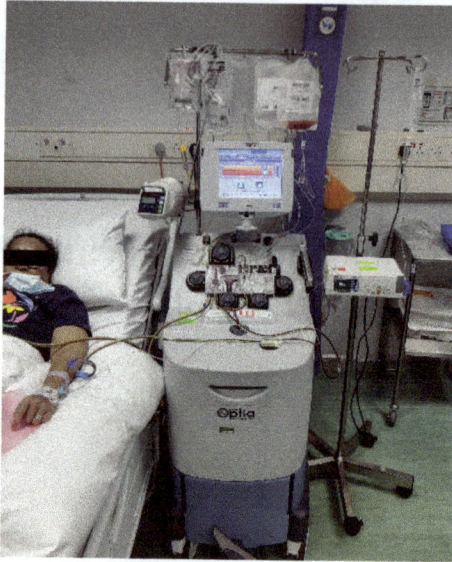

Fig. 14.1. Peripheral blood apheresis for planned autologous stem cell transplantation. In this patient, CD34+ stem cells have been mobilised into peripheral blood circulation by the prior administration of G-CSF. These cells are harvested through an automated continuous mononuclear cell collection programme using a cell separator.

umbilical cord blood, although this is often reserved for paediatric transplants due to the limited number of stem cells in single units of cord blood. Stem cells are administered intravenously and find their way to the bone marrow of the recipient. Following engraftment, they proliferate, differentiate and repopulate the marrow with haemopoietic cells. However, for 2–3 weeks following transplantation, the patient is profoundly cytopenic and in need of red cell and platelet transfusions, antibiotics and nutritional support. There are two types of haemopoietic stem cell transplantation (HSCT): autologous, whereby the patient's own stem cells are collected and later reinfused into them; and allogeneic, in which stem cells are derived from a donor.

Autologous Stem Cell Transplantation

Autologous stem cell transplantation is a method of intensifying chemotherapy in refractory malignant diseases. The patient is given chemotherapy and G-CSF to mobilise stem cells, which are harvested and stored. Intensive chemotherapy is then administered, following which the stored stem cells are reinfused. The full blood count recovers within approximately two weeks of the infusion, which is significantly faster than it would have been without the administration of stem cells. Autologous stem cell transplantation has been primarily applied to multiple myeloma and relapsed or refractory lymphoma. Some non-haematological malignancies are also treated using this method, such as refractory germ cell tumours, which are often sensitive to chemotherapy but may require greater dose intensities to achieve cure.

Additionally, autologous stem cell transplantation is used to treat certain autoimmune diseases, such as multiple sclerosis. The principle here is to administer intensive immunosuppressive therapy with the goal of eradicating pathogenic lymphocytes, and then allow for immune reconstitution by reinfusing previously collected myeloid and lymphoid stem cells. More recently, the principles of autologous stem cell transplantation are also being applied to gene therapy; for example, in thalassaemia major, the patient's own DNA is modified before reinfusion of the stem cells into the patient.

Allogeneic Stem Cell Transplantation

The purpose of allogeneic transplantation may be either to provide normal haemopoietic or lymphoid stem cells when they are lacking, to replace abnormal haemopoietic cells, or to rescue a patient from bone marrow failure after intensive chemotherapy for leukaemia, lymphoma or a related condition. In the treatment of haematological malignancies by allogeneic transplantation, there can also be a benefit from an immune attack on leukaemic cells by transplanted immune cells, known as the graft-versus-leukaemia (GVL) or graft-versus-tumour effect. Some of the current indications for allogeneic transplantation are shown in Table 14.1.

Donor selection and matching

Donor stem cells may come from a sibling or other close relative, an unrelated donor or a bank of cryopreserved umbilical cord blood stem cells. Donor histocompatibility antigens (in particular, the human leukocyte

Table 14.1.   Some indications for allogeneic haemopoietic stem cell transplantation.

Indication	Principle
Aplastic anaemia	Provision of haemopoietic stem cells
Severe combined immunodeficiency	Provision of lymphoid stem cells
β thalassaemia major	Replacement of genetically abnormal stem cells
Sickle cell anaemia	Replacement of genetically abnormal stem cells
Acute myeloid and acute lymphoblastic leukaemia	Replacement of stem cells after intensive chemotherapy has destroyed both leukaemic cells and residual normal stem cells; elimination of any residual leukaemic cells by GVL effect
Chronic myeloid leukaemia if refractory to tyrosine kinase inhibitors	

class I and II antigens, HLA) are matched as closely as possible to those of the host. This is required to prevent not only the rejection of the transplanted cells by the host's residual immune cells but also an attack on the host's tissues by donor lymphocytes, an attack that gives rise to graft-versus-host disease (GVHD). Acceptance of the transplanted cells by the host is facilitated by 'conditioning' to reduce host immune responses. Conditioning can be achieved through chemotherapy and/or radiotherapy. Less stringent matching is needed for cord blood cell transplantation, as lymphocytes are immunologically naïve.

The balance between donor and host: Graft-versus-host disease

Unless the transplant is from an identical twin, there will always be some histoincompatibility. Donor lymphocytes are transplanted together with donor haemopoietic stem cells and serve to reconstitute the immune system. However, donor lymphocytes can recognise host histocompatibility antigens, leading to GVHD, which manifests clinically particularly in the skin, gastrointestinal tract and liver (Fig. 14.2). Immunosuppressive treatment (e.g. ciclosporin and methotrexate) is routinely administered post-transplant in an attempt to reduce the incidence of GVHD. Additional doses of chemotherapy (such as cyclophosphamide) can also be administered several days

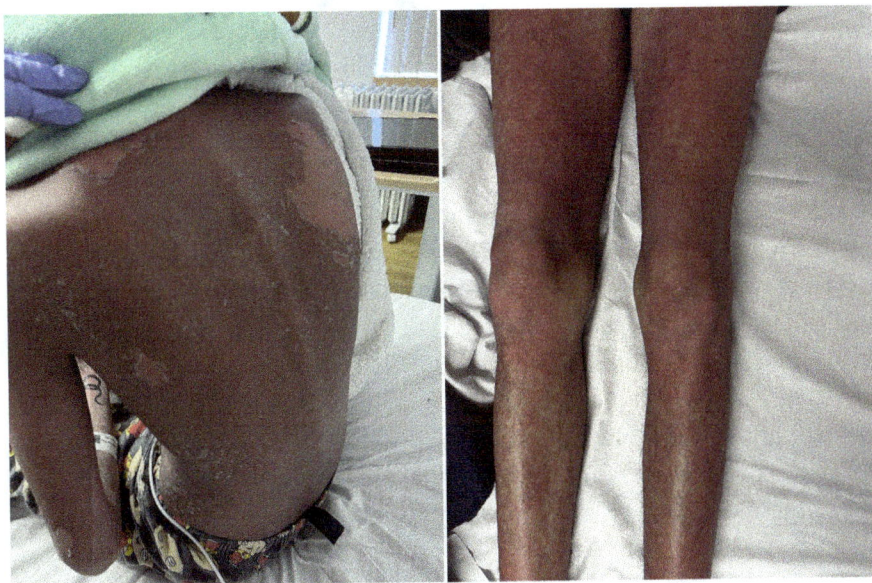

Fig. 14.2. Acute cutaneous graft-versus-host disease. This patient developed a widespread erythematous maculopapular rash with areas of desquamation on day +32 of an unrelated donor allogeneic HSCT after having forgotten to take ciclosporin for two days.

after stem cell infusion so as to deplete the highly proliferative alloreactive T-cells that cause GVHD. This approach has allowed transplants from less stringently matched donors and has therefore expanded the accessibility of allogeneic stem cell transplantation in recent years. If GVHD occurs despite these prevention measures, then further immunosuppression, such as by using corticosteroids, may be required. Cord blood stem cell transplantations result in a lower incidence of GVHD compared to transplantations of adult stem cells.

When transplantation is performed for a benign condition, such as thalassaemia major, it is not necessary to eliminate all host haemopoietic cells, so conditioning can be milder. When transplantation is performed for a malignant condition, intensive chemotherapy is usually preferred. However, it is also possible to use 'reduced-intensity conditioning' and rely on the graft-versus-leukaemia effect to eliminate any residual leukaemic cells. If all leukaemic cells have not been eliminated (as shown, for example, by molecular studies) or if an overt relapse occurs, the GVL effect can be enhanced by the infusion of donor lymphocytes.

Morbidity and mortality of transplantation

Allogeneic transplantation is associated with significant mortality, ranging from 10% to 40%, depending on the age and general health of the recipient and the closeness of tissue matching. Death may result from a bacterial, fungal or viral infection, GVHD or relapse. It is also associated with significant morbidity.

Reduced-intensity conditioning transplantation is associated with lower morbidity and mortality. Thus, this has made transplantation available over a wider age range and therefore also for diseases that particularly affect the elderly, such as myelodysplastic syndromes and chronic lymphocytic leukaemia.

CAR-T Cell Therapy

Arguably, the most promising advance in oncology in the past two decades has been the development of immune effector cell therapies — in particular, chimaeric antigen receptor (CAR)-T cells — to treat relapsed or refractory haematological malignancies. CAR-T cell therapy is a form of adoptive cell-transfer immunotherapy, developed by genetically modifying T-cells to express CARs. CARs are designer molecules consisting of several components: an extracellular domain that binds to a specific cancer antigen (which is usually derived from the variable domain of a monoclonal antibody, scFv); a transmembrane domain that anchors the CAR to the T-cell surface; and an intracellular signalling module, which mediates T-cell activation resulting in selective tumour cell killing (see Fig. 14.3).

The current CAR-T cell therapies in clinical use are autologous, i.e. using patients' own T-cells collected by peripheral blood apheresis. After collection, the T-cells are genetically engineered to express CARs through transduction using a virus that encodes a DNA construct. The CAR-T cells are then expanded and subsequently reinfused into the patient. Patients are usually treated with chemotherapy just prior to receiving the CAR-T cells to reduce their own endogenous lymphocytes (a process

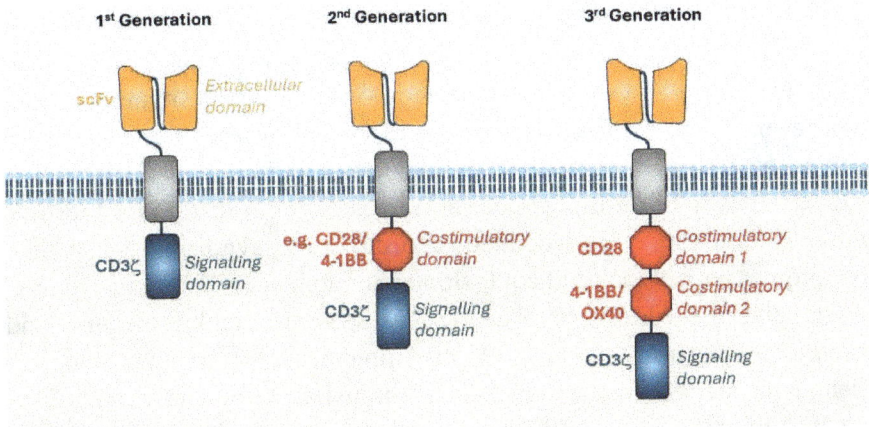

Fig. 14.3. Generations of chimaeric antigen receptor (CAR) construct designs. All CARs comprise an extracellular antigen-binding domain and a transmembrane domain. The first-generation CARs contain only the CD3ξ signalling domain. Second-generation CARs include a costimulatory domain (e.g. CD28 or 4-1BB), which serves to enhance the cytotoxicity, expansion and persistence of CAR-T cells. Third-generation CARs include a second costimulatory domain, which further enhances T-cell expansion and persistence.

called lymphodepletion). This helps to improve the efficacy of the CAR-T cells by reducing competition and promoting their expansion and persistence in the patient's body. Research is currently underway to develop allogeneic ('off-the-shelf') CAR-T cell products, which may potentially improve access to this treatment for patients in the future.

The greatest clinical advance has been the development of CARs directed against the B cell surface marker CD19. CD19-CAR-T cells can induce durable remissions in a range of cancers, including B-lymphoblastic leukaemia and non-Hodgkin lymphomas (notably diffuse large B-cell lymphoma and mantle cell lymphoma). CAR constructs targeting a number of other cancer antigens are in development, such as B cell maturation antigen (BCMA) directed CAR-T cells to treat relapsed multiple myeloma.

Adverse effects of CAR-T cell therapy

Although highly effective, CAR-T cell therapy is not without risks. The most commonly observed toxicity is cytokine release syndrome (CRS).

This occurs because of immune activation leading to the release of inflammatory cytokines; it usually coincides with peak CAR-T cell expansion (a few days after cell infusion). CRS typically manifests with high fevers and, in severe cases, can lead to cardiovascular or respiratory compromise or other organ dysfunctions. Another frequent adverse effect of CAR-T cells is a form of central nervous system disturbance termed immune effector cell-associated neurotoxicity syndrome (ICANS). Symptoms can include mild confusion or somnolence, dyspraxia and dysphasia, and in severe cases, it can lead to seizures, cerebral oedema and coma. Patients are therefore closely monitored for any neurological changes in the weeks after CAR-T cell infusion. Fortunately, both CRS and ICANS are usually self-limiting and can be treated if necessary with immunosuppressive medications (such as tocilizumab and steroids). Other common complications of CAR-T cell therapy include infections and cytopenias, which can occasionally be prolonged and require months of transfusion support.

Conclusions

Haemopoietic stem cell transplantation has been an important therapeutic advance. It is a potentially hazardous procedure, requiring meticulous medical and nursing care.

CAR-T cell therapy is a promising new field of immunotherapy which can induce durable remissions in refractory haematological malignancies; however, it is associated with unique toxicities.

Test Case 14.1

A 24-year-old man with acute myeloid leukaemia achieves remission after two cycles of combination chemotherapy. He then undergoes an allogeneic stem cell transplant from an HLA-matched sibling donor. On Day 26 post-transplant, he develops anorexia, bloody diarrhoea and a widespread erythematous desquamating skin rash.

Questions

1. What is the likely diagnosis and what is the most appropriate initial treatment?
2. In transplant practice, what measures are routinely taken to reduce the risk of the complications experienced in this case?
3. When a patient with acute leukaemia achieves a remission after chemotherapy, what are the main factors to consider when deciding on an allogeneic stem cell transplant?

Write down your answers before checking the correct answer (page 409) or re-reading any relevant part of the chapter.

15

Haematology in Obstetric Medicine

Andrew Godfrey

What Do You Need To Know?

☞ Common changes in haemostasis during pregnancy
☞ The role of thromboprophylaxis in pregnancy
☞ The management of thrombocytopenia in pregnancy

Haemostasis During Pregnancy

Pregnancy induces a number of changes over the nine months of gestation as the maternal physiology adapts both to the presence of the fetus and in preparation for delivery, where there is a genuine risk of maternal mortality from bleeding. This adaptation includes a significant increase in procoagulant factors, such as factor VIII and the von Willebrand factor (vWF), and a significant decrease in anticoagulant factors, such as protein S.

The thrombotic risk to the mother increases progressively over the course of the pregnancy, in line with gestational age, and does not return to baseline for 6–12 weeks after delivery.

An overview of the changes in clotting factors by trimester is shown in Table 15.1.

Table 15.1. Clotting factor changes in pregnancy. Other procoagulant and anticoagulant factors are not significantly changed by pregnancy.

Clotting factor	First trimester	Second trimester	Third trimester
Factor VIII	↔	↑	↑↑↑
Factor VII	↔	↑	↑
vWF	↑	↑↑	↑↑↑
Fibrinogen	↔	↑	↑↑
Factor X	↔	↔	↔
Protein S	↔	↓	↓
D-dimer	↔	↑	↑↑

Note: vWF stands for von Willebrand factor.

Thrombosis in Pregnancy

The overall relative risk of thrombosis throughout the whole pregnancy period is estimated to be 4–10 times the baseline risk. This is not only because of the changes in haemostasis but also because of the increased risk of venous obstruction in the pelvis as the fetus grows.

Thrombosis during pregnancy is the fifth-most common cause of maternal mortality in the UK. The complications of both deep vein thrombosis (DVT) and pulmonary embolism (PE) are the same during and after pregnancy, and anticoagulation is achieved with low-molecular-weight heparin (LMWH). Neither direct-acting oral anticoagulants (DOACs) nor vitamin K antagonists are suitable during pregnancy, as both cross the placenta. Vitamin K antagonists are also teratogenic, although data regarding the safety of DOACs during pregnancy are lacking.

There is little evidence on which dosing regimen for LMWH is best; however, most centres use a twice-daily dosing schedule based on either the patient's weight at booking or their current weight, whichever is higher.

There has been much debate regarding the role of inferior vena cava (IVC) filters in patients presenting at a late stage of pregnancy; however, current practice recommends against their routine use, although they may be considered in specific cases.

Systemic thrombolysis and thrombectomy carry considerable risks to the mother and fetus and, as such, should be reserved for life-threatening thrombosis after discussion between the patient, an obstetrician, an anaesthetist and a haematologist.

Anticoagulation continues throughout pregnancy and is reassessed at delivery. Most commonly, women will be offered a further six weeks of treatment after delivery or the completion of a minimum of three months of anticoagulation treatment, whichever is longer.

Delivery and epidural analgesia while on anticoagulation represent unique challenges, as at the point of delivery, the risk of both haemorrhage and thrombosis is highest. The decisions regarding the mode of delivery and the timing of intervention should be made by an obstetrician, a haematologist and an anaesthetist in a multidisciplinary team (MDT) environment.

The role of thromboprophylaxis in pregnancy

Due to the increased risk of thrombosis, some women benefit from a prophylactic dose of LMWH to reduce this risk. The decision regarding the use of prophylaxis should be made by an obstetrician or midwife during the booking visit. It is rare that thromboprophylaxis is required before this since the majority of the prothrombotic changes occur later in the course of the pregnancy (see Table 15.1).

Women with a previous history of unprovoked or hormone-provoked thrombosis are offered thromboprophylaxis throughout the pregnancy. In other cases, thromboprophylaxis is given either throughout pregnancy or from week 28, depending on the number of risk factors, as listed in Table 15.2.

LMWH is the preferred choice for thromboprophylaxis; however, in patients who are allergic, fondaparinux is a suitable alternative.

LMWH should be given at a prophylactic dose based on the patient's weight at the time of booking (noting that obesity is a risk factor).

Patients on thromboprophylaxis do not usually require additional precautions or planning for delivery; they are simply advised not to take additional LMWH once they enter labour. The timing of when epidural analgesia may be appropriate is usually determined based on when the last dose of LMWH was administered.

Table 15.2.   Pregnancy-associated risk factors for thrombosis.

Permanent risk factors	Transient risk factors
Obesity (BMI >30 kg/m^2)	Dehydration
Age >35 years	Hyperemesis
Parity >= 3	COVID-19/systemic infection
Smoker	Hospitalisation
Gross varicose veins	Long-distance travel
Current pre-eclampsia	
Immobility	
Family history of unprovoked or hormone-associated VTE	
Low risk of thrombophilia	
Multiple pregnancy	
IVF/ART	

Note: IVF/ART stands for *in vitro* fertilisation/assisted reproductive technology.

Source: Adapted from the Green Top Guidelines 37a of the Royal College of Obstetrics and Gynaecology, www.rcog.org.uk.

Management of Thrombocytopenia During Pregnancy

A fall in the platelet count is a common finding during pregnancy and represents a physiological change. Although the platelet count often reduces slightly, the mean platelet volume increases, resulting in a higher total platelet volume; consequently, patients are often prothrombotic.

The lower limit of normal platelet count in the third trimester of pregnancy is 100×10^9/L, and values above this do not require further investigation. This is termed gestational thrombocytopenia.

Of the documented cases of thrombocytopenia in pregnancy, approximately 85% are gestational.

The safe platelet level for epidural anaesthesia is 80×10^9/L, and for either vaginal delivery or caesarean section, a platelet count of 40–50×10^9/L is considered acceptable. If the cause of thrombocytopenia is unknown, it should be determined before administering platelets, although in an emergency, attaining a safe platelet count for intervention should be the primary goal.

Where the platelet count drops below 100×10^9/L, gestational thrombocytopenia remains the most likely cause (85% of cases), however pre-eclampsia needs to be excluded. Pre-eclampsia represents about 15% of such cases (platelet count below 100×10^9/L). Pre-eclampsia is a common complication of late-stage pregnancy and is managed with antiplatelet drugs and delivery of the baby. Pre-eclampsia is characterised by hypertension and proteinuria, with red cell fragmentation frequently observed in the blood film. A grave form of pre-eclampsia that indicates urgent delivery is the haemolysis, elevated liver enzymes and low platelets (HELLP) syndrome.

The serious haematological causes of thrombocytopenia in pregnancy represent less than 1% of cases. Management involves an MDT approach involving clinicians experienced in these conditions.

16

Things You Need to Know Before You Graduate

Barbara J. Bain

What Do You Need To Know?

☞ How to take a clinical history

☞ How to perform a physical examination

☞ How to request laboratory tests

☞ How to interpret laboratory tests and initiate further investigation of abnormal results

☞ How to prescribe blood components

☞ How to prescribe and monitor heparin and oral anticoagulants

☞ When to suspect a haematological disorder and how to recognise a haematological emergency

☞ How to acquire information you do not have

☞ How to relate to a patient

There are some parts of haematology that you need to know by the time you graduate and commence medical practice. There are others that you do not need to know in any detail. For example, you will need to know how to prescribe blood components and how to manage anticoagulant therapy, since you are likely to be responsible for these, but you do not need to know how to treat acute myeloid leukaemia. You need to know how to acquire and assess new information when the circumstances require and when to ask for help. Here are some of the things you need to know.

How to Take a Clinical History

As in all branches of medicine, taking a clinical history can be of crucial importance. Features in the history that may be of particular relevance to haematological conditions are shown in Table 16.1. In assessing haemostasis, a careful clinical history is a better diagnostic tool, e.g. pre-operatively, than a coagulation screen.

The history should include a dietary history as well as of bowel function, which may be of relevance to an iron, vitamin B_{12} or folic acid deficiency. A history of adverse reaction to fava beans should be specifically sought if glucose-6-phosphate dehydrogenase (G6PD) deficiency is possible.

Table 16.1. Features in the clinical history of particular relevance in patients with haematological disorders.

Feature in clinical history	What haematological abnormality may be indicated
Fatigue, dyspnoea, ankle swelling	Anaemia
Recurrent infection	Neutropenia, defective neutrophil function, inherited or acquired immune deficiency (possible acute leukaemia, myelodysplastic syndrome, multiple myeloma)
Bruising, epistaxis, bleeding gums, menorrhagia, bleeding following surgery or trauma, any other abnormal bleeding	Thrombocytopenia, inherited or acquired coagulation defect or defect of platelet function
Jaundice	Haemolysis or ineffective haemopoiesis
Dark urine	Haemolysis
Fever, night sweats, weight loss	Lymphoma
Alcohol-induced pain or cough	Hodgkin lymphoma
Pruritus	Lymphoma or polycythaemia vera
Bone pain	In a child, possible acute lymphoblastic leukaemia; in an adult, possible multiple myeloma

A drug history should be routinely taken and should include a history of 'alternative' medications (which may include toxic or pharmacologically active substances). Of particular relevance are the intake of drugs that interfere with platelet function (such as aspirin), that cause macrocytosis (such as zidovudine or methotrexate), and the recent intake of drugs that can cause haemolysis. Alcohol intake should always be documented and is important in assessing macrocytosis, cytopenia and coagulopathy. Cigarette smoking should likewise be documented, since this may be the cause not only of a high haemoglobin concentration but of an increased neutrophil or lymphocyte count.

In many clinical circumstances it is important to assess the likelihood of exposure to the human immunodeficiency virus (HIV), hepatitis B and hepatitis C. All of these can cause haematological abnormalities and be relevant to the treatment that is given for an unrelated condition.

A travel history should be taken. It is particularly relevant to the assessment of eosinophilia and can indicate that the blood film should be examined for malaria parasites.

A family history should include a history of anaemia (including, specifically, sickle cell disease, thalassaemia and G6PD deficiency), jaundice and any bleeding disorder. It should include a history of the health of parents and siblings and because of the possibility of autosomal recessive or X-linked inheritance in various haematological disorders, a history of the health of cousins and male relatives on the mother's side of the family. The possibility of consanguinity should be explored when this might be relevant.

The ethnic origin should be specifically documented since it may be relevant but not obvious. For example, Mediterranean ancestry might suggest thalassaemia or G6PD deficiency.

How to Perform a Physical Examination

The physical examination should be thorough so that all organ systems are evaluated. Features of particular relevance to haematological disorders include pallor, purpura, hepatomegaly, splenomegaly, lymphadenopathy and jaundice. Glossitis, angular cheilosis and koilonychia should also be noted. Joint or muscle swelling may be indicative of a bleeding disorder and swelling around the small bones of the hands and feet in children may indicate sickle cell disease.

How to Request Laboratory Tests

You should know how to complete requests for laboratory tests, whether on paper or electronically. Providing accurate clinical details can be very important in helping laboratory staff to assess test results and give you an informed opinion. For example, if the patient has been recently transfused, assays of serum B_{12} and red cell folate will be invalid as will testing relevant to thalassaemia or haemoglobinopathies; if the patient has been transfused at another hospital it is highly unlikely that the laboratory staff will discover this unless you tell them. Don't forget to tell the laboratory that a patient is on warfarin, direct oral anticoagulants or heparin, otherwise resources may be wasted in investigating a 'coagulation defect'.

Meticulous completion of a request form is particularly important in blood transfusion; not only must identifying details be totally correct but previous pregnancies or blood transfusion must be documented. It is important to know whether the patient is currently pregnant (for example, pregnant women receive cytomegalovirus-negative blood), so don't forget to give this information if the patient is attending somewhere other than the antenatal clinic. If the patient is attending the antenatal clinic, remember to note the period of gestation as this is relevant to when tests for atypical blood group antibodies are done.

How to Interpret Laboratory Tests

You should understand the concept of a reference range and a normal range and be able to interpret tests in relation to a range provided. You should be aware of the influence of age, gender, ethnic origin and pregnancy on common haematology tests. You should be able to assess whether an abnormal test result is likely to indicate a serious disorder and whether investigation is indicated. If further investigation is indicated, you should be able to plan a cost-effective and clinically relevant sequence of testing.

How to Prescribe Blood Components

You should understand when it is appropriate to prescribe blood components and be able to do so. This includes obtaining consent for transfusion.

How to Prescribe and Monitor Anticoagulant Therapy

You should know how to prescribe unfractionated and low molecular weight heparin and oral anticoagulants, and how to monitor and adjust the dose of unfractionated heparin and vitamin K antagonists. This will usually be done according to guidelines available in individual hospitals but you should understand the principles.

Don't forget to plan ahead if a patient on anticoagulant therapy is going to require surgery.

When to Suspect a Haematological Disorder and How to Recognise a Haematological Emergency

There are a small number of haematological emergencies that must be recognised since delayed diagnosis can be very detrimental to the patient. These include acute promyelocytic leukaemia and other causes of disseminated intravascular coagulation and very high grade lymphomas (such as Burkitt lymphoma). If there is reason to suspect these conditions, ask for advice immediately; don't wait till the next morning. Severe thrombocytopenia also needs to be dealt with urgently but not necessarily by platelet transfusion. If the cause might be immune, i.e. autoimmune, thrombocytopenic purpura or thrombotic thrombocytopenic purpura, seek advice immediately.

Neutropenic sepsis is also a medical emergency. This may occur following cytotoxic chemotherapy in haematology or oncology patients. The units responsible will have therapeutic guidelines as to the choice of antibiotics, but if you are responsible for the immediate care of the patients (e.g. out-of-hours) make sure that there is no delay in taking specimens for culture and instituting antibiotic therapy. Starting treatment in such patients should take precedence over less urgent matters as death can occur rapidly when the body's defences are inadequate.

Generally you will be aware when a haematological disorder is likely but there are some conditions that are overlooked because they are uncommon. Don't forget that swelling of a joint may be the result of undiagnosed haemophilia rather than septic arthritis, osteomyelitis or trauma. Think of haemophilia also if you are considering a diagnosis of non-accidental injury in a child who presents with bruising or bleeding. You must request a blood film in any child presenting with renal impairment, particularly if there is also jaundice, since this may be haemolytic uraemic syndrome. In an adult presenting with acute renal failure, don't forget that multiple myeloma is responsible for a significant proportion of cases. In an adult any combination of anaemia, backache and renal impairment may be due to myeloma. In any patient presenting with jaundice, remember that this may represent haemolysis rather than hepatic or post-hepatic jaundice.

How to Acquire Information You Do Not Have

Your medical course should have equipped you to acquire new information when there is something you do not know. This will include obtaining information from more experienced colleagues: not only medical colleagues but also nursing staff, pharmacists and laboratory scientists. A modicum of humility does not go amiss in dealing with non-medical colleagues; they will often know a great deal that you do not know.

You should also know how to acquire specific information — from textbooks, journals and websites. You should be aware of reliable sources of information, such as the British National Formulary and the guidelines provided by the National Institute for Health and Clinical Excellence (NICE) and various professional groups (e.g. The British Society for Haematology guidelines). Although you will not initially be making major clinical decisions unaided, you should be able to assess the validity and clinical relevance of published trials and know how to evaluate and make use of systematic reviews including meta-analyses. In assessing original articles and systematic reviews, it is important not only to assess the quality of the publication but also to ask yourself two questions. Are there results applicable to my patients? Are any benefits demonstrated worth the potential harm and the cost?

How to Relate to a Patient

All patients should be treated with respect. Patients, particularly elderly patients, may not wish to be addressed by their first names. Be careful not to discuss clinical matters in lifts, hospital canteens or any other place where you may be overheard. Be honest with your patients but don't force on them more information that they wish to receive. Try to present information in an optimistic manner but without concealing the truth — a difficult balance to strike. Don't be afraid to say that you don't know.

Conclusions

The skills you need to deal with haematological disorders are exactly the same skills that you need for any other branch of medicine. However, it is important to know how to deal with common haematological disorders, how to recognise an emergency and when to suspect an uncommon but important condition.

17

Further Reading

This list is provided for reference purposes and for in-depth reading on selected topics. It will be most useful to students in the later years of their medical course.

General

American Society of Hematology website: https://Hematology.org.
British Society for Haematology website: https://b-s-h.org.uk/.
Hoffbrand AV, Higgs DR, Keeling DM and Mehta AB (eds). *Postgraduate Haematology*, 7th Edn., Wiley-Blackwell, Oxford, 2016.

Chapter 1 Physiology of the Blood and Bone Marrow

Crispino JD. Introduction to a review series on hematopoietic stem cells. *Blood.* 2023;142(6):497.

Chapter 2 The Blood Count and Film

Bain BJ, *A Beginner's Guide to Blood Cells*, 3rd Edn., Wiley-Blackwell, Oxford, 2017.
Bain BJ, *Blood Cells*, 6th Edn., Wiley, Oxford, 2022.
Bain BJ and Leach M. *Immunophenotyping for Haematologists*. Wiley-Blackwell, Oxford, 2021.

Leach M and Bain BJ. *From the Image to the Diagnosis*. Wiley-Blackwell, Oxford, 2022.

Roberts I and Bain BJ, *Neonatal Haematology: A Practical Guide*, Wiley-Blackwell, Oxford, 2022.

Chapter 3 Microcytic Anaemias and the Thalassaemias

Bain BJ and Rees DC. *Haemoglobinopathy Diagnosis*, 4th Edn., Wiley-Blackwell, Oxford, 2025. (Includes thalassaemias.)

Camaschella C. Iron deficiency. *Blood*. 2019;133(1):30–39.

Hokland P, Daar S, Khair W, Sheth S, Taher AT, Torti L, *et al*. Thalassaemia-A global view. *Br J Haematol*. 2023;201(2):199–214.

Chapter 4 Macrocytic Anaemias

Green R. Vitamin B(12) deficiency from the perspective of a practicing hematologist. *Blood*. 2017;129(19):2603–2611.

Chapter 5 Haemoglobinopathies and Haemolytic Anaemias

Luzzatto L, Ally M, Notaro R. Glucose-6-phosphate dehydrogenase deficiency. *Blood*. 2020;136(11):1225–1240.

Makani J, Nkya S, Collins F, Luzzatto L. From Mendel to a Mendelian disorder: Towards a cure for sickle cell disease. *Nat Rev Genet*. 2022;23(7):389–390.

Thein SL, Howard J. How I treat the older adult with sickle cell disease. *Blood*. 2018;132(17):1750–1760.

Chapter 6 Miscellaneous Anaemias, Pancytopenia and the Myelodysplastic Syndromes

Bain BJ. *Leukaemia Diagnosis*, 6th Edn., Wiley-Blackwell, Oxford, 2024. (Includes myelodysplastic syndromes.)

Hellstrom-Lindberg ES, Kroger N. Clinical decision-making and treatment of myelodysplastic syndromes. *Blood*. 2023;142(26):2268–2281.

Young NS. Aplastic Anemia. *N Engl J Med*. 2018;379(17):1643–1656.

Chapter 7 Leucocytosis, Leucopenia and Reactive Changes in White Cells

Young LS. Epstein-Barr virus at 60. *Nature*. 2024;627(8004):492–494.

Chapter 8 Blood Cancer Pathology: Lymphoma and Acute Leukaemia

Ansell SM. Hodgkin lymphoma: 2023 update on diagnosis, risk-stratification, and management. *Am J Hematol*. 2022;97(11):1478–1488.

Eichhorst B, Robak T, Montserrat E, Ghia P, Niemann CU, Kater AP, *et al*. Chronic lymphocytic leukaemia: ESMO Clinical Practice Guidelines for diagnosis, treatment and follow-up. *Ann Oncol*. 2021;32(1):23–33.

El Chaer F, Hourigan CS, Zeidan AM. How I treat AML incorporating the updated classifications and guidelines. *Blood*. 2023;141(23): 2813–2823.

Matutes E, Bain BJ and Wotherspoon A. *Lymphoid Malignancies: An Atlas of Investigation and Diagnosis*. 2nd Edn., EBN Health, Oxford, 2020.

Chapter 9 Myeloproliferative Neoplasms

Cazzola M. Introduction to a review series on classic myeloproliferative neoplasms. *Blood*. 2023;141(16):1897–1899.

Smith G, Apperley J, Milojkovic D, Cross NCP, Foroni L, Byrne J, *et al*. A British Society for Haematology Guideline on the diagnosis and management of chronic myeloid leukaemia. *Br J Haematol*. 2020; 191(2):171–193.

Chapter 10 Multiple Myeloma

Kyle RA, Larson DR, Therneau TM, Dispenzieri A, Kumar S, Cerhan JR, Rajkumar SV. Long-term follow-up of monoclonal gammopathy of undetermined significance. *N Engl J Med*. 2018 Jan 18;378(3):241–249.

van de Donk NWCJ, Pawlyn C, Yong KL. Multiple myeloma. *Lancet*. 2021 Jan 30;397(10272):410–427.

Chapter 11 Platelets, Coagulation and Haemostasis

Bannow BS, Konkle BA. How I approach bleeding in hospitalized patients. *Blood.* 2023;142(9):761–768.

Nogami K, Shima M. Current and future therapies for haemophilia: Beyond factor replacement therapies. *Br J Haematol.* 2023;200(1):23–34.

Chapter 12 Thrombosis and Its Management: Anticoagulant, Antiplatelet and Thrombolytic Therapy

Akpan IJ, Hunt BJ. How I approach the prevention and treatment of thrombotic complications in hospitalized patients. *Blood.* 2023;142(9):769–776.

Arachchillage DJ, Mackillop L, Chandratheva A, Motawani J, MacCallum P, Laffan M. Thrombophilia testing: A British Society for Haematology guideline. *Br J Haematol.* 2022;198(3):443–458.

Chapter 13 Blood Transfusion

British Blood Transfusion Society. Take a look — NHSBT blood components app. https://www.bbts.org.uk/blog/nhsbt_blood_components_app.

Independent Report. Guidelines from the expert advisory committee on the Safety of Blood, Tissues and Organs (SaBTO) on patient consent for blood transfusion. Published 17 December 2020. https://www.gov.uk/government/publications/blood-transfusion-patient-consent.

Lise J. Estcourt, Janet Birchall, Shubha Allard, Stephen J. Bassey, *et al.* BSH Guidelines for the use of platelet transfusions. *Br J Haematol.* 2017 Feb;176(3):331–502.

NHS Blood and Transplant. Who can give blood. https://www.blood.co.uk/who-can-give-blood/.

NICE. Blood transfusion. Quality standard [QS138] in 15 December 2016. https://www.nice.org.uk/guidance/qs138/resources/blood-transfusion-pdf-75545425760965.

Qureshi H, Massey E, Kirwan D, Davies T, Robson S, White J, Jones J, Allard S. British Society for Haematology. BCSH guideline for the use of anti-D immunoglobulin for the prevention of haemolytic disease of the fetus and newborn. *Transfusion Med.* 2014 Feb;24(1):8–20.

The Blood Safety and Quality Regulations. UK Statutory Instruments 2005 No. 50. https://www.legislation.gov.uk/uksi/2005/50.

White J, Qureshi H, Massey E, Needs M, Byrne G, Daniels G, Allard S. British Committee for Standards in Haematology. Guideline for blood grouping and red cell antibody testing in pregnancy. *Transfusion Med.* 2016 Aug;26(4): 246–263.

Chapter 14 Haemopoietic Stem Cell Transplantation and CAR-T Cell Therapy

Carreras E, Dufour C, Mohty M, Kröger N, editors. *The EBMT Handbook: Hematopoietic Stem Cell Transplantation and Cellular Therapies.* 7th Edn., Cham (CH): Springer; 2019.

Mitra A, Barua A, Huang L, Ganguly S, Feng Q, He B. From bench to bedside: The history and progress of CAR-T cell therapy. *Front Immunol.* 2023 May 15;14:1188049.

Morris EC, Neelapu SS, Giavridis T, Sadelain M. Cytokine release syndrome and associated neurotoxicity in cancer immunotherapy. *Nat Rev Immunol.* 2022 Feb;22(2):85–96.

Muraro, P., Martin, R., Mancardi, G. *et al.* Autologous haematopoietic stem cell transplantation for treatment of multiple sclerosis. *Nat Rev Neurol.* 13, 391–405 (2017). https://doi.org/10.1038/nrneurol.2017.81.

Shlomchik, W. Graft-versus-host disease. *Nat Rev Immunol.* 7, 340–352 (2007). https://doi.org/10.1038/nri2000.

Singh AK, McGuirk JP. Allogeneic stem cell transplantation: A historical and scientific overview. *Cancer Res.* 2016 Nov 15;76(22):6445–6451.

Sterner, R.C., Sterner, R.M. CAR-T cell therapy: Current limitations and potential strategies. *Blood Cancer J.* 11, 69 (2021). https://doi.org/10.1038/s41408-021-00459-7.

Chapter 15 Haematology in Obstetric Medicine

Middeldorp S, Ganzevoort W. How I treat venous thromboembolism in pregnancy. *Blood.* 2020;136(19):2133–2142.

Self-Assessment

18

Preparing for Exams and Self-Assessment

Barbara J. Bain and
Donald Macdonald

Preparing for Exams and Self-Assessment

☞ Basic multiple-choice questions
☞ More advanced, single best answer multiple-choice questions
☞ Extended matching questions
☞ Answers to questions

Preparing for Exams

Remember that what you are really preparing for is a lifetime commitment as a medical practitioner. You may view examinations as a barrier on the way, but if they are well designed, they will be testing the core knowledge and skills that you need. Only some of these skills can be tested in a paper-based examination, and that is all that can be dealt with here.

Work out ways that you find useful to tabulate and store basic knowledge for quick reference and revision. This is likely to be in electronic format, although some people find lightweight cards to be useful. Base your learning from actual patients. This makes knowledge more meaningful and therefore easier to remember. When you see a patient, familiarise yourself with the history and results of the physical examination. Work out the differential diagnosis and the relevant tests, and when the test results become available, make sure that you can interpret them. Do some extra reading on the subject, and see how theoretical knowledge can be applied to a clinical situation.

Ward rounds, outpatient clinics and clerking patients are all important. In the later years of your course, make sure that you learn how to manage anticoagulant therapy and blood transfusions. Shadow the junior medical staff.

Self-Evaluation Questions

By the end of your haematology course, you should know the approximate normal range in men and women for haemoglobin concentration (Hb), mean cell volume (MCV), white cell count (WBC) and platelet count. If you need to refer to normal ranges for the full blood count and differential count to answer these questions, see Tables 2.1 and 2.2.

Other useful ranges and some abbreviations are shown in Table 18.1. The most straightforward self-evaluation questions in this chapter are the basic multiple-choice questions. The most difficult questions, requiring some clinical knowledge, are the extended matching questions; by the end of your medical course, you should know the answers to almost all of these.

Table 18.1. Normal ranges (NR) in adults.

Test	95% range
Vitamin B_{12}	180–640 ng/l
Serum folate	3–20 μg/l
Serum ferritin	15–300 μg/l
Serum iron	10–30 μmol/l
Serum transferrin	1.7–3.4 g/l
Erythrocyte sedimentation rate (ESR)	<10 mm in 1 hour (men), <15 mm in 1 hour (women)
Reticulocyte count	$50–100 \times 10^9$/l
Haemoglobin A_2	2.0–3.5%
Prothrombin time (PT)	12–14 seconds
International normalised ratio (INR)	0.8–1.2

Table 18.1. (*Continued*)

Test	95% range
Activated partial thromboplastin time (APTT)	30–40 seconds
Thrombin time (TT)	15–20 seconds
Fibrinogen assay	1.8–3.6 g/l
D-dimer	<0.50 mg/l
Serum bilirubin	<17 μmol/l
Alanine transaminase (ALT)	5–42 iu/l
Alkaline phosphatase	100–300 iu/l
Creatinine	60–125 μmol/l
Lactate dehydrogenase	200–450 iu/l
Calcium	2.20–2.60 mmol/l

Basic Multiple-Choice Questions

The number of true statements may be between one and five.

Question 1

An FBC sample is received by a laboratory with no clinical information provided. The test results are: Hb 82 g/l, MCV 82 fl, reticulocytes 15×10^9/l (NR 25–100), WBC 1.4×10^9/l, neutrophils 0.2×10^9/l, lymphocytes 0.9×10^9/l and platelets 15×10^9/l. Which of the following conditions should be included in the differential diagnosis?

1. Acute lymphoblastic leukaemia (ALL)
2. Aplastic anaemia (AA)
3. Pernicious anaemia
4. Chronic myeloid leukaemia (CML)
5. Immune thrombocytopenic purpura (also known as autoimmune thrombocytopenic purpura, ITP)

Question 2

An 8-year-old child with known sickle cell disease is found to have Howell–Jolly body red cell inclusions, seen on a blood film. He recently arrived in the UK with no record of previous medical supervision. Which of the following should be recommended?

1. Vitamin B$_{12}$ supplementation
2. Pneumococcal vaccination
3. *Pneumocystis jirovecii* prophylaxis
4. Penicillin V prophylaxis
5. Meningococcal vaccination

Question 3

Which of the following conditions commonly present with generalised lymphadenopathy and hepatosplenomegaly?

1. Primary myelofibrosis
2. Chronic lymphocytic leukaemia
3. Chronic myeloid leukaemia
4. Acute lymphoblastic leukaemia
5. Follicular non-Hodgkin lymphoma

Question 4

Which of the following causes of thrombocytopenia are associated with an increased risk of thrombosis?

1. Immune thrombocytopenic purpura
2. Heparin-induced thrombocytopenia (HIT)
3. Post-transfusion purpura
4. Neonatal alloimmune thrombocytopenic purpura
5. Thrombotic thrombocytopenic purpura (TTP)

Question 5

A high Hb could be the result of:

1. Renal carcinoma
2. Renal failure
3. Chronic obstructive pulmonary disease
4. Polycythaemia vera
5. Full and partial thickness burns over half the body

Question 6

A 53-year-old woman is found to have an Hb level of 101 g/l and an MCV of 107 fl. This could be the result of:

1. Early iron deficiency
2. Excessive alcohol intake
3. Myelodysplastic syndrome
4. Vitamin B$_{12}$ deficiency
5. Hyperthyroidism

Question 7

An increased neutrophil count with toxic granulation is a likely result of:

1. Pneumococcal pneumonia
2. Gangrene of the foot
3. Infectious mononucleosis
4. Ethnic variation
5. Postpartum period

Question 8

A blood film might be expected to show spherocytes in:

1. Hereditary elliptocytosis
2. Autoimmune haemolytic anaemia
3. Delayed haemolytic transfusion reaction
4. Pregnancy
5. Iron deficiency anaemia

Question 9

A patient of blood group A Rh D-positive could safely receive a transfusion of red cells resuspended in SAGM from a donor who is:

1. Group AB Rh D-positive
2. Group A Rh D-negative
3. Group O Rh D-positive (with high-titre antibodies excluded)

4. Group B Rh D-positive
5. None of the above

Question 10

A 5-year-old boy presents with a haemarthrosis of the left knee. Coagulation studies show PT of 14 seconds, APTT of 55 seconds and TT of 18 seconds (control: 19). Possible explanations for the coagulation defect include:

1. A defect in the intrinsic system
2. A defect in the extrinsic system
3. A defect in the common pathway
4. Thrombocytopenia
5. Hypofibrinogenaemia

(If necessary, refer to Fig. 11.4 to work out your answer.)

Question 11

An 18-year-old man presents with a gastrointestinal haemorrhage. Coagulation studies show: PT 13 seconds, APTT 48 seconds, TT 18 seconds (control 20), fibrinogen concentration 3.7 g/l and D-dimer 38 mg/l (NR < 50). Likely explanations include:

1. Haemophilia A
2. Von Willebrand disease
3. Liver failure
4. Anticoagulant overdose
5. Disseminated intravascular coagulation

Question 12

Patients with long-standing, difficult-to-control rheumatoid arthritis have an increased incidence of anaemia due to:

1. Iron deficiency
2. Felty syndrome
3. Folic acid deficiency
4. Vitamin B_{12} deficiency
5. Anaemia of chronic disease

Question 13

A pregnant woman is blood group A Rh D-positive, and her partner is group O Rh D-positive. The baby could be:

1. Group O Rh D-positive
2. Group O Rh-D negative
3. Group A Rh D-positive
4. Group A Rh-D negative
5. Group AB Rh-D negative

Question 14

A male surgical patient is blood group B Rh-D negative. He has never received a transfusion. The antibodies expected in his plasma are:

1. Anti-A
2. Anti-B
3. Anti-O
4. Anti-D
5. Anti-d

Question 15

A high reticulocyte count could be due to:

1. Aplastic anaemia
2. Recent blood loss
3. Haemolysis
4. Chronic myeloid leukaemia
5. Untreated iron deficiency anaemia

Question 16

An 18-year-old student is febrile, and his blood film shows numerous atypical lymphocytes. This could be due to:

1. Toxoplasmosis
2. An allergic reaction to a drug
3. A primary human immunodeficiency virus (HIV) infection
4. A primary cytomegalovirus (CMV) infection
5. A primary Epstein–Barr virus (EBV) infection

Single Best Answer Multiple-Choice Questions

Question 1

A 37-year-old woman is referred to a combined obstetric haematology clinic. She is in the second trimester of pregnancy, and following assessment she is determined to be at an intermediate risk of venous thromboembolism (VTE). Which antenatal VTE prophylaxis management would you recommend?

1. Aspirin
2. Aspirin and clopidogrel
3. Low-molecular-weight heparin (LMWH)
4. Rivaroxaban
5. Warfarin

Question 2

Chimaeric antigen receptor T cell (CAR-T) therapy, directed against the epitope CD19, is an effective therapy for which haematological cancer?

1. Chronic myeloid leukaemia
2. Acute T-cell leukaemia lymphoma
3. Diffuse large B-cell lymphoma
4. Sézary syndrome
5. Acute myeloid leukaemia

Question 3

In a patient with newly diagnosed Hodgkin lymphoma, the PET CT scan indicates disease involving the following sites only: supraclavicular fossa, mediastinum, inguinal nodes and spleen. Which anatomical stage (Ann Arbor staging) is this?

1. Stage 0 disease
2. Stage 1 disease
3. Stage 2 disease
4. Stage 3 disease
5. Stage 4 disease

Question 4

A 62-year-old man with myeloma has responded well to first-line treatment. He now presents with a six-week history of increasing shortness of breath and severe dependent oedema. The laboratory results are: IgGλ paraprotein 12 g/l, serum free λ light chain 29 mg/l (5.7–26), serum free κ light chain 3.2 mg/l (3.3–19), creatinine 125 μmol/l (60–120), albumin 21 g/l (35–50), brain natriuretic peptide (BNP) 600 pg/ml (<100) and urine protein 6.3 g/24 hr.

A renal biopsy is performed. What is the most likely histological finding?

1. AL amyloidosis
2. Focal segmental glomerulosclerosis
3. Myeloma kidney (cast nephropathy)
4. Nephrocalcinosis
5. Renal papillary necrosis

Question 5

Acute graft versus host disease post-allogeneic haemopoietic stem cell transplantation is mediated by which cell type?

1. Donor B lymphocytes
2. Donor T lymphocytes
3. Recipient B lymphocytes
4. Recipient NK lymphocytes
5. Recipient T lymphocytes

Question 6

A newborn baby becomes jaundiced and is found to be anaemic, with a positive direct antiglobulin test (Coombs test) and spherocytes on a blood film. His mother is blood group A Rh-D negative, while he is group O Rh-D positive. What is the most likely diagnosis?

1. ABO haemolytic disease of the newborn
2. Glucose-6-phosphate dehydrogenase deficiency
3. Hereditary spherocytosis

4. Rh haemolytic disease of the newborn
5. Immature neonatal hepatic function

Question 7

Which of the following decreases during pregnancy?

1. D-dimer
2. Factor VIII
3. Fibrinogen
4. Protein S
5. Von Willebrand factor

Question 8

In obstetric practice, the maximum risk of fatal maternal thrombo-embolism occurs at which stage of pregnancy?

1. First trimester
2. Post-amniocentesis
3. Postpartum
4. Second trimester
5. Third trimester

Question 9

Regarding acute myeloid leukaemia, which statement is true?

1. It has a similar prevalence at all ages
2. It has reduced in prevalence in recent decades
3. It increases in incidence with increasing age
4. It is more common in females than males
5. It is the most common form of leukaemia in children

Question 10

A 29-year-old woman suffers an amniotic fluid embolism during labour. She becomes unwell with hypotension, accompanied by ongoing vaginal blood loss plus oozing from cannula sites. The coagulation results are: INR 1.9 (NR: 0.8–1.2), APTT 53 seconds (22–41), fibrinogen 0.8 g/l (2–4.0) and D dimers 210 mg/l (<50). What is the most likely haematological diagnosis?

1. Thrombotic thrombocytopenic purpura
2. Lupus anticoagulant
3. Disseminated intravascular coagulation (DIC)
4. Von Willebrand disease
5. Factor 8 inhibitor

Question 11

A 66-year-old man, who was being monitored for hypercholesterolaemia, had a blood count done and was found to have a lymphocyte count of $15.4 \times 10^9/l$, with the blood count being otherwise normal. The most likely diagnosis is:

1. Infectious mononucleosis
2. Cytomegalovirus infection
3. Acute lymphoblastic leukaemia
4. Pertussis
5. Chronic lymphocytic leukaemia

Question 12

A 23-year-old woman presents with a nosebleed and is found to have petechiae. A blood count shows a platelet count of $7 \times 10^9/l$, a white cell count of $5.2 \times 10^9/l$ and an Hb level of 120 g/l. The blood film does not show any platelet clumps or any other abnormalities. A coagulation screen is normal. The most likely diagnosis is:

1. HIV infection
2. Acute lymphoblastic leukaemia
3. Aplastic anaemia
4. Immune thrombocytopenic purpura
5. Acute promyelocytic leukaemia

Question 13

A 35-year-old Scottish woman has a history of Crohn disease with a recent worsening of her symptoms. Her laboratory tests show: WBC $11.3 \times 10^9/l$, neutrophil count $9.3 \times 10^9/l$, lymphocyte count $1 \times 10^9/l$, monocyte count $1 \times 10^9/l$, Hb 97 g/l, MCV 76 fl, platelet count $480 \times 10^9/l$, ESR 44 mm in 1 hour, serum iron 8 μmol/l (NR 10–30), serum transferrin 1.5 g/l (NR 1.7–3.4) and serum ferritin 520 μg/l (NR 15–300). The most likely cause of the anaemia is:

1. Vitamin B_{12} deficiency due to Crohn disease of the terminal ileum
2. Anaemia of chronic disease
3. Iron deficiency
4. Recent gastrointestinal blood loss
5. Folic acid deficiency

Question 14

A Greek couple, both with a family history of thalassaemia, opt for pre-conceptual testing. They are both found to be heterozygous for β thalassaemia. The likely outcome of pregnancy for this couple is:

1. No risk of thalassaemia major
2. A 25% chance of thalassaemia major
3. A 50% chance of thalassaemia major
4. A 75% chance of thalassaemia major
5. Almost certain thalassaemia major

Question 15

A 25-year-old Nigerian man requires emergency surgery following a road traffic accident that caused multiple fractures. A blood count and sickle solubility test are performed. His Hb level is 120 g/l, the sickle solubility test is positive, and the blood film shows some target cells. Which of the following statements is true?

1. He has sickle cell heterozygosity, which is of no significance
2. He has sickle cell anaemia, and surgery should not be undertaken

3. He has sickle cell heterozygosity, and care must be taken to avoid hypoxia, dehydration and acidosis
4. No diagnosis can be made without further tests, so surgery should be delayed
5. He has sickle cell anaemia, and surgery should not be undertaken without an exchange transfusion

Question 16

A 56-year-old man presents with numbness in his feet and is found to have reduced vibration sense and joint position sense. Plantar responses are upgoing. A blood count shows an Hb level of 118 g/l and an MCV of 103 fl. The most likely explanation is:

1. Diabetic neuropathy
2. Folic acid deficiency
3. Multiple sclerosis
4. Spinal cord compression
5. Pernicious anaemia

Question 17

The normal intravascular life span of a neutrophil is about:

1. 1 hour
2. 7 hours
3. 24 hours
4. 10 days
5. 120 days

Question 18

A 35-year-old Indian woman, who is vegetarian and has three young children, complains of fatigue and is found to have an Hb level of 80 g/l. Her blood film shows hypochromia, microcytosis and pencil cells (elliptocytes). The most likely diagnosis is:

1. Hereditary elliptocytosis
2. Vitamin B_{12} deficiency

3. Iron deficiency anaemia
4. Lead poisoning
5. Folic acid deficiency

Question 19

An Eritrean refugee is investigated for iron deficiency anaemia and is found to have hookworm. His blood film is most likely to show:

1. Neutrophilia
2. Eosinophilia
3. Basophilia
4. Lymphocytosis
5. Monocytosis

Question 20

A 50-year-old man suffers crushing central chest pain radiating to his left shoulder. The following day, he is found to have leucocytosis (WBC: $13 \times 10^9/l$) and neutrophilia (with a neutrophil count of $8.5 \times 10^9/l$). The Hb and platelet counts are normal. The most likely explanation of the abnormality in the blood count is:

1. Chronic myeloid leukaemia
2. Myocardial infarction
3. Pneumococcal pneumonia
4. Splenic infarction
5. Aortic dissection

Question 21

An accident and emergency department requires fresh frozen plasma for a 66-year-old man of unknown blood group, who appears to exhibit severely impaired liver function and is bleeding from oesophageal varices. Which group plasma should be chosen?

1. O
2. A
3. B

4. AB
5. None of the above

Question 22

A 46-year-old woman presents with weight loss and abdominal enlargement. She has also noticed that she is sweating more than normal, and
her temperature is 38°C. She has been found to have an enlargement of
the liver 2 cm below the right costal margin and of the spleen 6 cm
below the left costal margin. Lymph nodes are not enlarged. FBC shows:
WBC $98 \times 10^9/l$, Hb 83 g/l and platelet count $504 \times 10^9/l$. A blood film
shows increased numbers of neutrophils, eosinophils and basophils. In
addition, white cell precursors are elevated, although blast cells are
infrequent.

The optimal treatment for this patient is likely to be:

1. Allogeneic stem cell transplantation
2. Combination chemotherapy
3. A tyrosine kinase inhibitor
4. Blood transfusion as required to relieve symptoms
5. Rifampicin and isoniazid

Extended Matching Questions

Question 1: Paediatric haematology

Options:

A. Acute lymphoblastic leukaemia
B. Acute myeloid leukaemia
C. Autoimmune thrombocytopenic purpura
D. Glucose-6-phosphate dehydrogenase deficiency
E. Haemolytic uraemic syndrome
F. Hereditary spherocytosis
G. Infectious hepatitis
H. Meningococcal septicaemia
I. Sickle cell anaemia

J.   Sickle cell heterozygosity

K.   Thrombotic thrombocytopenic purpura (TTP)

For each clinical description provided in the following, select the most likely diagnosis from the list of options above. Each option may be used once, more than once or not at all.

1.   A 5-year-old Caucasian child who has recently suffered an upper respiratory tract infection presents with bruising and bleeding from his mouth. His full blood count shows: WBC 6.4×10^9/l, neutrophils 4.4×10^9/l, lymphocytes 2.0×10^9/l, Hb 112 g/l and platelet count 12×10^9/l.

2.   A 10-year-old Caucasian girl presents with fever and a reduced level of consciousness. She appears quite unwell, with multiple petechiae. Her FBC shows: WBC 15×10^9/l, neutrophils 12.3×10^9/l, Hb 150 g/l and platelet count 30×10^9/l. Her blood film confirms the low platelet count and shows toxic granulation in the neutrophils; however, RBC morphology appears normal.

3.   A 5-year-old child who recently arrived from Nigeria presents with recurrent limb and chest pains. His mother says that his eyes sometimes appear yellow. His haemoglobin concentration is found to be 62 g/l.

4.   A 6-year-old Caucasian boy presents with pallor, pain in his legs and bruising. He is found to have small volume lymphadenopathy, and his spleen is palpable 2 cm below his left costal margin. His full blood count shows: WBC 64×10^9/l, Hb 82 g/l and platelet count 20×10^9/l.

5.   A 6-year-old Italian boy becomes jaundiced while being treated for a urinary tract infection. A blood film shows numerous irregularly contracted cells and polychromasia.

Question 2: Haematological cancer diagnosis

Options:

A.   Acute myeloid leukaemia

B.   Acute promyelocytic leukaemia

C.   Adult T-cell leukaemia/lymphoma

D. B-cell acute lymphoblastic leukaemia

E. Burkitt lymphoma

F. Chronic lymphocytic leukaemia

G. Chronic myeloid leukaemia

H. Enteropathy-associated T-cell lymphoma

I. Mantle cell lymphoma

J. Multiple myeloma

K. T-cell acute lymphoblastic leukaemia

For each clinical scenario provided in the following, select the most likely diagnosis from the list of options above. Each option may be used once, more than once or not at all.

1. A 42-year-old woman presents with abdominal pain and massive splenomegaly. Her FBC shows: WBC $65 \times 10^9/l$, neutrophils $48 \times 10^9/l$, myelocytes $12 \times 10^9/l$, basophils $3 \times 10^9/l$, Hb 102 g/l and platelet count $460 \times 10^9/l$.

2. A 72-year-old woman presents with a history of severe back pain. Her FBC shows: WBC $1.8 \times 10^9/l$, neutrophils $0.3 \times 10^9/l$, Hb 87 g/l and platelet count $30 \times 10^9/l$. Her blood film shows rouleaux. Her serum-corrected calcium level is 3.1 mmol/l, and she has an IgG kappa paraprotein with a concentration of 62 g/l.

3. A 56-year-old Afro-Caribbean man presents with weight loss and confusion. His FBC shows: WBC $25 \times 10^9/l$, neutrophils $2.5 \times 10^9/l$, lymphocytes $20 \times 10^9/l$, Hb 97 g/l and platelet count $60 \times 10^9/l$. His blood film shows lymphocytes with multi-lobulated nuclei. His serum-corrected calcium level is 3.2 mmol/l (2.2–2.6), and he has antibodies to the HTLV-1 virus.

4. A 66-year-old man attends a routine health check. His FBC shows: WBC $29 \times 10^9/l$, neutrophils $2.5 \times 10^9/l$, lymphocytes $24 \times 10^9/l$, Hb 101 g/l and platelet count $97 \times 10^9/l$. His blood film shows mature lymphocytes, with many smear cells.

5. A 25-year-old male presents with a headache, a deteriorating level of consciousness and widespread bleeding. His FBC shows: WBC $7 \times 10^9/l$, neutrophils $0.5 \times 10^9/l$, Hb 81 g/l and platelet count $15 \times 10^9/l$. His blood film shows circulating myeloid precursor cells with large

granules and many Auer rods. *PML::RARA* fusion transcripts are detected in peripheral blood by RT-PCR analysis.

Question 3: Red cell abnormalities

Options:

A. Aplastic anaemia
B. Beta thalassaemia major
C. Beta thalassaemia trait
D. Folic acid deficiency
E. Glucose-6-phosphate dehydrogenase deficiency
F. Hereditary spherocytosis
G. Iron deficiency anaemia
H. Pernicious anaemia
I.   Sickle cell anaemia
J. Sickle cell trait

For each clinical history provided in the following, choose the single most likely diagnosis from the above list of options. Each option may be used once, more than once or not at all.

1. A 10-year-old Afro-Caribbean girl requires urgent surgery for suspected appendicitis. Pre-operative haemoglobin concentration is normal, but a sickle solubility test is positive
2. A 23-year-old West African man with malaria is given quinine, followed by primaquine. Having initially experienced only a mild fever, he becomes jaundiced and severely anaemic, and his urine turns dark. His blood film shows no malaria parasites but shows irregularly contracted cells
3. An adolescent girl with coeliac disease refuses to comply with a gluten-free diet. She develops pallor and lethargy and is found to have an Hb level of 83 g/l and an MCV of 113 fl
4. A 5-year-old African boy has recurrent limb pain and mild jaundice. His Hb level is 64 g/l, and haemoglobin electrophoresis shows 95% haemoglobin S and 5% haemoglobin F

5. A 50-year-old man requires a cholecystectomy for gallstones. A pre-operative blood count and film show an Hb level of 110 g/l, spherocytes, polychromasia and an increased reticulocyte count

Question 4: Blood transfusion

Options:

A. ABO-incompatible transfusion
B. Allergic reaction to foreign protein in donor blood
C. Bacterial contamination of transfused blood
D. Delayed haemolytic transfusion reaction
E. Immediate haemolytic transfusion reaction due to Rh D antibodies
F. Post-transfusion purpura
G. Pulmonary embolism
H. Transfusion-induced graft-versus-host disease
I. Transfusion-related acute lung injury (TRALI)
J. Transfusional haemosiderosis
K. Viral hepatitis

For each clinical situation provided in the following, choose the single most appropriate answer from the list above. Each option may be used once, more than once or not at all.

1. A 24-year-old male, who was diagnosed with thalassaemia major at the age of 13 months, presents to the outpatient clinic complaining of malaise and erectile dysfunction; he is noted to have increased skin pigmentation
2. A 54-year-old male smoker is seven days post-operative after the repair of an abdominal aortic aneurysm. He presents with fever and jaundice, and his haemoglobin concentration has dropped
3. A 33-year-old man was admitted after a serious road traffic accident. He required a transfusion of six units of blood. Four hours later, he developed a fever and a dry cough and became increasingly breathless

4. A 22-year-old African woman with sickle cell anaemia presented 15 minutes after a donor blood transfusion with a diffuse, itchy, erythematous rash on both forearms. She responded well to cetirizine

5. A 33-year-old patient with myelodysplastic syndrome receives transfusions regularly every four weeks. She is admitted as a day case, and 10 minutes after starting a blood transfusion, she develops loin pain and feels distressed. Her blood pressure drops, and she is tachycardic. The next urine specimen she passes is positive for blood (as determined by a urine dipstick test)

Question 5: Coagulation tests

Options:

A. Activated partial thromboplastin time (APTT)
B. Anticardiolipin antibody
C. Anti-Xa assay
D. Factor II assay
E. Factor VIII assay
F. Factor V Leiden genotype
G. Fibrinogen assay
H. Haematocrit
I. International normalised ratio (INR)
J. No testing required
K. PFA 200 (platelet function analyser) test
L. Thrombin time

For each clinical scenario provided in the following, choose the single most appropriate test from the list of options above. Each option may be used once, more than once or not at all.

1. A 29-year-old woman with a family history of thrombosis suffers from unprovoked deep vein thrombosis. To investigate the possibility of recurrence, which test would be most useful?

2. A 66-year-old man, post-cardiopulmonary bypass, receives an intravenous infusion of unfractionated heparin

3. A 29-year-old woman with a family history of easy bruising experiences severe menorrhagia and recurrent epistaxis

4. A woman receives prophylaxis with LMWH following a caesarean section
5. A young man with end-stage renal failure (dialysis dependent) receives a therapeutic dose of LMWH for deep vein thrombosis

Question 6: Abnormalities of white cells

Options:

A. Acute lymphoblastic leukaemia
B. Acute myeloid leukaemia
C. Acute promyelocytic leukaemia
D. Chronic lymphocytic leukaemia
E. Chronic myeloid leukaemia
F. Follicular lymphoma
G. Hodgkin lymphoma
H. Multiple myeloma
I. Reactive lymphocytosis
J. Reactive neutrophilia

For each clinical history provided in the following, choose the most appropriate and specific diagnosis from the list above. Each option may be used once, more than once or not at all.

1. A 54-year-old man presents with weight loss and increased sweating. His spleen is palpable 8 cm below his left costal margin. His blood count shows: WBC $111.2 \times 10^9/l$, Hb 95 g/l and platelet count $540 \times 10^9/l$. A differential count shows a marked increase in neutrophils and neutrophil precursors, but blast cells are infrequent. Eosinophils and basophils are also elevated
2. A 4-year-old boy is noted by his mother to be pale and listless. His general practitioner finds him to have cervical and inguinal lymphadenopathy and several bruises on his legs. FBC shows: WBC $49.5 \times 10^9/l$ with 85% blast cells, Hb 85 g/l and platelet count $48 \times 10^9/l$. The blast cells have no granules
3. A 75-year-old man presents with herpes zoster. FBC shows: WBC $18 \times 10^9/l$, Hb 155 g/l, platelet count $200 \times 10^9/l$ and lymphocyte count $12.3 \times 10^9/l$. The blood film shows mature small lymphocytes

4. A 50-year-old woman presents with pallor and bruising. Her spleen is palpable 2 cm below her left costal margin, and some petechiae are noted. She is febrile and exhibits moist sounds at both lung bases. FBC shows: WBC 16.8 × 10⁹/l, Hb 85 g/l and platelet count 80 × 10⁹/l. The blood film shows that about 50% of leucocytes are blast cells, some of which contain Auer rods

5. A 48-year-old woman has previously been treated for carcinoma of the breast by removal of the breast lump, radiotherapy and chemotherapy. She presents six years later with epistaxis, extensive bruising and haemorrhage into the soft tissues of her arms. Her FBC shows: WBC 6.3 × 10⁹/l, Hb 116 g/l and platelet count 45 × 10⁹/l. Her blood film shows small numbers of immature cells that are packed with brightly staining granules. A coagulation screen shows prolonged PT, APTT and TT. Fibrinogen concentration is reduced, and fibrin degradation products are increased

Question 7: Renal disease

Options:

A. Glomerulonephritis
B. Haemolytic uraemic syndrome
C. Hyperparathyroidism
D. Loss of renal concentrating ability
E. Monoclonal gammopathy of undetermined significance
F. Multiple myeloma
G. Renal cell cancer
H. Renal failure due to recurrent infarction
I. Thrombotic thrombocytopenic purpura
J. Wegener granulomatosis

For each clinical history provided in the following, choose the most appropriate diagnosis from the list above. Each option may be used once, more than once or not at all.

1. A 4-year-old girl presents with jaundice and pallor following an episode of diarrhoea. Her FBC shows: WBC 11.2 × 10⁹/l, Hb 84 g/l and

platelet count $352 \times 10^9/l$. Her blood film shows numerous red cell fragments and polychromasia. Her creatinine and potassium levels are elevated

2. A 44-year-old woman presents with fever, purpura and mental confusion. There is no lymphadenopathy or hepatosplenomegaly. FBC shows: WBC $13.8 \times 10^9/l$, Hb 87 g/l and platelet count $52 \times 10^9/l$. The blood film shows numerous schistocytes. Creatinine level is elevated

3. A 45-year-old man has a lifetime history of sickle cell anaemia. FBC shows: WBC $6.8 \times 10^9/l$, Hb 50 g/l and platelet count $243 \times 10^9/l$. The blood film shows sickle cells, target cells and Howell–Jolly bodies. Creatinine level is elevated, and reticulocyte count is not increased

4. A 56-year-old man presents with fatigue and haematuria. A mass is found in the right loin. FBC shows: WBC $12.8 \times 10^9/l$, Hb 185 g/l and platelet count $400 \times 10^9/l$. The blood film is reported as showing a 'packed film'.

5. A 63-year-old man presents with backache, which has been troubling him for several months. No specific abnormality is found on a physical examination. His FBC shows: WBC $6.7 \times 10^9/l$, Hb 96 g/l and platelet count $145 \times 10^9/l$. His blood film shows rouleaux and increased background staining, and his ESR is 78 mm in one hour. He has elevated levels of calcium and creatinine

Question 8: Coagulation tests

Options:

A. APTT
B. Anticardiolipin antibody
C. Anti-Xa assay
D. Factor VIII assay
E. Factor V Leiden genotype
F. INR
G. No testing required
H. Thrombomodulin assay
I. Thrombin time
J. Von Willebrand factor antigen

For each clinical scenario provided in the following, choose the single most appropriate test from the list of options above. Each option may be used once, more than once or not at all.

1. A 23-year-old woman has an unprovoked lower limb DVT. The APTT is prolonged.
2. A 66-year-old woman has recurrent epistaxis and menorrhagia, the APTT is prolonged. There is a family history of bleeding problems.
3. A 77-year-old woman with atrial fibrillation receives warfarin for anticoagulation.
4. A woman taking regular DOAC medication with no bleeding problems.
5. A young man has an abnormal fibrinogen level but no clinical symptoms.

Question 9: Sickle cell disease

Options:

A. Acute chest crisis
B. Dactylitis
C. Osteomyelitis
D. Painful crisis
E. Parvovirus-induced red cell aplasia
F. Pneumococcal pneumonia
G. Septic arthritis
H. Splenic infarction
I. Splenic sequestration
J. Splenic vein thrombosis

For each patient with sickle cell anaemia, select from the option list above the most likely explanation of the clinical picture. Each option may be used once, more than once or not at all.

1. A 2-year-old child presents with pallor and marked lethargy, an Hb level of 40 g/l and enlargement of the spleen extending below the umbilicus
2. A 7-year-old girl and her 5-year-old sister present with pallor and lassitude. Both are found to have experienced a drop in Hb levels, and their reticulocyte counts are considerably below the normal range

3. A 2-year-old presents with acute swelling of one hand and one foot. She is crying with pain

4. A 4-year-old child has pain in his left upper quadrant and left shoulder tip. His spleen is palpable on inspiration and is tender

5. A 10-year-old child presents with rib and abdominal pain, with no specific localising signs

Question 10: Splenomegaly

Options:

A. Acquired immune deficiency syndrome (AIDS)
B. Acute lymphoblastic leukaemia
C. Amyloidosis of the spleen
D. Biliary cirrhosis
E. Chronic lymphocytic leukaemia
F. Haemochromatosis
G. Hodgkin lymphoma
H. Metastatic carcinoma
I. Portal cirrhosis
J. Primary myelofibrosis

For each clinical history, select the most likely diagnosis from the option list above. Each option may be used once, more than once or not at all.

1. A 32-year-old HIV-positive engineer presents with fever, night sweats and itch. He is diagnosed with generalised lymphadenopathy (with nodes of 1.5–2 cm), and his spleen is palpable 3 cm below the left costal margin. FBC and biochemical tests show normocytic normochromic anaemia, with the biochemical features of anaemia of chronic disease. He has eosinophilia, and his ESR is elevated

2. A 65-year-old accountant consults his general practitioner regarding impotence. He does not smoke and rarely consumes alcohol. He is noted to be heavily pigmented; his liver is abnormally firm, and his spleen is palpable just below the left costal margin. There is no lymph node enlargement. An FBC shows anaemia and thrombocytopenia. His blood film shows no specific abnormalities

3. A 67-year-old retired schoolteacher presents with abdominal enlargement and bruising. He is found to be pale, with an enlargement of the spleen 8 cm below the left costal margin. An FBC shows: WBC 3.8×10^9/l, Hb 90 g/l and platelet count 82×10^9/l. The blood film is leuco-erythroblastic and shows anisocytosis and poikilocytosis, including teardrop poikilocytes

4. A 69-year-old retired man, under follow-up for hypertension, is found to have generalised lymphadenopathy, with lymph nodes up to 1.5 cm in diameter. His spleen is palpable 2 cm below the left costal margin. An FBC shows: WBC 54×10^9/l, lymphocyte count 48×10^9/l, Hb 110 g/l and platelet count 110×10^9/l. The lymphocytes are small and mature, and smear cells are present

5. A 54-year-old former stockbroker presents with abdominal enlargement. He smokes 15 cigarettes and consumes 5–6 units of alcohol a day. He is found to have ascites, splenomegaly, a firm irregular liver edge, gynaecomastia and testicular atrophy. There are no palpable lymph nodes. FBC shows mild pancytopenia and macrocytosis; blood film shows no abnormal cells

Question 11: Anaemia

Options:

A. Anaemia of chronic disease
B. Autoimmune haemolytic anaemia
C. Glucose-6-phosphate dehydrogenase deficiency
D. Hereditary spherocytosis
E. Iron deficiency anaemia
F. Megaloblastic anaemia
G. Myelodysplastic syndrome
H. Sickle cell anaemia
I. Sickle cell heterozygosity
J. Thalassaemia intermedia

For each clinical history, select the most likely diagnosis from the option list above. Each option may be used once, more than once or not at all.

1. A 50-year-old North European Caucasian man who experiences altered bowel function is found to have an Hb level of 88 g/l and an MCV of 70 fl. His diet is normal.

2. A 16-year-old African man presents with haematuria. His WBC is $4.5 \times 10^9/l$, Hb level is 125 g/l and platelet count is $423 \times 10^9/l$. His blood film shows target cells. A sickle solubility test is positive.

3. A 34-year-old North European woman with a history of systemic lupus erythematosus presents with jaundice and fatigue. She is found to exhibit elevated levels of unconjugated bilirubin and lactate dehydrogenase, an Hb level of 95 g/l, spherocytes and an increased reticulocyte count. Her direct antiglobulin test is positive.

4. A 23-year-old Italian man was given antibiotics for a urinary tract infection. A few days later, he presents with an acute onset of jaundice, pallor, fatigue and breathlessness. He is found to have an Hb level of 62 g/l, an increased reticulocyte count and a blood film showing numerous irregularly contracted cells.

5. A 53-year-old woman presents with fatigue and is found to have an Hb level of 88 g/l and an MCV of 110 fl. Neutrophils show reduced segmentation (known as pseudo-Pelger–Huët anomaly) and are hypogranular. Platelet count is $60 \times 10^9/l$. Vitamin B_{12} and folic acid assays are normal.

Answers to Questions

Basic multiple-choice questions

Question 1

1 and 2 are correct. This is pancytopenia, which suggests a bone marrow disorder such as AA or ALL. In a proportion of ALL cases, lymphoblasts may be present in the peripheral blood, resulting in a raised WBC count. Pernicious anaemia may cause pancytopenia, but with a raised MCV.

Question 2

2, 4 and 5 are correct. This child is hyposplenic and requires pneumococcal and meningococcal vaccinations (consult local guidelines for full vaccine recommendations) and prophylactic penicillin V.

Question 3

2 and 5 are correct. Lymphoproliferative neoplasms may present with lymphadenopathy and hepatosplenomegaly. ALL primarily involves the

bone marrow and blood and lymphatic tissue may also be involved; however, generally, bone marrow failure ensues before there is time for significant lymphadenopathy to develop. Myeloproliferative disorders are associated with hepatosplenomegaly but rarely lymphadenopathy.

Question 4

2 and 5 are correct. Both HIT and TTP are associated with thrombosis. The mechanism is described in relevant chapters. Thrombocytopenia, due to most other causes, is associated with skin (petechiae) and mucosal bleeding.

Question 5

1, 3, 4 and 5 are true. Renal failure causes a low Hb level.

Question 6

2, 3 and 4 are correct. Iron deficiency causes microcytosis. It is hypothyroidism that can cause macrocytic anaemia, not hyperthyroidism.

Question 7

1, 2 and 5 are correct. Infectious mononucleosis causes an increase in atypical lymphocytes, and neutropenia rather than neutrophilia is an ethnic variation.

Question 8

2 and 3 are correct. The spherocytosis in autoimmune haemolytic anaemia is caused by the removal of antibody-coated red cell membrane sections by splenic macrophages.

Question 9

2 and 3 are correct; however, remember that it would generally be preferable to keep A D-negative red cells for D-negative recipients.

Question 10

1 is correct. This can only be a defect in the intrinsic system since the PT is normal. The likely diagnoses are haemophilia (factor VIII deficiency) and factor IX deficiency.

Question 11

The defect can be localised to the intrinsic pathway. Either 1 (haemophilia A) or 2 (von Willebrand disease) is likely. In von Willebrand disease, the prolonged APTT is due to the associated reduction in factor VIII clotting activity.

Question 12

1, 2 and 5 are true. The likelihood of iron deficiency is increased because the patient may have been taking aspirin, non-steroidal anti-inflammatory drugs or corticosteroids, any of which could cause chronic gastrointestinal blood loss. Felty syndrome is a complication of rheumatoid arthritis in which both hypersplenism and autoantibodies contribute to anaemia and cytopenia (particularly neutropenia).

Question 13

1, 2, 3 and 4 are true. Remember that group A may be genetically OA and group D may be genetically Dd.

Question 14

1 is true. Only anti-A is expected. Anti-O and anti-d do not exist, and anti-D is not expected in a man who has never received a transfusion.

Question 15

2 and 3 are true. In the other conditions, the bone marrow is unable to produce an appropriate response to anaemia.

Question 16

All statements are true.

Single best answer multiple-choice questions

Question 1

LMW heparin (3) can be used during pregnancy and has a relatively short half-life, which is important peripartum in view of the risk of obstetric haemorrhage. Warfarin is teratogenic in the first trimester. Rivaroxaban is not used during pregnancy. Aspirin and clopidogrel alter platelet function and are used to prevent arterial thrombosis.

Question 2

Diffuse large B-cell lymphoma (3). CD19 is expressed on B lymphocytes, both normal and malignant. It is not expressed on myeloid cells (1 and 5) or on T lymphocytes (2 and 4).

Question 3

Stage 3 disease (4). There is disease above and below the diaphragm but it is confined to the lymphatic system (with the spleen being considered a lymphatic site). Disease that has spread beyond the lymphatic system, commonly to the liver and/or bone marrow, constitutes stage 4.

Question 4

AL amyloidosis (1) is a rare complication of myeloma, often presenting with nephrotic syndrome and cardiac failure due to amyloid deposition in the kidney and heart. Other organs may also be affected. In myeloma practice, cast nephropathy is the commonest renal complication, presenting with renal failure in the presence of high levels of serum-free light chains.

Question 5

Graft versus host disease is mediated by donor-derived T lymphocytes (2).

Question 6

Rh haemolytic disease of the newborn (4). Options 2, 3 and 5 may cause jaundice, but the DAT would be negative. Option 1 is incorrect because, although IgG class, anti-B antibodies may rarely occur and can cross the placenta, the newborn baby is blood group 0.

Question 7

Protein S (4). Pregnancy is associated with a decrease in anticoagulant proteins and an increase in procoagulant proteins.

Question 8

Postpartum (3)

Question 9

The incidence of AML increases with age (3). The other statements are false.

Question 10

Disseminated intravascular coagulation (DIC) (3).

Question 11

The most likely diagnosis is chronic lymphocytic leukaemia (5). None of the other conditions is likely to cause lymphocytosis in an asymptomatic middle-aged man.

Question 12

The most likely diagnosis is ITP (4), as the other diagnoses are less likely to cause isolated, very severe thrombocytopenia. The only other diagnosis that should be seriously considered is acute promyelocytic leukaemia, but the normal Hb level and the normal coagulation screen make this less likely than ITP.

Question 13

The anaemia is most likely anaemia of chronic disease (2), as a result of her inflammatory bowel disease. This is suggested by the low levels of iron and transferrin and the raised ferritin level.

Question 14

There is a 25% chance of β thalassaemia major (2) with each conception in this couple.

Question 15

The mild anaemia is consistent with blood loss. The near-normal Hb level and the fact that the blood film shows only target cells make sickle cell anaemia highly unlikely. The most likely diagnosis is sickle cell trait (3), which requires particular care in administering anaesthesia.

Question 16

The most likely diagnosis is pernicious anaemia (5). Patients who present with neurological features may exhibit only mild haematological abnormalities.

Question 17

The normal intravascular lifespan of a neutrophil is about 7 hours (2). Ten days is the life span of a platelet, while 120 days is the life span of a red cell.

Question 18

Vegetarians, particularly women who have had a number of pregnancies, are much more likely to have iron deficiency (3) than vitamin B_{12} deficiency, and neither B_{12} deficiency nor folic acid deficiency would explain the blood film. Some elliptocytes can be seen in iron deficiency, and hereditary elliptocytosis would not explain the hypochromia and microcytosis. Lead poisoning can cause microcytic anaemia but is quite uncommon.

Question 19

His blood film is most likely to show eosinophilia (2).

Question 20

The most likely explanation is a myocardial infarction (2) causing reactive neutrophilia.

Question 21

Group AB plasma (4) would be selected for a patient of an unknown group requiring urgent correction of a coagulation defect.

Question 22

This is a complex question since it requires the correct diagnosis to be made so that the optimal treatment can be selected. The patient is likely to have CML, and the optimal treatment is therefore a tyrosine kinase inhibitor (3), such as imatinib.

Extended matching questions

Question 1

1C, 2H, 3I, 4A, 5D

Question 2

1G, 2J, 3C, 4F, 5B

Question 3

1J, 2E, 3D, 4I, 5F

Question 4

1J, 2D, 3I, 4B, 5A

Question 5

1F, 2A, 3K, 4J, 5C

Question 6

1E, 2A, 3D, 4B, 5C (Note that 5B is also correct; however, you are asked for the most appropriate **and specific** diagnosis.)

Question 7

1B, 2I, 3H, 4G, 5F

Question 8

1B, 2J, 3F, 4G, 5G

Question 9

1I, 2E, 3B, 4H, 5D

Question 10

1G, 2F, 3J, 4E, 5I

Question 11

1E, 2I, 3B, 4C, 5G

19

Answers to Test Cases

Barbara J. Bain and
Donald Macdonald

Test Case 3.1

There is nothing to suggest any chronic infection or active inflammation, and the borderline elevation of the erythrocyte sedimentation rate (ESR) and C-reactive protein (CRP) is evidence against this possibility. This is, therefore, likely to be iron deficiency anaemia. The next test to be conducted is serum ferritin, which was performed and subsequently confirmed the iron deficiency. The patient can be treated with oral ferrous sulphate, but his treatment must also include determining the cause of the iron deficiency. He has been taking aspirin regularly, so chronic blood loss from the stomach is possible. However, for a man of this age, the possibility of colonic carcinoma must not be neglected. He requires a colonoscopy. This was performed and showed a carcinoma of the ascending colon. This may be the reason for the slight elevation of the CRP (which has been found to be elevated, on average, in patients with colonic cancer).

Test Case 4.1

The most likely diagnosis is pernicious anaemia since the neurological symptoms are consistent with a vitamin B_{12} deficiency, and there is also macrocytosis. Pernicious anaemia is the most likely cause of an overt vitamin B_{12} deficiency in a middle-aged or elderly Caucasian woman with a normal diet. Although excessive alcohol intake can cause peripheral neuropathy, consuming 1–2 units a day is not sufficient for this effect. Some patients under-report their alcohol intake, but the normal liver function in this patient makes alcohol overconsumption unlikely. Hypothyroidism has not been excluded as a cause of the macrocytosis; however, it would not explain the neurological abnormalities.

Serum vitamin B_{12} and serum folate should be assayed, and intrinsic factor antibodies should be sought. The serum B_{12} level is very likely to be low, and the folate level may also be reduced. It is quite likely that intrinsic factor antibodies will be detected. If intrinsic factor antibodies are not found, parietal cell antibodies support the diagnosis but are not as definitive as intrinsic factor antibodies.

The patient is likely to be treated with parenteral hydroxocobalamin, starting with a dose of 1,000 μg daily in view of the neurological deficit. Her maintenance dose will be 1,000 μg every three months.

Test Case 5.1

Gallstones are surprising at this age and are the result of increased bilirubin production caused by chronic haemolytic anaemia. The most likely diagnosis is hereditary spherocytosis. Spherocytosis could also be due to autoimmune haemolytic anaemia; however, this is unlikely for two reasons. First, it is unlikely that the patient has had an undiagnosed autoimmune haemolytic anaemia for such a long time that gallstones have developed. Second, the direct antiglobulin test is negative; therefore, there is no evidence of immunoglobulin or complement on the red cell membrane. A demonstration of reduced red cell binding of eosin-5-maleimide (EMA binding) would confirm your provisional diagnosis.

Test Case 5.2

The very low reticulocyte count and the lack of polychromasia are not something that we would normally expect in sickle cell anaemia since the marrow responds to the shortened red cell lifespan by an increased output of erythrocytes. This suggests a failure of erythropoiesis. Megaloblastic anaemia is unlikely because folic acid is being taken regularly and both the white cell and platelet counts are normal. This is most likely pure red cell aplasia as a result of a parvovirus B_{19} infection. Since the anaemia is severe, blood transfusion is needed after first taking a blood sample to test for antibodies to parvovirus. Immunoglobulin M antiparvovirus antibodies would confirm a recent infection.

Test Case 6.1

The first thing to consider is whether the patient has pancytopenia as a result of bone marrow metastases. However, the blood film is not leucoerythroblastic, and there are no biochemical abnormalities to suggest widespread metastases. What the blood film does show is dysplastic neutrophils plus red cell features, which suggest sideroblastic erythropoiesis and occasional blast cells. The most likely diagnosis is myelodysplastic syndrome, resulting from previous chemotherapy. The patient's medical history is certainly relevant. She should undergo a bone marrow aspiration, and cytogenetic analysis should be performed. Further, the nature of the condition and the prognosis should be discussed with her. As her anaemia is symptomatic, a trial of erythropoietin could be considered a first step.

Test Case 7.1

The red cell indices suggest that the patient has iron deficiency anaemia. The eosinophil count is high. Hookworm infection would provide an explanation for both the iron deficiency and the eosinophilia. Being an asylum seeker from an impoverished country, there might also be dietary deficiencies. In a Somali, schistosomiasis could also be considered a cause of eosinophilia. If you looked up the normal range for the neutrophil count, you might conclude that this patient has a low neutrophil count. However, in a Somali, it could be normal, i.e. an ethnic neutropenia.

Test Case 7.2

The patient has carbimazole-induced agranulocytosis. The carbimazole should be stopped immediately, blood and throat swabs should be taken for culture, and antibiotics should be prescribed. Agranulocytosis is a serious illness, and if the patient is febrile, hospitalisation is recommended. Administration of granulocyte colony-stimulating factor could be considered, as it may shorten the period of agranulocytosis.

Test Case 8.1

The findings pertain to chronic lymphocytic leukaemia (CLL). A clone of kappa-positive B cells is present, weakly expressing surface membrane immunoglobulin. There are a small number of lambda-positive normal B cells, and 10% of the cells are T cells. CD5 is expressed on the great majority of cells and is hence clearly expressed on ~85% of clonal B cells as well as T cells. The neoplastic cells therefore expressed CD5, CD23 and weak immunoglobulin, but not FMC7 or CD79b. The patient has an early-stage disease, so he does not need any CLL-directed therapy. However, he should be vaccinated against pneumococcus, SARS-CoV-2 and seasonal influenza. He will require regular follow-up to determine whether, in the future, he might need CLL-targeted therapy.

Test Case 8.2

The findings suggest B-cell acute lymphoblastic leukaemia (ALL). The FBC with an extremely high WBC, mainly blasts, is indicative of acute leukaemia. In childhood, ALL is more common than AML, and the immunophenotype of the blasts confirms that this is B-ALL. The important further diagnostic tests are BM aspiration for cytogenetic and molecular studies to check for the presence of recurrent genetic aberrations. Other investigations to aid management are biochemical screening (to test for renal and liver function and the levels of uric acid, calcium and phosphate), coagulation studies, blood group test and antibody screening. A lumbar puncture and a cytological examination of the CSF are required to determine whether CNS disease is present at diagnosis.

Test Case 9.1

The raised Hb and haematocrit levels indicate polycythaemia. We need to consider whether this is a result of his COPD or an unrelated abnormality. Aquagenic pruritus can occur in polycythaemia vera (PV), thereby offering a clue. The key investigation is to test for the presence of the *JAK2* V617F gene mutation. (Note that testing for the *JAK2* exon 12 mutation should be conducted if the V617F mutation is not detected.) If a PV diagnosis is confirmed, then there is a risk of thrombotic complications, such as a cerebrovascular accident. The most appropriate management for this patient would be cytoreductive therapy using hydroxycarbamide. Low-dose aspirin therapy is also required. In a younger patient with no other comorbidities, venesection plus aspirin may be a treatment option.

Test Case 10.1

The diagnosis of myeloma is often delayed, as symptoms such as fatigue, backache and recurrent infections may be wrongly attributed to old age. One must be alert to the diagnosis; of concern in the clinical and laboratory findings are backache with new neurological symptoms, a raised IgG level, immune paresis, hypercalcaemia and anaemia. The laboratory investigations required are protein electrophoresis to determine if this is a monoclonal IgG paraprotein (M band), serum-free light chain concentrations and renal function tests. A bone marrow biopsy is needed to determine plasma cell numbers. In due course, a whole-body MRI or CT scan to identify bone lesions will be needed. The clinical picture is one of a myeloma emergency with possible spinal cord compression. The management plan requires an urgent spinal MRI and neurosurgical review. If cord compression is confirmed and surgery is not indicated, then dexamethasone and urgent radiotherapy to the site of cord compression would be the likely plan.

Test Case 11.1

The clinical picture and laboratory findings are indicative of chronic disseminated intravascular coagulation (DIC). This condition can be associated with either bleeding or an increased thrombotic risk. Adenocarcinoma cells, in some cases, may release procoagulant factors into the blood, leading to the activation of coagulation and fibrinolysis. The increased consumption of clotting factors may be partially compensated for by increased production. There is increased fibrinolysis, which explains the raised D-dimer levels.

Test Case 11.2

There is a history of mucosal bleeding, an apparent autosomal dominant inheritance and a deficiency of factor VIII and the von Willebrand factor in the woman. This points to a diagnosis of von Willebrand disease. Platelet function is likely to be abnormal since, when a blood vessel is damaged, the von Willebrand factor binds platelets to the exposed subendothelial collagen. Factor VIII is low because the von Willebrand factor stabilises it and increases its half-life in the plasma.

Test Case 12.1

The combination of spontaneous venous thrombosis and prolonged APTT suggests a lupus anticoagulant. There is a suspicion that the patient may actually have systemic lupus erythematosus, in view of the history of arthritis and the presence of neutropenia and thrombocytopenia. Laboratory tests relevant to the antiphospholipid syndrome (APS), anti-cardiolipin and anti-β2 glycoprotein 1 antibodies are needed. She also requires investigation for underlying lupus erythematosus with tests such as antinuclear activity and anti-double-stranded DNA (or anti-ds DNA) antibodies. Renal function should be checked, and the urine should be tested for albumin. The patient requires anticoagulation, which could initially be a DOAC; however, if APS is confirmed by repeat testing 12 weeks later, this treatment should be reviewed by a haematologist. Any underlying connective tissue disorder should be diagnosed and treated.

Test Case 13.1

An ABO-incompatible transfusion should be suspected. Stop the transfusion immediately, but keep the drip open and maintain blood pressure and urine output by infusing normal saline. Check the patient's identity and verify the details on the blood bag by comparing them with those in the wristband and the blood request form. If you find that the wrong blood bag was being used for the transfusion, check immediately that the bag intended for this patient is not being given to another patient in the daycare ward. Inform the transfusion laboratory, and return the blood bag immediately to the laboratory together with a further blood sample from the patient, which will be used to confirm the group. Repeat the antibody screen and perform a direct antiglobulin test. At the same time, take a sample to check liver and renal functions, electrolytes and coagulation status. Ask the nursing staff to test the next urine sample that the patient passes for haemoglobin to detect haemoglobinuria resulting from intravascular haemolysis. Contact a member of the hospital transfusion team or a consultant haematologist for advice and help.

Test Case 14.1

The patient has acute GVHD, which can be of variable severity and commonly involves: skin (ranging from palmar erythema to severe widespread bullous skin disease with desquamation), gut (ranging from anorexia to profuse intractable bloody diarrhoea) and liver (intrahepatic cholestasis). The initial treatment is with corticosteroids. Standard measures to prevent or reduce the risk of GVHD include the use of stem cells harvested from fully HLA-matched donors and the routine administration of immunosuppressants, such as methotrexate and ciclosporin, during the early post-transplant period.

Regarding the role of allogeneic stem cell transplant in acute leukaemia, as this procedure has a 10–40% treatment-related mortality, it is reserved for clinical scenarios where the prognostic factors (generally, the leukaemia-associated molecular or cytogenetic findings) predict a high risk of post-chemotherapy relapse. Additional factors to consider include the patient's age, performance status and the availability of a fully HLA-matched donor.

Index

www.ingramcontent.com/pod-product-compliance
Lightning Source LLC
Chambersburg PA
CBHW061614220326
41598CB00026BA/3757